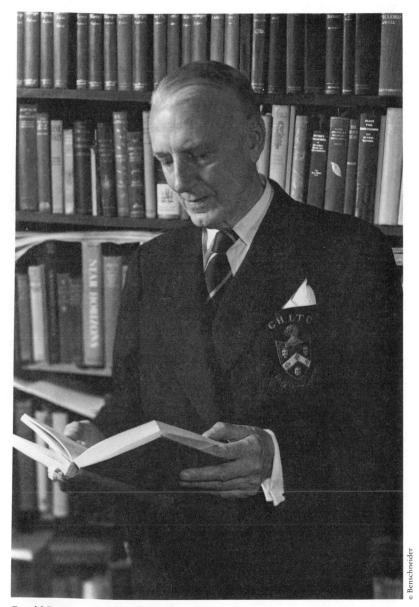

© Benschneider

Gerald Bertram Webb M.D. 1871–1948

Dr. Webb of Colorado Springs

HELEN CLAPESATTLE

Dr. Webb of Colorado Springs

COLORADO ASSOCIATED UNIVERSITY PRESS
BOULDER, COLORADO

This book was made possible by a generous grant from the Webb-Waring Lung Institute

Copyright © 1984 by Colorado Associated University Press
Boulder, Colorado 80309
International Standard Book Number 0-87081-050-2
Library of Congress Catalog Card Number 84-070852
Printed in the United States of America
Designed by Bruce Campbell
Set in type by Columbia Publishing Company, Inc.

Contents

List of Illustrations

Prologue: Who Was Dr. Webb?

Herodotus said he wrote of the ancient Greeks to secure for them "the honor of remembrance."

Americans today, engrossed with the whirl or the humdrum of their daily lives, are not good at stopping to remember even their nearest forebears. Outside the publicized arenas of politics, sports, and show business, we let our heroes go unsung, especially if their endeavor was in an arcane field such as science and medicine. Who among us remembers Nobel Prize winners in science, say, beyond the day or week their awards are announced? Persons with lesser accolades, no matter how much they may have benefited their fellow men, are allowed to slide swiftly into the pool of the forgotten.

To these belongs "Dr. Webb of Colorado Springs." His christian names were Gerald Bertram but these were not needed even in initials to identify him when during the first half of this century he was one of the most widely known and genuinely respected physicians in the nation.

"Dr. Webb's the best there is for what you've got," an eminent New York doctor told a patient whom he had diagnosed as a victim of tuberculosis, at that time the world's terrifying number one killer. Scores of doctors the country over were of the same opinion and sent their tuberculous patients by the hundreds to be treated by Dr. Webb in his little city at the foot of Pikes Peak.

The chief of the division of medicine at the University of Colorado told a commencement audience in 1938 that "in our medical world Colorado Springs is synonymous with Dr. Webb." And a decade later a historian of the Springs community estimated that fully a quarter of the new residents and new houses since 1900 were there because of the work and reputation of Dr. Webb.

Yet today you can search the maps and walk the streets of Colorado Springs looking in vain for some sign that the man is remembered there. All you will find, hidden away in Glockner-Penrose Hospital, is a medical library named in his honor.

You must go to Denver, to the Health Sciences Center of the University of Colorado, to find a worthy memorial to Dr. Webb. One of the buildings there, housing a complex of research laboratories, is named the Webb-Waring Lung Institute. But even there few of the laboratory doctors, busy with their studies and experiments, know much if anything about the man whose name stands first in the hyphenated rubric under which they work.

As for the immunologists who tower so tall in the medical landscape today, they remember Dr. Webb not at all. Ask them about him and they look at you blankly and say gruffly, "Never heard of him." Yet it was he who named their specialty and their prestigious American Association of Immunologists, of which he was a founder and the first president. When the science of immunity was still in its infancy he was prophesying that "the doctor of the future will be an immunologist."

Dr. Webb was a first-rate practitioner, superbly able to inspire absolute trust and respect in his patients. He believed in encouraging the body to heal itself instead of drugging it or cutting it up, and he practiced his own preachment, that it was a physician's duty to minister to the mind and spirit as well as to the body. During the long years of the rest cure for tuberculosis, before the development of antibiotics and chemotherapy, he sought to divert his patients from gloom and despair by engaging them in occupations and interests that could endure as worthwhile hobbies when health returned. He brought them armfuls of good books to read, led them into birdwatching, taught them to play chess. And those who got well he guided into suitable ways of earning their living again.

But his passion was research. His god was Pasteur, his creed Pasteur's assurance that the discovery of microbes and of vaccines had placed it within the power of man to eradicate infectious diseases from all the earth. Dr. Webb's conviction that this blessing could be achieved made him one of the early fathers of vaccination in the United States. It also set the goal of his own research: to develop a vaccine against tuberculosis.

Far, far away from the resplendent research laboratories that philanthropy was bringing to birth in the East, Dr. Webb established his own laboratory in a small addition he built onto his house. In experiments there he was the first in the United States to recognize lymphocytes as primary agents in inducing immunity and the first to make a prolonged study of those mysterious wandering cells that today are considered the architects and builders of the immune system.

Compared with the mature state of the art in immunology today, Dr. Webb's investigations were groping, his conclusions stumbling, but they impressed his contemporaries, few of whom ever tried to do more than prescribe at the bedside. Harvard University and the University of Michigan both offered him research professorships on their medical faculties. Several national medical societies elected him their president. The National Tuberculosis Association also awarded him its highest honor, the Trudeau Medal.

Through all this, Dr. Webb was no perpetually frowning sobersides. He was "a big, warm, beautiful man," in the words of a New York journalist who became his patient. Born and reared an Englishman, he of course thought many forms and frequent periods of diversion were essential to a productive life. He loved music and drama, excelled in several sports and games, enjoyed hiking and climbing in the mountains, studied birds and wildflowers, butterflies and trees. He roamed the world of books, reading widely in three languages and collecting what a Boston colleague called "one of the great libraries" in medical history and biography.

It has been a stirring and stretching experience for me to piece together the story of this extraordinary man. If I have succeeded in restoring flesh to his bones and recapturing his wit and spirit, it should be a quickening encounter to read about him in the pages that follow, thus doing him for a time "the honor of remembrance."

Dr. Webb of Colorado Springs

I

A Guy's Man

FOR YOUNG GERALD WEBB life turned suddenly, dizzyingly topsy turvy in 1894.

He began the year in London, buoyantly confident of his future. He was getting on well in his chosen study of medicine and surgery at Guy's Hospital. He was newly married to a lovely, spirited girl he adored and had income enough to support her in modest comfort. "I am *so* happy," he wrote his mother.

But when the year ended he was adrift in the pine barrens of the American state of Georgia, dependent on his wife's family for money to meet expenses, apprehensively uncertain of what lay ahead of him.

Gerald was then twenty-three years old. Only three years removed from the shelter of a large and enfolding family, he was still tender to the world. Life in that family was vibrant and nourishing, although it was often made stormy by the caprices of an erratic but magisterial father whom even a plucky and protective mother could only circumvent, not control.

William John Webb, the father, was a highly intelligent but unstable person, a dreamer, an eccentric, eventually an alcoholic. According to family legend his father was the illegitimate son of the heir of the Duke of Norfolk and Elizabeth Webb, the beautiful daughter of the duke's bailiff. Whether fact or fantasy, this tale of noble ancestry undoubtedly helped to shape William's self-image and aspirations and so contributed to his sense of frustration and defeat.

His boyhood ambition was to become an actor. Why he did not the records do not show. They are utterly blank about him from the notation of his birth on 19 March 1821 until he emerged from two years at Burrage Academy in Woolwich at the age of fourteen, and blank again for twelve years thereafter.

3

His father had done exceedingly well for a bastard. He had climbed from the registry status of "laborer" to that of "gentleman," from penury to ownership of a china and glass factory in Greenwich plus several houses in the county of Kent. When he sold his business he bought a large and well-known inn, the Queen's Head, in Chislehurst and spent his declining years there with his daughter Sophia and her family. When he died in 1858 he left all these freehold properties, plus "effects" of £3,000, to Sophia and her brother William John.

So, however and wherever, William John got a good education. He spoke and wrote excellent English and French, played the piano well, had got by heart "half the plays of Shakespeare" and long passages from Molière, Milton, Keats, and other favorite poets, and had traveled away from home enough to become thoroughly familiar with London and Paris.

At the age of twenty-six, in 1847, William received from his father enough capital to go into business for himself. The venture he chose was a dealership in coal—"black diamonds" he called it—in the municipal borough of Cheltenham, in Gloucestershire, ninety miles northwest of London.

It was in character for William to choose Cheltenham. Not only was the town a busy commercial center for the shipping of agricultural produce and livestock down the Severn River to Gloucester and Bristol; it was also a popular health resort with a glamorous past. King George III had journeyed often with his entourage to its mineral springs, and the bath and assembly buildings of the Royal Spa still stood in use at the end of a sixteen-mile promenade arched with chestnut and sycamore trees. Enough personages of wealth and noble lineage and enough traveling troupes of entertainers still came to the spa to make the place attractive to romantic William.

His black diamonds proved a good investment and William John an able business man. By 1855 he could afford to marry the petite, hazel-eyed Frances Susannah LePlastrier of London and install her as mistress of a fourteen-room house with added kitchens, pantry, and storage cellars below stairs and on the grounds a conservatory, flower gardens, a tennis lawn, and capacious stables. The address was 19 Tivoli Place.

The capable, spunky Frances Susannah was vainglorious about her own heritage. On her father's side she was descended from a Huguenot family of wealthy goldsmiths who, stripped of all their possessions in Rouen, fled to London during the persecutions following the revocation of the Edict of Nantes in 1685. They prospered again in England but foolishly squandered all they earned on a prolonged legal battle to regain the fortune they had left behind in France.

Her mother Jane Agate came from an old family of country gentry who owned large estates, moved to London for "the season" each year, and otherwise hobnobbed on the fringes of the nobility. Two of her mother's cousins were considered "the best architects in England since Wren": Sir Charles Barry, who designed the Houses of Parliament, and Sir Wolfe Barry, who drew the plans for Tower Bridge.

Extant letters show that William John and Frances Susannah were a truly loving couple at first, but as the marriage matured it developed unbridgeable fissures. One grating rub was this matter of pride in family. Frances Susannah would scoff at William's belief in his noble lineage, he at her boast that her family ranked far above anyone "in trade." Didn't Jane Agate and her sisters get their riches from London trade in timber and furs? he would taunt. The two came to hate each other's relatives so bitterly that to keep a semblance of peace between them they cut all connections on both sides.

In due course nine children, four girls then five boys, came along to fill the big house at 19 Tivoli Place. They were Fanny Sophia (Sophie), Eleanor Jane Mary (Nell), Amy Laura Constance, Ida Nicola, Harold Arthur, Roland Julian (Roly), Wilfred LePlastrier, Gerald Bertram, and Francis William John (Frank). By the time Gerald Bertram, born on 24 September 1871, was growing out of babyhood, William found the house too full and bought another, smaller one down the block which he turned into a dormitory with play and study rooms for the boys.

All the Webb girls got their schooling at Ellenborough House, a "young ladies school" in Cheltenham, and the boys at Cheltenham Grammar School—until the first classes began at the Dean Francis Close Memorial School in May 1886, when Gerald and Frank were immediately enrolled in the smaller and more exclusive institution, Gerald as a junior, Frank two years behind.

From the few grammar school reports for Gerald that survive it is difficult to tell what kind of pupil he was, the judgment of the masters varied so. Some of them rated him "a diligent little boy" and his "conduct and progress" good or satisfactory, but others found him "talkative and idle" and "needing a little more application" to improve. The application must have been forthcoming because his masters at the Dean Close School considered him a superior student—"the best and brightest boy in his class," the headmaster called him some years later. He won the first prize in chemistry, a copy of Charles Kingsley's *Madame How and Lady Why*.

Gerald received much of the most useful and enduring parts of his education outside the classroom. From his mother—"a proper lady" he called her—he absorbed strict moral standards, habits of thrift, the English conventions of courtesy, and warm and winning ways. Helping her tend her gardens, he learned to sow and till and weed. Best of all, he thought, "she taught me to be resourceful, never to say a thing could not be done but rather to figure out how it could."

Nature shaped him further. Rippling along the horizon in a half circle around Cheltenham were the Cotswold Hills, gorse-covered sanctuaries for songbirds and wildflowers. Gerald loved to ramble through those hills and spent many hours learning to know the birds and the flowers. From the top of Leckhampton Hill, tallest of the summits to the west, he could look north across twenty miles of elm-shaded meadows to the Malvern Hills and south beyond Gloucester to the glistening estuary where the Severn joined the sea. Solitary hours dreaming and reading in that favored spot implanted in him the habit of seeking strength in times of stress by escape to lonely wilds.

More gregariously, Gerald picked up varying degrees of competence in a remarkable range of skills: boating along the wide reaches of the Severn; swimming in the river and the heated waters of the spa; hockey, rugby, and cricket from play with schoolmates in the nine-acre schoolhouse yard; riding on horses from the family stables; tennis from fiercely competitive games with his brothers on the tennis lawn behind his mother's garden; chess from neighborhood friends in a community that doted on the game.

At home, along with his brothers and sisters, he learned to enjoy music, to play the violin and the piano, and to sing. And willy-nilly he acquired a taste for poetry and drama. The dinner hour provided William Webb, sometimes called Pater but more often "the Governor" by his children, with the audience he craved, and he subjected the family evening after evening to vigorous declamations

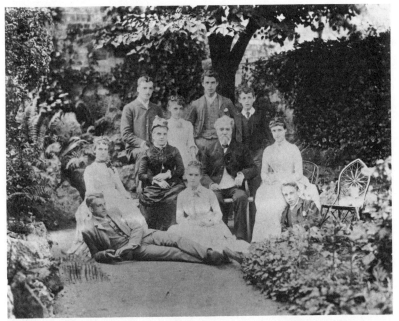

Webb family in the garden at Heimat. Grouped around Mater and Pater are (*left* to *right*, beginning in bottom center): Amy, Roland, Sophie, Harold, Ida, Wilfred, Frank, Nell, and Gerald

of entire scenes from Shakespeare or verses from his favorite poets.

The children often grew bored and restless but they were compelled to listen and they learned in spite of themselves. Gerald never caught as much feel for rhythm and cadence or swelled to the excitement of high drama as did his brother Frank, but he absorbed enough to make poetry and plays necessary pleasures throughout his life.

William's mealtime monologues were supplemented by more ambitious performances at every opportunity. Touring theatrical companies playing the spa at Cheltenham usually were invited to 19 Tivoli Place for a late night of impromptu acting—which all too often degenerated into drunken roistering that rocked the house till dawn, making the occasion a sore trial for the children and Mater, as they called their mother. Tension ran high in the house for days thereafter.

William directed his own "troupe" too. He assembled the youth of family and neighborhood and coached them for amateur theatricals and recitals which he staged at his home. The elaborately printed "Programme" for one of these, on 6 April 1887, is extant.

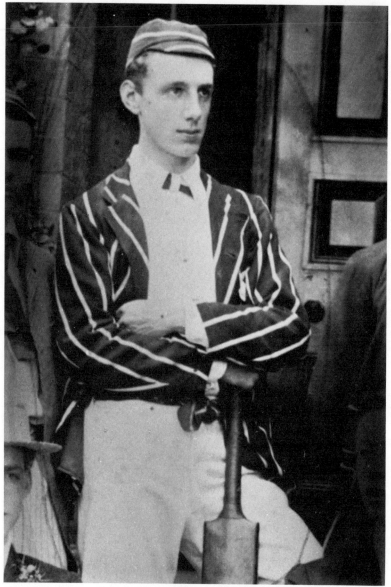

Gerald as captain of the cricket team at the Dean Close School

Part I presented "The Ethiopian Serenaders," a blackface chorus with soloists singing songs from the American South. Part II began with Haydn's *Toy Symphony* and concluded with a miscellany of dramatic recitations. The performers, numbering twenty-two in all, included all nine of the Webb children.

The following spring Gerald went to London to take the all-England examination for matriculation at Oxford University. He was the only Dean Close senior to pass the examination that year, although he was at the same time captain of both the school's cricket eleven and its rugby team.

His success in the examination renewed a perennial family battle. William John was stubbornly set against higher education for any of his children. Neither their pleas nor their mother's fierce arguments could budge him.

He did permit Ida to study singing at the Royal Conservatory of Music in London but when Harold won a scholarship to Cambridge University the Governor would not let him accept it and finally forced him, along with Roland in his turn, to join in the coal business, to which the manufacture of bricks had been added. Wilfred his father apprenticed to an engineer in Gloucester, and Frank, who wanted desperately to be an artist, he articled for five years to a firm of solicitors, also in Gloucester. As it turned out, he chose wisely for Wilfred but Frank he condemned to a lifetime in an uncongenial occupation.

Gerald, supported vigorously by his mother and the Dean Close masters, argued and pleaded for permission to go to Oxford, or failing that, for a chance to study medicine. This seemed a likely alternative. Gerald was known for his insatiable curiosity about insects and small animals and his persistent efforts to dissect all the dead specimens he could find. He was even suspected of spiriting away some of the neighborhood cats to satisfy his curiosity about their innards.

Also, tagging along on boat trips, perhaps with the coal and the bricks, down the Severn to Berkeley, he often played in the old home of Edward Jenner, the naturalist-physician who had originated vaccination against smallpox, and was fascinated by what he learned of Jenner's combined study of birds and medicine.

But the only concession that Gerald and Mater could win from William was that the boy might become a dentist instead of a maker of bricks. So Gerald began to learn the craft of "stopping" teeth with a Cheltenham dentist as preceptor.

William's attitude, given his own education and literary interests, is hard to explain. It was not a matter of money; he could easily have afforded the university education his sons wanted. Indeed, he willingly gave them, and the girls too, a thousand pounds sterling apiece, each at an appropriate time or occasion in his or her development. He was especially obdurate about Gerald's studying medicine because, like his beloved Molière, he contemned all doctors.

Gerald did not give up. He was tenacious and patient. After two years he re-opened the question, again with Mater's support. He knew now that preceptorship was considered only the beginning of a truly professional education in dentistry, and that the best dental schooling in England was offered as an adjunct to the famous program in medicine at the College of Guy's Hospital in London. The introductory courses were the same in both programs. He proposed to his father that he complete his dental training at Guy's Hospital.

Victory was not easily won, but William, growing old now, in poor health, and somewhat softened by Gerald's hard work with his preceptor, at last agreed. Made suspicious, though, by the proximity of medical studies at the hospital, he sternly exacted from Gerald an unconditional pledge that he would be a dental student in the College and would take the L.D.S. (Licentiate of Dental Surgery) degree.

Triumphantly, on 29 September 1891, five days after his twentieth birthday, Gerald moved his books (including the multivolume *Complete Works of Shakespeare* that Mater had just given him as a birthday gift), his chess set, tennis racquet, and violin into a room at 44 Trinity Square, Newington, in southeast London, and set off to explore his new milieu at Guy's Hospital.

He was then a tall (six feet two inches), lanky but good-looking young man. As the result of a childhood injury while playing in his father's coal yard, he walked with his left foot turned slightly inward, just enough to give him a distinctive gait. His blond hair was bleached almost white by summer hours on the Cotswolds. From beneath his fair skin shone the English rosy glow, and in his narrow, oval face his hazel eyes, a heritage from the LePlastriers, were set wide above a long, straight nose, a firm mouth, and a cleft chin.

In manner he was quiet and shy, but friendly, candid, trusting—

"a thoroughly good fellow" in the opinion of Mr. Lansdale, his landlord.

William by no means let loose of his son. He arranged to pay for Gerald's room and board by quarterly checks for £20 each and received in return regular reports from Mr. Lansdale on the boy's progress and wellbeing. Gerald's letters home reported to his father how much he had spent for books and dental equipment, enclosed the receipts, and asked for a check to reimburse him. Sending the requested check, William felt it necessary to instruct the fledgling, "You must write your name on the back of the cheque in order to get the money."

Gerald elected a heavy schedule for himself at Guy's, enrolling in both dentistry and medicine, which required, in addition to many hours in laboratories and the dental clinics and wards, frequent classes and extensive reading in anatomy, physiology, biology, chemistry, physics, and metallurgy. His Cheltenham schooling, with no university education to supplement it, was found wanting in the sciences, so that he was also required to take in that first year the preliminary scientific course in the College.

One by one he passed the requisite examinations, winning an impressive second place in both anatomy and physiology. With the basic science work behind him, he was able in his second year to add to his dental studies the beginning courses in medicine, surgery, and midwifery. He became known at Guy's as a brilliant, ambitious student and a disciplined worker.

He also, to his dismay, gained a reputation for uncertain health. Fatigue or unwonted stress was likely to show quickly in his face, making him pale and sunken-eyed. Boardinghouse food kept him excessively thin, and he was quite often laid up for two or three days with pleurisy or an ailment he called "hospital throat." His teachers and classmates were constantly urging him to slow down and predicted that he would "go into consumption" if he didn't take care. Each time he went to Dr. Shaw, dean of the College at Guy's, for a physical checkup, the doctor warned him that he had "a weak chest" and must guard against "lung disease."

Yet he felt himself to be well and strong. In true British fashion he always found time for ample recreation. He played tennis and cricket on occasion for London neighborhood clubs and was a regular member of the tennis team at Guy's. When in a victory against Cambridge he won his tennis blue and the right to wear the hospital insignia on his blazer for life, he considered himself to be a true "Guy's man."

The London theaters, when faced with a small audience, often sent free tickets to be used by Guy's students to fill the stalls. Gerald always took advantage of the opportunity. In this way he saw at the Savoy Theatre many of the premier performances of the light operas of Gilbert and Sullivan and became a life-long fan of those witty masters.

The whole family felt only release when William John died suddenly in May 1893. Any love or rapport between him and his children had long since vanished under the burden of his alcoholic tantrums. The two youngest, Gerald and Frank, had come to fear his rages and to hate his surly, scowling presence as he sat for hours hunched in silent brooding in his chair by the fire.

Perhaps in consequence they loved their protective mother all the more. "Little lady of the glorious hair," Gerald called her. She was bustling and cheery and always full of ambitious plans. She was also determined and opinionated and sometimes pushed them too hard in her wish to see them successful in a profession and thus enter a social class above those who earned livings in trade, but they adored her.

Their oldest brother Harold was in many ways a surrogate father to the boys. He taught them to ride and to play tennis, and he told them lively tales of the adventures he had when his parents, fearing that a persistent cough presaged consumption, sent him off to spend a year on an Australian ranch. He nursed the sick when smallpox swept the ship, evaded quarantine at the dock, was a cowpuncher in the outback, returned home by way of America, and got caught in a gale on the Atlantic that sent his ship drifting helplessly south to the equator. An Australian doctor had cured his cough by whacking off an overlong uvula in his throat.

Harold and Roly also made life exciting for the family, and for Cheltenham as well, by leasing the Montpellier Gardens and Winter Gardens of the spa and turning themselves into first-rate impresarios. Among the stars they brought to town were Madame Adelina Patti, Mrs. Patrick Campbell, Buffalo Bill Cody, and Tex Austin. More thrilling for Gerald were the exhibition matches by the Allen brothers and the Renfraw brothers, England's tennis heroes. Harold also introduced Gerald to golf and let him help lay out a nine-hole course at the Gardens.

William John's death brought to each member of the family a measure of financial independence: to Mater a lifetime income and tenancy of the house at 19 Tivoli Place, which they all now called Heimat, the German word for home; to Harold and Roland the coal and brick business; to each of the other children some £5,000 — said to be the equivalent of about £50,000 today — not affluence but a comfortable cushion.

A rash of travel now broke out in the family. Roland and Amy toured Russia. Wilfred roamed the Continent. Harold and Sophie set sail for Australia. Ida and Frank crossed the Atlantic and went west as far as the Rocky Mountains; Frank journeyed on to adventures in Japan while Ida turned back for home alone. "Timid little thing, indeed! That took some courage," Frank wrote Gerald about their sister.

Gerald prudently asked Wilfred, the executor of William John's estate, to invest the bulk of his legacy in British consols (government bonds) so he could live off the interest. He did move away from the watchful eye of Mr. Lansdale into diggings with a fellow student named Trixie Finch nearer the Spit, as the Guy's men called the hospital; he bought himself a piano; and he paid £160 for a lifetime ticket to hospital practice at Guy's. Then, when his summer holiday of 1893 began, he sailed to America to visit Miss Jenny Raphael Kenney of Philadelphia.

It was his brother Roland who first met Jenny. In his pursuit of knowledge about the making of bricks, Roland went to see George Dickson of Liverpool, manager of the English branch of the New Jersey Asbestos Company. He was soon courting George's daughter Lilian and followed her to America when she went to visit her relatives in New Jersey. She introduced him to Jenny. When he learned Miss Kenney was planning a trip to London, he urged her to visit his sister Ida, who was still studying music in London. Ida invited her to tea and asked Gerald to come from Guy's Hospital to join them.

The Kenneys were a large, united, wealthy clan. Jenny's mother died when the girl was small, and her father Robert fled west, leaving Jenny in the care of his sister Beade, who was then unmarried.

By the time Robert had settled in Wahoo, Nebraska, and remarried, Jenny was a young lady with a mind of her own and she

decidedly preferred Aunt Beade to her stepmother and lively Philadelphia to sleepy Wahoo. So she lived on with Beade in the old
family home, becoming the pet of the clan and a favorite member
of a fashionable younger set that danced dizzily from Philadelphia
to New York to the Jersey Shore to Europe and back again.

After graduating from Wellesley College Jenny became engaged
to a dashing young millionaire named Frederick Brokaw. In 1892,
only weeks before they were to be married and take charge of the
Brokaw white marble mansion on Fifth Avenue at Seventy-ninth
Street in New York City, Frederick drowned while swimming at
Monmouth Beach.

By this time Beade, a devout churchwoman, had married the
Reverend Andrew J. Myers of the Methodist Episcopal Church
and established her own home in Asbury Park, New Jersey. In the
spring of 1893 she took the grieving Jenny with her to Philadelphia
to dismantle and sell the beloved old Kenney house.

Needing distraction, Jenny planned a trip to London. And
there, at Ida Webb's flat, she met Gerald.

Jenny was something new in Gerald's experience: beautiful,
vivacious, teasingly flirtatious, well schooled in the social graces
American style, always dressed in the latest fashion, yet highly intelligent and well read. Gerald was attracted, fascinated, and soon
in love.

With equal speed Jenny lost her heart to the handsome, engaging
young Englishman. She was sure she would not at all mind exchanging her gay life in the American social whirl for love in a cottage with him. Besides, she was certain that with her help he would
quickly become a great and famous man, well able to support her
in the style to which she had been reared. In any case, later on they
would have plenty of money because she knew she had been named
heir to Beade's fortune.

Gerald must see her country and meet her relatives. He was
received warmly by the Reverend and Mrs. Myers and traveled
with them and Jenny on a circuit of Pennsylvania, back to Asbury
Park, and on to nearby Ocean Grove for a Methodist camp meeting. He was wide-eyed at the luxury of travel in America, at all the
"huge, palatial houses, on account I suppose of space being unlim-
ited," and at finding even small towns "so up-to-date with electricity and street-cars." He described the novel experience at Ocean
Grove in letters home:

"This is a queer sort of place we're in now. If you haven't heard of it you ought, for it's worldfamed for religion. They have tremendous camp meetings and religious services of all kinds, to which Jenny and I go you bet!! They occupy all Mrs. Myers' time morning noon and night.... The meetings are held all day long from 6 in the morning to 10 at night. Thousands of people attend and at each performance some ten or so are 'converted' or 'saved,' standing up and giving their experiences. I have 'said a few words' and been saved this morning for the 9th time—being nine in the family I thought you would like one each. As a rule, though, Jane [as he often called her] and I prefer beach-meeting in this squeezing heat."

Another diversion from the preaching moved him to enthusiasm: "Went to West End Wednesday and saw another aunt, Mrs. Bates. That day we spoke to no one but millionaires—lunched with one of the Vanderbilts. My word, I have had a gorgeous time." Mrs. Bates was Jenny's Aunt Sally, the wife of D. Homer Bates, a New York banker and head of the John M. Bradstreet company.

Gerald and Jenny were engaged and hoping soon to be married when he sailed for home on 30 August. He had stayed weeks longer than he had intended (and had spent a good deal more too, having cabled twice to "Webb Bros." for additional funds) and now must study doubly hard for the qualifying examination in dentistry that was coming up in November.

In counterpoint to his reading—much of which he did at the College of Surgeons Museum, "rather a jolly place in Lincolns Inn Fields"—he gave restless thought to ways of increasing his income. Once he asked Mater, "What do you think of my starting in practise at dentistry near the hospital in partnership with one of the dental staff? He's offered it to me if I get through. Being near the Spit I could work on and finish the medical course and at the same time be earning money."

He got through readily. From Examination Hall on the Victoria Embankment on 16 November he sent a hurried scrawl to Mater: "Passed LDS. Just waiting to sign Diploma and be admitted before Examining Board. Had a jolly time of it and did quite well. Will come to Cheltenham in a day or so."

At Cheltenham he found Heimat deserted. Sophie and Amy were roaming in Wales and Mater had gone to stay with Nell, who was now married to a clothing manufacturer in Leicester. So he

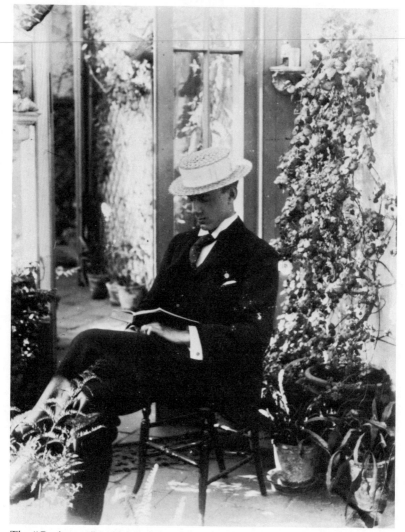

The "Guy's man" in Heimat's conservatory

spent the afternoon alone on the summit of Leckhampton Hill, came back to have dinner with Harold and his wife (Harold had been married while Gerald was in America), and then sat down at Heimat to write his mother. He had applied for a post as house dental surgeon at Guy's, he told her, but "I want to have a long talk with you about my future. I am in doubt about which to practise, dental or medical, and about America too."

Mater counseled patience and delay. He must not give up his medical studies, and he must not saddle himself with so much work and responsibility that his health would suffer. Besides, was he sure that Jenny was the proper wife for him? Mater did not believe a girl reared to the extravagant tastes and giddy ways of an American social butterfly could ever endure the quiet and frugal domesticity that would be her lot as the wife of a serious medical student with a limited income. Would not a nice English girl soundly trained in housewifery be more suitable?

Gerald was too smitten to entertain such questions when Jenny was arguing persuasively for immediate marriage. Word that he had won not only the appointment as house dental surgeon but another as clinical clerk in surgery, both carrying respectable stipends, settled the matter. In late November from a Liverpool hotel, on the eve of sailing again for America, he wrote his mother an exuberant letter only lightly tinged with penitence:

"Cheer up, my dear mother. Your prodigal will be home for Xmas when we'll have a jolly time. Do not fret or worry about me. I have a most brilliant future and what I am doing now will not damage it in the least, for I am more ambitious than ever, and have gold medals to carry off yet. Fancy, LDS I have started with, shortly MRCS and LRCP to add, and then MS, FRCP to follow, and I'm going to get the lot. You will think I am the luckiest johnny ever when I return, and Jane will help to brighten your life."

Across the Atlantic all was flurry. Jenny's host of relatives and friends must all be present to see her married and meet her wonderful English bridegroom. Invitations from the Reverend and Mrs. Myers named the date of the wedding as 19 December, the time six in the evening, the place "Brightside" in Frankford near Philadelphia, the elegant country home of one of Jenny's cousins.

Gerald was upset by the late date Jenny had fixed upon. Apologetically he wrote Mater that they could not after all spend Christmas at Heimat—"fancy, the first one I have missed"—they would have to celebrate the day on the ocean, for they must sail on the twenty-third to get him back at Guy's in early January.

Still in a euphoric daze from the round of elaborate wedding festivities Jenny's folks had put them through in Philadelphia and New York, Gerald upon landing in England sent Jenny to Cheltenham to stay with Mater while he hurried to London to begin his duties at Guy's and find a place for them to live.

It was just as well that Jenny never saw the hasty note marked "Private" that he penned at once to Mater: "You will find Jenny a sweet, loving girl with any amount of good sense, and anything you do not like in her please tell me now and I will alter it. You must please talk to her about wearing wool next her skin, she is naughty and will not. You, Mater, must insist."

Gerald had fixed upon Blackheath as the best place for them to live, since it was only twenty minutes from the hospital and he, being a member of the tennis club there, knew nice people in the district who would be friends for Jenny. When a quick look around the area turned up no suitable quarters he could afford, he resorted to the temporary expedient of renting a room in a boardinghouse in Russell Square.

The arrangement must have been a shock to Jenny, but she cheerfully left at Heimat her trunks full of gowns and hats and all their gorgeous wedding gifts of silver, china, glassware, and linens and settled down to shiver in the cold and drafty boardinghouse while she wrote thank-you notes and bread-and-butter letters. London had greeted their arrival the evening before "in a nightdress of dense fog," she told Mater, "and even today she has not troubled to change her costume." Gerald added that it was certainly nice to have a secretary now to answer all the fifty letters he had found awaiting him.

At Guy's he had been greeted with the gratifying news that he had won his appointment as house dental surgeon by a staff vote of 19 to 1 and that his assignment for the surgical clerkship was to look after eleven beds in the wards. Although "how I shall do the two together I do not know yet," he was jubilant because this was the first time a student had won two such appointments and the first time "a dental" had been given surgical wards.

The jubilation faded into dogged persistence as he established a wearing daily schedule: Up at 7:00, breakfast at 7:30, arrival by bus at Guy's 8:50, departure for home 5:00 or 5:30, dinner 6:00 or 6:30, then three hours of study while Jenny sat near him sewing or reading.

Each morning at the hospital he examined the mouths of some forty outpatients in the dental clinic, decided on the work to be done in each case, allotted it to one of the students, then supervised their efforts. Difficult fillings, extractions, abscess excisions, and the like he did himself, on some days administering gas to half a dozen or more patients who needed such procedures. One night

journey was by express train instead
the time for study.

Restless Jenny, prowling around i
decided within a month that they we
accommodations and so transferred t
few blocks nearer the station. Here G
down from Guy's; here Mater came
some of her homemade jams that G
from here, when Gerald wangled a tv
hospital before beginning his work in
brother Wilfred for a merry tour of I

Not all was roses of course. Gerald l
folk. Mater, growing old and weary,
apron strings. She complained becaus
dom now and was not placated by his
ties at Guy's. She fretted constantly a
once moving him to real annoyance by
having seen him in London, reported

He wished Nell would mind her ov
tually he was very fit, being told repe
how much better he was looking, not
so often a year ago. He had gained e
tops were all too small.

Mater sniffed that of course she had
she knew he no longer needed her advi
not to be foolish, that there were man
would want her counsel. She was ups
worrying that the long daily trips wou
autumn approached she urged them t
the winter, and remained unconvinced
ald would need the fresh sea air more
the noxious atmosphere of the dissect

Mater was still suspicious that Jenny
extravagant wife. She was certain it v
taken them to live in a seaside resort an
by the girl's meticulous household accou
When Roland and Lilian were married
Jenny were sending along their mite to
ding gifts, Mater wrote in outrage on

he gloatingly reported to Jenny that he had that day pulled twenty-five teeth for a patient under chloroform.

In the afternoons he looked after patients in the dental and surgical wards, changing their dressings and attending to other details of their postoperative care. He liked this ward work but was glad when it ended in March; the clinic duties were enough. Still, when Mr. Fripp, the surgical anesthetist assigned to the dental division on Wednesday mornings, found the work not to his liking and asked Gerald to do it for him, Gerald agreed because, he told Mater, the extra twenty cases a week would add to his experience and the favor might win the anesthetist's support for further surgical appointments.

He kept thinking ahead and raising his sights for how fast and in what order he should take the examinations for the M.R.C.S. (Member of the Royal College of Surgeons), the L.R.C.P. (Licentiate of the Royal College of Physicians), and the academic M.B. (Bachelor of Medicine). He was determined to have passed them all by the summer of 1895.

After June 1894 he was through with dentistry at Guy's. Two more members of the dental staff had offered him partnerships in private practice but he refused both offers. His heart was set on medicine, especially surgery.

He was therefore overjoyed when he was appointed assistant surgical dresser to Mr. L. A. "John" Dunn, his favorite teacher, for the summer term and assistant demonstrator of anatomy for the fall quarter. (The chief demonstrator was the Mr. Fripp whose work he had added to his own in dental anesthesia; the favor apparently *had* paid off!) He had intended to do a lot of dissection that term anyway, he told Mater, because a thorough knowledge of anatomy "is so important to a good surgeon," but now he would be saved the cost of body parts and be paid £15 besides.

He reported in the fall that all was going swimmingly. "The appointment is by far the nicest I have ever done. It's the best thing to have in the hospital and I was very lucky to get it, considering there were only two vacancies and nine applicants, all good men. There are something like two hundred students dissecting and I get called around to dive for some nerve or muscle they cannot find and then to teach them the parts they cannot grasp. If you were to come

round the dissecting room you
with my diagrams and drawing

Jenny called the dissecting rc

Gerald and Jenny were living
searches in Blackheath and els
their means that was not "disgu:
on in Russell Square. But Jenny
own, however modest, where s
and cozy for Gerald to study. A
where there are no people you
naturally gregarious.

On a weekend excursion to F
by the idea of living there beside
away from the dirt and smoke c
small rooms in a "cotlet" just tw
seven minutes' from the station,
tance more than they were alrea
straightaway.

The landlady, who according
of "howling swells," agreed to c
if Jenny would do the shopping
said he would be content to live
it became a point of pride with
would permit good nourishing n
She sent to Heimat for their wedc
that arrived from America for h
covers and a Wedgwood tea set,
tively their own.

"I get up at 6:30 to see that G
boasted to Mater. "He thinks it a
things I have never done in my li
such things."

"It's simply ripping living here
Gerald. "Guy's men abound her
timate as people are such a both

He reveled in a quick bathe in
leisurely swim before dinner, lc
beach or a band concert on the
seventy minutes instead of twent

sending it on to Nell that the "mite" was "a case of solid silver tea-spoons and sugar tongs!" She guessed that the lavish gift was Jenny's doing.

The American bride was in fact making her difficult adjustment admirably. Not only in style of living and spending but, more pain-fully, in manner of speaking and behaving. She was quickly made aware that her lively spirits, pert banter, and ritual flirtations, all so admired at home, were not appreciated by the Victorian female members of the Webb family. On early visits to Heimat she cried herself to sleep more than once after sharp rebukes from one or an-other of the ladies.

Gerald would have remonstrated on her behalf but she forbade him, preferring to keep peace in the family. Instead she learned to rein her tongue and her impulses to carefree fun. In her letters spon-taneity and frankness gave way to fulsome blandishment, and American slang like "P.D.Q." (pretty damn quick) disappeared, along with playful endearments and fanciful names like "Rolandi-no" and "Frankincense."

She did not enjoy the constraint: "It is a great loss, this of the old independence of speech and action. It oppresses me to 'be careful'; I like being *myself*, and somehow I *cannot* be. I have been shocked into a reticence that I cannot overcome."

At first Jenny welcomed the quiet life as a restful change, though she responded eagerly on the rare occasions when Gerald, feeling fed up with his grind, suggested a night at the theater or opera or attendance at a tennis or cricket match. But as the year proceeded the long days she spent alone and the nights of silence while Gerald studied wore her down. To help speed the hours Gerald got her a poodle pup. She named him Gerry and whiled away much time training and grooming him.

But she could not always keep her spirits high. When Mater hinted that it was Jenny who enjoyed Brighton so much, she replied more candidly than usual: "I never observe that the sun shines every day—all I feel is that it *sets*. HE is here then.... As I cannot live in the one place I care to live, it makes no difference where I am. Brigh-ton is very uninteresting to me except for the bracing air and the sea."

Depression sometimes came upon her from illness and fatigue. In London she had suffered frequent colds, owing in part no doubt to her stubborn refusal to exchange her dainty silk underclothing

"Thursday—in the midst of turmoil" was the heading on Jenny's farewell letter to Mater. "Believe me, mother," she wrote, "I should not go a step of this journey were it not that Gerald needs renewed vigor as much as I." She confessed that at last she had surrendered and was wearing woollen underwear.

Gerald added that "naturally after the anxiety of the last few days I am broken up" but that Mater need not worry about money matters; Uncle Homer had cabled that he would look after their expenses until Jenny was well again. They would not be gone long, he promised her. Jenny's family were planning a communal journey to England next May and he and Jenny would return with them.

When they landed in New York in early December, they found that Uncle Homer had taken charge. He had reserved a big, airy room for them at the Savoy Hotel on Fifth Avenue near Fifty-ninth Street, across from the William and Cornelius Vanderbilt homes and next door to the Langham Hotel, where the Bateses were living and where Jenny and Gerald were to have their meals "in terrible howling style." Uncle Homer was not there, having set off on a tour of the South looking for the best place for them to go; they were to stay in New York until he returned.

Gerald was again bemused by the wealth and splendor that surrounded them and by the hordes of callers and invitations that descended upon them. "They all just worship Jenny," he told Mater.

Amusingly he described the elegance of the two hotels and their patrons, the Metropolitan Club for millionaires only in which a friend of Jenny's had got him a membership while he was in the city, the extreme ladies' fashions ("those d———d bustles are in again!"), the theaters, the opera house "which licks Covent Garden into fits for size and magnificence," the fancy and superabundant food, including the juicy fresh oysters on which he was gorging himself.

His preferred companions were Jenny's Cousin Homer and his two partners in the law firm of Bostwick, Morrell, and Bates. The three were young, rich bon vivants, "so lively and larky," and Gerald felt at home with their enthusiasm for amateur theatricals.

He was keeping his eye on Jenny, who at first seemed better back in old haunts with old friends; her cough disappeared entirely. But Gerald did not like the nervousness, high fevers, and profuse night sweats which the constant excitement produced in her. It took her an hour to dress for each social event and there were sometimes four of them a day. "Her family just doesn't realize how ill she is, and want to keep her on the go all the time," he fretted to Mater; "at present their kindness only kills."

He finally forbade all visitors and refused all invitations, staying alone with Jenny in their hotel room, reading the medical books he had brought with him and concealing as best he could his impatience for Uncle Homer's return and his growing doubt about the wisdom of taking Jenny south; here in New York everyone seemed to think the West was the best place for consumptives.

He must have considered staying in Jenny's beloved Philadelphia, for he wrote to the University of Pennsylvania asking how long, with the training he already had, it would take him to get an American degree in medicine. One year, the officials replied. That was too long; he expected to return to England come spring.

(He might have thought twice about this if he had known that Pennsylvania offered the best education in medicine to be had in America at this time, a training more attuned to the future than his cherished Guy's was providing. Young Dr. Simon Flexner was shortly to become professor of pathology at the Pennsylvania school and, through his mentors William Henry Welch and William Osler, would establish its strong ties with the new Johns Hopkins University medical school—the fount from which progress and preferment in medicine would flow for decades.)

It was a welcome diversion from Gerald's anxious uncertainties when he took Jenny to spend Christmas at Brightside, the country house near Philadelphia at which they had been married a year ago. There Gerald was half dazzled, half appalled at the spectacle of lavishly tinseled trees and gaily clad packages. "Xmas cards you scarcely see here," he told Mater; "all friends send costly presents."

The smothering display of elaborate toys in the nursery moved him to outspoken protest: "I called it wicked extravagance" and said the whole monstrous lot ought to be carted away to the children's hospital.

"You may have it all," was Gerald's conclusion about the glittering life he was witnessing. "I am by no means blasé, but this grandeur is not in my line. My tastes are plain. Our simple rooms in Brighton were better. For these people the sole object in life is money, and they think a man must be a confounded idiot not to get it. They cannot understand a man's being content with a couple of hundred pounds a year to support him in a life of science, sports, and education."

Jenny wonderingly concurred: "I had almost forgotten how more than royally these people live. What millions they spend! Under everything is money—just money. Once I was wedded to all this fashion and luxury and fast living, but now I feel a bit afraid of it all, a bit overpowered by the rush of it, and I look toward the modest, quiet, old-fashioned home life of England and find more comfort in it."

Uncle Homer returned just after Christmas and summoned Gerald to New York to hear his authoritative recommendation that the young couple go to a resort in Thomasville, Georgia, just across the state line from Florida. Having explored the southern residences for invalids all the way west to New Orleans, he rated this one the best and had reserved accommodations there for the Webbs. Florida proper he thought too swampy, too malarious.

Obediently and gratefully, Jenny and Gerald on 29 December left a Philadelphia blanketed in snow and, after twenty-six hours on the train, rode in summertime warmth along the shaded road through dense forests that led to the Piney Woods Hotel.

II

Health-Seekers

THE YOUNG WEBBS had now joined a migrant throng that supported a sizable industry in America as well as in Europe: the merchandising of climate, location, and services to those wandering the world in search of health.

It was more than twenty centuries old, the belief that the exchange of one kind of air or temperature or water for another could cure or alleviate the ills of man—everything from a broken heart or aching bones to paralysis, dyspepsia, and consumption. And for almost as many centuries every spot on earth that could claim some therapeutic advantage, from hot or mineral springs to dry air, had sought to lure the traveling invalids to its hostelries and land. The traffic was encouraged by the doctors, who, as ignorant as their patients of any facts in these matters, followed ancient customs or the prevailing fashion about what place was good for the relief of what ailment.

The advantages ascribed to Thomasville, Georgia, were abundant warmth and sunshine in winter and the supposedly health-giving exhalation of turpentine from a vast acreage of surrounding pines.

The idea that there was healing power in pine trees had persisted through the ages. In the first century Pliny the Elder had recommended pine groves for phthisical patients and in the middle of the nineteenth Hermann Brehmer, a German botanist who recovered from phthisis in the Himalaya Mountains, established the first sanatorium for consumptives in the midst of a pine forest at Görbersdorf in the Prussian province of Silesia.

To its aromatic setting the Piney Woods Hotel, seven miles into the forest from Thomasville, added luxurious ease of living, an elaborate cuisine, and a plethora of choices for recreation. There were tennis courts and golf links on its grounds; the woods afforded excellent hunting of small game; extending in a cogwheel arrangement from the hotel were enough roads canopied by pines to permit a different walk, carriage ride, or exercise in "wheeling" every day for a month.

Indoors the hotel provided card rooms for euchre and whist, a spacious floor for dancing to the music of an excellent orchestra that played till past midnight each evening, and in the lobby, as well as on the two piazzas, long rows of rocking chairs for people-watching. These chairs were occupied the afternoon the Webbs arrived and Gerald was tickled by the whisper of "Honeymooners!" that ran down the gauntlet with them all the way to the desk.

They lived a pleasant life the next few weeks. After a gargantuan breakfast at nine o'clock — "I had an orange, cheese omelette, roast quails on toast, veal cutlets, and then! Flannel cakes with maple syrup!! 12 of them. Lovely!" — Gerald played tennis, took lessons in golf, or improved his skill in hunting while Jenny read *Trilby* or did needlepoint under a parasol on the piazza.

In the afternoons Jenny napped and Gerald practiced pistol shooting on the hotel range before taking a walk or carriage ride together through the redolent pines.

In the evenings they might do some dancing, which Jenny loved but Gerald did not enjoy because he felt himself no good at it, but most often they played whist, about which they admitted going halfway mad.

Scrupulously observing the English canon of good manners not to speak to strangers until spoken to (lest you obtrude upon someone in a higher social class than your own), the Webbs were pleased to be taken up by the socially prominent guests. By no means all of these were invalids; some had come to Piney Woods for a few weeks of good hunting, others merely to escape the rigors of winter in the North. Even the health-seekers were, like Jenny, fully ambulatory; Piney Woods did not invite the presence of advanced or terminal cases whose suffering might detract from the pleasure of other guests.

Gerald's English speech made him a magnet for several rabid Anglophiles in the group. With wry humor he asked the family to send him a Debrett for reference: "These people know all about even our minor nobility and I don't even know the royal family."

Jenny was getting better with each passing day, but Gerald grew tired of his aimless hours. Once again he pulled his textbooks from the trunk and resumed his reading. He wrote to the University of Georgia as he had to Pennsylvania and got a similar reply. "[The American degree is] not worth much when you've got it, I suppose," the cocky Guy's man commented to sister Nell, "but might just as well get it to passer le temps."

On second thought, Piney Woods was almost as good as a hospital for clinical material. So Gerald improved his acquaintance with the hotel doctor, Morton by name, and presently was discussing with him the symptoms and treatment of each of his current cases: Bright's disease, Bell's palsy, a hip-joint disorder, melancholia, nervous prostration, alcoholism, asthma, bronchitis, consumption.

Gerald also played at being "a business johnny." His British consols were on the rise and Wilfred was planning to sell them for him when they peaked, so he was looking around for another investment. Mortgage money at 8 percent made him whistle — and advise his family to sell out in England, move to Georgia, and "double your income."

He was intrigued by an offer of a one-third interest in a Georgia factory that made cigars from imported Cuban tobacco but was prudent enough to consult Uncle Homer, who promptly sent him a "no good" rating of the firm from Bradstreet's. Mr. Bates suggested instead that he invest safely in the family's Gamewell Company, manufacturers of the familiar red street-corner fire-alarm boxes.

All such considerations came to an abrupt end in early February. The constant sunshine with temperatures in the 90s gave way to days of torrential rains followed by a record-breaking dip to 14 degrees and a heavy snowfall. Jenny caught a severe cold which progressed rapidly into pneumonia plus pleurisy. Her condition grew critical.

Gerald became her nurse and, the hotel not being equipped against such weather, struggled to warm the room by keeping a fire of pinewood roaring in the small fireplace. Dr. Morton came in to help as often as he could, prescribing one ounce of brandy every hour with periodic injections of morphine to deaden the pleurisy pain.

Gerald did not see how Jenny could live. Twice he and Dr. Morton thought her dead and marveled to see her begin to breathe again. Only when the doctor at last took the risk of tapping her chest and drawing off the pleuritic fluid did she come slowly out of danger and begin to recover.

From the first Gerald had been sending daily telegrams to Uncle Homer, who passed the bulletins on to the rest of the family. They were all frantic because none of them could get to Jenny's bedside; the record storm had produced in the North a raging blizzard that piled snow six or more feet high and stalled all trains.

When Aunt Beade at last got through and took over the nursing, Gerald was soon wishing she had not come. The family might consider her a cheery, comforting "good angel," but she did not please Jenny now. He turned the situation into dialogue for Mater:

She keeps worrying Jenny with religion, and me too, and you know Jane can't stand it.

    Mrs. Myers—You must pray to the Lord, Jenny. He will stop your pain.

    Jenny—I think he's a very *cruel* God to make me suffer so much. *Do* shut up, Beade.

Consternation of Mrs. Myers!!! She calls me outside the room.

    Mrs. Myers—Why, Gerald! I never knew any of our family to be dying without calling on God.

    Gerald—Oh, it's alright, Beade. You let her alone. If any girl ever went to heaven, she will—if there is one.

Then again—

    Mrs. Myers—What time did she recover from her attack of heart failure last Sunday?

    Gerald—About 12 o'clock at night.

    Mrs. Myers—Oh! *Exactly the time* Rev. Myers and I were praying to God to spare her a little longer—and my! I never heard a man pray so eloquently.

Poor Jane suffering agony all the time, you can imagine how cross this would make her. But then, Beade is very kind in other ways. If only she wouldn't force her religion down your throat.

Letters of concern and hopeful wishes came from everywhere, including a rare note from Jenny's father in Wahoo. It showed "Papa and Mama" to be as given to piety and prayers as was Aunt Beade.

Jenny's convalescence progressed slowly. Not until April was she strong enough to sit again, pale and thin, in the sun on the piazza. If she had not guessed before, she knew now for whose sake they were traveling and what her disease was, for in her lap lay the telltale sign, her handkerchief stained with blood-flecked sputum.

A week later she wrote her first letter to Mater: "I want to write you from this place where I have been so very near never writing you again. . . . We shall leave Thomasville for Washington this week. . . . All our friends and the doctor advise our going at once to Colorado. I cannot bear the thought, it is so far west and I dislike the west. But I leave the plans to Gerald. Perhaps he is wiser than I."

Gerald was not making the decision lightly. Returning to England this spring was now out of the question and Dr. Morton would not predict how soon it might be possible. Jenny would never recover in the sea-level dampness of Georgia, he told Gerald; the pleurisy had collapsed her diseased left lung and the only place to expand it properly again was in the dry, light air of the Colorado mountains.

Uncle Homer was urging them to settle in Washington, D.C., where he was sure the climate would be mild enough and where they would be within easy reach of Jenny's family in case of another such ordeal. But it seemed to Gerald that Washington's air would be much the same as Georgia's without the pines, and the book he was reading about Colorado's health resorts was persuading him that the consumptive probably fared best in someplace high and dry.

His mind was not fully made up when they left Georgia for Washington, traveling by way of St. Augustine, Florida, partly to break the journey for Jenny and partly to take a look for themselves at the place Dr. Goodhart in London had prescribed.

How was it possible that areas so diverse in climate as Florida and Colorado could be recommended with equal conviction for the same disease? Because, simply, no science and few facts underlay the traditions of climate therapy.

Of all the treatments prescribed for consumption through the ages, change of place and climate had been the most persistent, but notions of just what climate was curative or palliative, and why, had shifted back and forth in succeeding centuries, even generations. By the nineteenth century physicians could choose at will among several traditional practices that had descended by skips and jumps from medical authorities of ancient India, Greece, and Rome. There were advocates of cold mountain heights, of warm southern climes, of long sea voyages, of moist air, of dry air. Common to all in some degree was the belief in exposure to sunlight; *Sol est remedium maximum* said Pliny the Elder.

Onto the roster of popular warm, sunny resorts had recently come the West Indies, especially Nassau in the Bahamas, and Cuba. When in the 1840s American physicians recognized that a similar climate was available nearer at hand, they, and soon their European colleagues, began sending patients to Florida.

From that time on, virtually every new American territory or state, seeking feverishly to people its empty acres, found some "salubrious" aspect of its air, waters, or topography to be touted as good for consumptives.

When the Civil War temporarily shut Florida and the West Indies out of the race, the state that took the lead in replacing them was, surprisingly, Minnesota. Its campaign for the favor of consumptives and their doctors was astonishingly successful. Among the thousands lured to its lakes and plains for cure were such notables as Edward Eggleston, Henry David Thoreau, Clara Barton, and Edward L. Trudeau.

A newspaperman from Cincinnati visiting the state in the late 1860s reported that "Minnesota all the year round is one vast hospital. All her cities and towns, and many of her farm houses, are crowded with those fleeing from the dread destroyer."

By that time Florida was re-entering the contest and during the succeeding decade the intense rivalry between the two states for the position of the nation's prime haven for consumptives produced a barrage of books, pamphlets, magazine articles, and newspaper reports throughout the country. These publications, many of them written by doctors, reveal vividly the preposterous mélange of myth and whim that determined the climatic treatment of consumption before, and for two or more decades after, the bacterial cause of the disease was discovered.

For example: Phthisis was then especially prevalent along the Atlantic Coast from Maine to Virginia, and the best explanation doctors could find for this geographic incidence was the northeast winds that blew chill and moisture-laden inland from the Atlantic Ocean. So firm became the belief in the unhealthiness of northeast winds that it was considered "no less than manslaughter" to lodge a person in a northeast bedroom. When consumption forced Ralph Waldo Emerson to close his school he went south, he said, "to escape the northeastern blasts."

In a debate between Harriet Beecher Stowe from Florida and one Dr. J. P. Little writing in *Lippincott's Magazine* the doctor stated an even more fanciful cause: "There are many feeble consumptives who suffer from a relaxed condition of the skin—who are always moist and easily thrown into profuse perspiration. For these a dry air is best."

The basic argument among doctors, reported frequently and at length in medical society *Proceedings* of the time, turned on the question of which was the more efficacious in the treatment of consumption, a warm or a cold climate. Many physicians thought the rigors of a northern winter entirely too much for an ailing body to endure. Exercise in the fresh air was essential to the cure of consumption, they insisted, and how could the patient walk and play outdoors in the frigid North?

The other side countered that a warm climate was enervating, *sedative* in its effects, whereas what the phthisical patient needed was a stimulating, *tonic* atmosphere, which only stinging cold could provide.

As the 1880s approached, Florida held its position and southern California rose to favor with the advocates of warm climates, but Minnesota yielded first place to the Adirondacks and Colorado's Rocky Mountains with those who sought invigoration for their patients. Texas, New Mexico, and Arizona drew custom from both camps, enough to permit a New Mexican writer to conclude that "Albuquerque has only two businesses, the Santa Fe Railroad and tuberculosis."

Edward L. Trudeau was largely responsible for the growing popularity of the Adirondacks. When a season in North Carolina and a year in Minnesota did his lungs no good, he resigned himself to his fate, decided to spend the months left to him in a place he enjoyed, and so returned to the East and set up a tent in the midst of pine forests on a slope of the Adirondacks. His health unexpectedly improved and he lived on to establish his famous sanatorium and research laboratory at Saranac Lake.

Colorado Territory, after the outpouring of publicity that attended the Pikes Peak gold rush of 1859, had become a last resort, largely self-prescribed, for a growing number of "lungers" who "roughed it" or took the "camp cure" in isolated shacks throughout the parks and valleys of its mountains.

But the territory (state after 1876) began its rise to national prominence as a health resort only when such prominence became an aim of government, railroad, and townsite promotion in the

1870s. The estimate is that 30,000 hopeful invalids had been lured to Colorado by 1880 and that within a decade this number had risen to 200,000. It is a reasonable guess that at least 75 percent of these migrants were consumptives.

In this resurgence of high-altitude therapy for phthisis (marked in Europe by the establishment of the famous sanatorium at Davos in the Swiss Alps that became the setting for Thomas Mann's *Magic Mountain*) a plausible explanation for the undeniable benefit of mountain living began to take shape. It was stated with vigor in the official *Colorado Gazetteer for 1871*:

"One of the curses of civilized life is the consummate stinginess with which people breathe. Here one *must* breathe, both more fully and more rapidly, or die of suffocation. The result is a permanent increase of the breathing capacity...and the appetite keeps pace with the respiration. The effect is a general awakening of all the vital powers that often seems like very magic, so that the patient is suddenly and substantially improved."

The man who refined this explanation, elevated it to a measure of medical respectability, and sent it circulating throughout the nation was Dr. Charles L. Denison of Denver.

In the winter of 1872–73 after a series of pulmonary hemorrhages Denison left his home in Hartford, Connecticut, to try the touted climate of western Texas. Feeling no better there he moved on to Colorado, where his health immediately improved and he eventually recovered.

This experience fixed his inquiring mind on the whys of climate therapy. He was appalled to discover how little was known on the subject and became intensely concerned for the welfare of consumptives who were being sent hither and yon on the basis of mere puffery. He began a crusade to collect facts about the effects of various climates on phthisis.

Dr. Denison kept reporting the information he assembled in papers read to his medical colleagues at their meetings and congresses, and these reports became the basis for his book entitled *Rocky Mountain Health Resorts: An Analytical Study of High Altitudes in Relation to the Arrest of Chronic Pulmonary Disease*, which was published in Boston in 1880.

This book remained for many years both an authoritative treatise among medical men and a descriptive guidebook for consumptives migrating to Colorado. In it Dr. Denison explained that the diminished amount of oxygen in the air at high altitudes forced an increase in respiratory activity; this not only expanded the lungs but improved circulation and digestion and alleviated insomnia. In addition, the thinner atmosphere made the healing sunlight more intense; the high-velocity mountain winds blew away putrid matter, keeping the air always fresh and pure; the sudden changes and daily variations in temperature that characterized mountain weather stimulated body responses and kept them flexible.

All this was mostly opinion and hypothesis still, but it was several degrees nearer physiological sense than was manslaughter by northeast winds or the debilitating effects of a relaxed skin.

Charles Denison's book may well have been the one Gerald Webb was reading in the Piney Woods Hotel.

Or he may have got hold of one even more widely known in the East, especially in nonmedical circles—Edward F. Tenney's *Colorado: Homes in the New West*, the book credited by Stewart Holbrook in *Yankee Exodus* with inspiring thousands of consumptives to move from New England to Colorado.

Tenney, a native of New Hampshire who had found health in Colorado, was a Congregational minister who became president of Colorado College in Colorado Springs in 1876. His forte was not statistics or medical explanations but enthusiasm and eloquence, and his book, first published in 1878, was several times reprinted in succeeding decades.

Whichever the book Gerald read, with resorts for consumptives available north and south from New York to California, and with a cacophony of claims and counterclaims filling the air, it was only chance that fixed the Webbs' attention on Florida and Colorado.

Florida they did not like at all. Gerald was captivated by the history of "the oldest city on the continent," he enjoyed its good sailing and swimming, he thought its palm trees an interesting novelty. But he judged all else about it dull and barren, even the citrus groves being mere stands of leafless sticks after the severe winter.

In Washington seven members of the Kenney clan had assembled to greet Jenny and were happily surprised to see her looking so well again. While the women busied themselves shopping for the six new dresses that were Aunt Sally's gift to Jenny, the men played golf and cards at a club in which Gerald had secured guest privileges through "a second secretary" with whom he was acquainted at the

British Embassy. It pleased him that *he* could be the man-of-the-world host this time.

By mid-May he had made his decision. "I have not heard Jane cough for a month," he told Mater. "We shall start for Colorado this week, and I think three months there of mountain air will quite set her up."

The journey west was not a happy one. Dark skies over Chicago turned into frightening storms on the prairies, the berths were cold and drafty, and the Webbs, low in spirits when they left Washington, sank further into gloom.

No matter what Jenny had been told about Colorado, her picture of the West remained that of the monotonous dusty plains of Nebraska, the crudities and boredom of Wahoo. She was leaving behind a life and people she treasured and could feel no hope of any good to come. Nor did it help that the sleeping car they rode in reminded her of John Sanger Pullman, a lively beau she had liked in the earlier carefree years.

For once Gerald could summon no cheer to comfort her. He was too conscious that every turn of the wheels was carrying him farther away from the England he loved and the career he wanted. He had heard that Trixie Finch was taking the examinations toward which he had been aiming. His sister Ida was giving song recitals in Cheltenham and Harold and Roly were setting the town afire with such innovative enterprises as introducing the telephone and electricity. Wilfred had invented a new kind of engine for which his Gloucester employers were paying him a handsome royalty. Even baby brother Frank would soon be a fully qualified solicitor. While here was he, Gerald, suspended in uncertainty, getting nowhere.

Jenny was exhausted and fretful and Gerald was aching and sniffling with a cold when they arrived at the Brown Palace Hotel in Denver in early June. His cold turned to tonsillitis and they spent their first days in Colorado being miserable in bed.

But the bright blue and gold of the sunny skies and the sophisticated comfort of the hotel were encouraging and they were in somewhat better spirits when they set off four days later on the seventy-five-mile trip to the popular resort in the mountains at Manitou.

Jenny whiled away the journey scribbling and rescribbling a birthday poem for Mater; Gerald was content to watch the passing scenes as the train rolled southward along the base of the Rockies.

He nudged Jenny to look too when majestic Pikes Peak, still wearing its winter cap of snow, came into view.

It was evening when they claimed their reservation at the Cliff House in Manitou, and, already feeling the need for sleep induced in newcomers by 6000 feet of altitude, they went early to bed.

Within a week, hope restored, Jenny was writing Mater enthusiastically about Manitou, "the most beautiful little spot imaginable — a tiny, hilly town nestling cozily among the giant peaks of these great rocky mountains. The air is delicious, the scenery superb."

She and Gerald became sightseers with the tourists who, now that "the season" had begun, poured into the town off each of the five trains arriving daily. Although Manitou claimed fewer than six hundred permanent residents, it was host to some five thousand guests each summer. All its hotels filled to capacity, private homes took in boarders, and summer cottages and tents perched like birds' nests in every available space on the hillsides.

Many of the visitors were health-seekers of course, and most of these were consumptives, but the resort was no dolorous collection of invalids huddled under shawls exchanging symptoms; the surroundings and activities outdoors were too inviting.

The Cliff House stood just across the street from a triangular park in which bubbled four of Manitou's seven natural springs. One of the four was the popular "soda spring" to which every visitor came. From their hotel verandah Jenny and Gerald watched the sick and well alike queue up, on foot or in carriages, to sip the sweet naturally carbonated water from long-handled tin ladles handed round by lads in rubber boots.

Jenny knew the taste well, for she had drunk "Original Manitou Water" poured from beautiful handblown green bottles at many a dinner party in Philadelphia and New York. And here, amid the springs, was the bottling works from which this water and the equally celebrated Manitou Ginger Champagne were shipped east and west in sixty-carload lots; the glass factory that produced the lovely bottles was just a stroll away on the edge of town.

A few hundred yards south of the soda spring lay the smelly sulphur spring called Shoshone, the bitter water of which was thought to have medicinal properties. Although many quaffed this water too with seeming pleasure, the Webbs forswore it after one taste.

Across from the Shoshone stood a two-storied bathhouse, complete with cornices, a widow's watch, and wide piazzas and balconies. Pipes carried both drinking and bathing waters from the springs to the parlors and bathing rooms on the first floor. Upstairs were reading rooms, lounges for the sociable, and the offices of an attending physician.

The whole buzzing human scene reminded Gerald irresistibly of the spa at Cheltenham, right down to the daily fashion parade. The ladies of rank and wealth came to Manitou as they did to Cheltenham with trunks full of elaborate high-fashion gowns which they donned and displayed in turn each afternoon in their ritual stroll down Ruxton Avenue, one block south of the Cliff House.

But Gerald admitted that Cheltenham offered nothing comparable to the scenic delights around Manitou. The prime attraction was the trip by cog railway up the valley of Ruxton Creek to the summit of Pikes Peak, with a stop a third of the way up for doughnuts and coffee at Half Way House. Gerald was not sure the added elevation, to 14,110 feet, would be safe for Jenny, and when he learned the excursion would cost them five dollars apiece he decided to wait and, like other sturdy souls, *walk* to the top sometime.

He and Jenny did indulge in some of the popular carriage trips: westward alongside leaping Fountain Creek to Rainbow Falls ("little Niagara" to the tourists); northward up the narrow yellow-walled corridor of Williams Canyon to the filigreed stalagmites and stalactites in Cave of the Winds; eastward past the castled estate called Briarhurst and then north to the awesome Garden of the Gods, where one could wander among gigantic uplifts of mellow red sandstone weathered by wind and time into eerie, mind-teasing shapes.

Just beyond the Garden another showplace mansion lay hidden in bewitching Glen Eyrie. Southward a scarily winding road climbed to exquisite Crystal Park, where John George Nicolay and John Hay had isolated themselves to finish their ten-volume biography of Abraham Lincoln and where Hay still lived in the intervals between his diplomatic missions.

Some five miles due east of Manitou sprawled the larger town of Colorado Springs. When the Webbs went exploring there, Gerald took along his diploma from Guy's Hospital, hoping to find a *locum tenens* in dentistry — a temporary post holding down the office for some dentist who wanted to get away for a while. He was amazed at how many of these there were. Several wanted him to take over their practice while they crossed to the southwestern slope of Pikes Peak to look after a claim or a mine in the Cripple Creek gold field eighteen miles away.

This was Gerald's introduction to the gold fever that was raging in Colorado Springs. "Never saw anything like it," he told Mater. "All these chaps wanted to talk about was gold mining, not dentistry. Everyone tackles me about some gold mine, but I have nothing to do with them—just say I am stone broke and come to make money (honestly if possible)."

To him there was something vaguely *dis*honest about this gold business and he shied away from it. He did not know that the Cripple Creek mines were no blue-sky speculation, that they were actually the richest gold field in America. Opened only four years before, they were already yielding ten million dollars annually and in a few years would be leading the world in gold production. The impressive business blocks downtown and the millionaires' residences on Wood and Cascade avenues in Colorado Springs were largely the product of the extractive operations at Cripple Creek.

The *locum* Gerald accepted was in the one office in which he heard no talk of gold, the office of Doctors F. C. and Anna D. Chamberlain, who wanted a brief rest together. He thought it "curious," a woman dentist practicing in partnership with her husband, but he agreed to look after their patients beginning the next day for "one-half the takings." He earned fifteen dollars the first day, twenty-five dollars for the week.

The Webbs saw plenty of health-seekers and tourists in Colorado Springs, which was as much a resort as Manitou, but Gerald became especially aware there of another element in the springs community, which he reported to Mater: "These parts simply *abound* with wealthy English people. Going to Colorado Springs you meet carriage after carriage of distinctly Englishers doing their shopping."

He might have added that the general sobriquet for Colorado Springs was "Little London." At that time more than two thousand emigrants from Great Britain were living in El Paso County, of which Colorado Springs and Manitou were the hub, and the customs these folks from abroad had brought with them prevailed throughout the community. Tea and crumpets at five, English styles of architecture, assorted varieties of British speech, and enthusiasm for sports and "culture" indelibly marked life around the springs.

The man chiefly responsible for transplanting these fragments of Great Britain to the foot of Pikes Peak was Dr. William A. Bell, who was shortly to become the patron of the Webbs.

Some twenty-five years earlier the young Dr. Bell, son of a fashionable and prosperous London physician, had come to the United States partly to represent his father at a medical congress in St. Louis and partly to seek a cure for his consumption. Hearing that the Kansas Pacific Railroad was just undertaking a survey to determine its route west from Kansas City, the ebullient Irish Bell forgot all about medicine, applied for a post on the survey, and was taken on as a photographer.

In charge of the survey was General William J. Palmer of Philadelphia, a veteran of the Civil War. The irrepressible Bell, aged twenty-six, and the stern, aloof Palmer, aged thirty, became close friends and explored the wilds of the Southwest together. When Palmer, having completed the Kansas Pacific rails to Denver, conceived the idea of a railroad to run south from that city through New Mexico into Mexico and organized the Denver and Rio Grande Railroad, Dr. Bell became its vice-president.

Traveling over the proposed route in a Concord coach one night, General Palmer stretched himself out to sleep under a blanket on the roof of the coach. Waking toward morning, he sat up to view the terrain in the moonlight. He must find sites for towns along the route to provide passengers and freight for the trains—and one of them must be someplace special that could become his home.

The coach was then a few miles south of the raucous gold-field service center called Colorado City, and suddenly Palmer was looking out upon a magnificent valley formed by the confluence of two rushing mountain streams. Above it in the distance hung the light-rimmed summit of Pikes Peak. There, he thought, there is the place for *my* town.

He took Dr. Bell to see the magic spot. Riding and tramping through the valley and its tributary canyons, the two men came upon the seven springs at the foot of Ute Pass and stopped to bathe in the tumbling waters. A few weeks later they organized the Colorado Springs Company with Palmer as president and Bell as vice-president and began arrangements to acquire the necessary acreage for the town. Bell's assignment was to bring both capital and settlers from England.

Emigration of money and people from the island kingdom was then at high tide. Millions of pounds sterling and thousands of restless farmers and workmen, younger sons, and family black sheep were spilling over into the American West. Bell went after a share of it all for the Pikes Peak region. He made annual recruiting trips to Britain, distributed the prospectuses of the Colorado Springs Company throughout Ireland and Scotland as well as England, and scattered alluring advertisements and glowing reports among British newspapers.

He was a clever press agent, quick to see and exploit opportunities. An example is the convalescence of Canon Kingsley:

Among the early comers to Manitou were Maurice and Rose Kingsley, son and daughter of Charles Kingsley, Canon of Westminster Abbey and author of *Westward Ho!* and *Water-babies*. Maurice was treasurer of the Colorado Springs Company for a year or so, while Rose in spinsterish tweeds tramped the mountainsides and canyons (Mount Rosa to the south of Colorado Springs was named for her) and introduced "culture" to the community by staging its first concert. When their celebrated father fell ill in San Francisco during a lecture tour of the United States, Rose took him to Manitou to recover.

He remained for a month, carefully ministered unto by Dr. Bell— who promptly informed Kingsley's adoring public in Great Britain that the Canon's sojourn amid the Pikes Peak springs was the highlight of his American journey and Manitou the only place in the land where a man could be made well in the British way: in bed with hot bricks to keep him warm and Earl Grey tea to soothe his miseries.

Bell blithely omitted the fact that Kingsley, testy in his illness, disliked Pikes Peak's thin air and abundance of rattlesnakes and was glad to get away.

Some of the first migrants helped Bell to sell Little London. Among the earliest investors in Palmer's railroad and townsite was a wealthy patient of the elder Dr. Bell, William Blackmore, brother of the author of *Lorna Doone*. Following his money to Colorado, Blackmore, who was addicted to Indian lore and to Longfellow's "Hiawatha," gave an Indian name to each of the seven springs and suggested Manitou, after the Algonquin god of healing, for the town platted around them. He also collected facts for an enthusiastic book, *Colorado as a New Field for Emigration*, which he published on his return to London.

Another helpful publicist was the suave and handsome young

physician, Samuel Edwin Solly. Son of a prominent Harley Street surgeon, a product of Rugby, and a diplomate of the Royal College of Surgeons, Solly had contracted phthisis and joined the wanderers in search of a cure. After making the rounds of European spas without benefit, he returned to London and there encountered William Bell, a boyhood acquaintance; their two fathers were professional friends. Persuaded by Bell's enthusiasm, Solly came at the age of twenty-seven to Manitou and there found health again.

Health *and* a golden opportunity. By boosting Manitou as heaven for invalids he could boost himself into a lucrative medical practice. Having learned from his experience all about resort promotion, he put his knowledge to use in a booklet for Dr. Bell's English market, *Manitou, Colorado, U.S.A., Its Mineral Waters and Climate*.

The author cast his net wide; if there was any human ailment that could not be cured by one or another of the seven springs, it was only because Solly had failed to think of it. Authorship worked so well for the doctor that he used it again a few years later in an elaborate guidebook, *The Health Resorts of Colorado Springs and Manitou*.

Dr. Bell was usually present to greet and help newcomers to the springs area. Having recovered his health in Colorado, he decided to live there. He bought twenty acres on the eastern edge of Manitou, brought over his English bride, Cara Georgina Whitemore Scovell, and built for her a large house of native stone modeled after an English castle. They christened the estate Briarhurst.

There the Bells raised their family of five children and assorted pets in a kind of cheerful bedlam. There they entertained incessantly at elaborate though often chaotic parties of all sizes and kinds for visitors and residents alike, making their home the undisputed center and themselves the arbiters of social life in Little London.

Dr. Bell made a huge fortune as an entrepreneur—in railroad, land, and townsite development, constructing hotels and business buildings, mining coal, milling iron, ranching. At one time he owned much of the land and most of the facilities in Manitou, plus substantial holdings in Colorado Springs and elsewhere in the state.

After some twenty years, in 1890 Dr. Bell took his family back to England to live on their second estate, Pendell Court at Bletchingley south of London, but they all returned to Briarhurst from time to time for lengthy visits.

Gerald and Jenny Webb within a few days of their arrival knew that Dr. Bell was the most important man in Manitou and that he and his family were currently in residence at Briarhurst. To American socialite Jenny it was obvious that they must go at once, as newly arrived visitors, to make the acquaintance of this wealthy compatriot of Gerald's. To reserved English Gerald doing such a thing would be unthinkably brash and rude. Jenny won the argument. Gerald recounted the sequel to his family:

"We hired a 'buggy' on Wednesday and with plenty of cheek drove up and called on a Mr. Wm. A. Bell, MB Cambridge, who has a lovely house and grounds. He started this place and is the most influential man in these parts. He and Mrs. Bell and their three girls have just returned from a long stay on their estate in Kent. Curiously we travelled from Omaha with their baggage, some 40 English trunks. All the family are howlingly *English*. Almost his first words were 'Are you a tennis player?' followed by an invitation to play the same evening. Of course he could not play much (age 50) so I walked him 6-love and got an invitation for the following night and again for Saturday.

"They are very nice people indeed. They brought back their English grooms, gardeners, and servants with them. Well, as I said, Bell is *the man* to know in these parts and *we* know him now. The rest will follow, for 'getting in' with him I shall make mean 'money.'"

Money was increasingly on the young man's mind. His enforced dependency on Uncle Homer was beginning to chafe and he was no longer always certain of the conclusion about wealth he had reached in New York.

Mater had not reared her children to dreams of riches, but these months of luxury and of hobnobbing with the wealthy were beginning to make money in substantial quantities seem desirable to Gerald. It appeared to be an essential adjunct of the "nice" people whose company and pursuits he enjoyed. Its importance to Jenny he could not doubt and was coming to understand. A tight budget she could make into a sort of adventure in England; among her own kind in America it hurt her pride and must be camouflaged or rationalized.

But economy, or the appearance of it, was still a necessity. Staying at the Cliff House was expensive and the food was not to their liking. Would it not be wise to rent a furnished cottage for two or three months so they could provide themselves good meals at less cost? There was a small five-room house on the grounds of Briar-hurst which Dr. Bell would rent them for little more than they had paid in Brighton. Having got Uncle Homer's approval, they moved into the Bell cottage before the month was out.

Jenny understood well the social advantage of this move, but she could not help feeling defensive about the house. Though it was several times the size of their quarters in Brighton, it was "small as American houses go," she told Mater. Someday, she dreamed, they would have a beautiful, very big house of their own.

Gerald thought the cottage bully. It was perched high on a hill-side, screened by trees from the Bells' manor house in the hollow below, with a glorious view from each of its three verandahs. The clematis vine in bloom at one corner of the front verandah stirred memories of the gardens at Heimat, and once he had got Jenny settled and busy training the village schoolteacher who had agreed to be their servant for the summer at fifteen dollars a month, he sought Dr. Bell's permission to break a patch of the virgin sod at the side of the house for a vegetable garden and another along the front for flowers.

Dr. Bell, delighted to have captured this congenial young man as a tennis partner, not only said yes but provided manure, hose for irrigating, and plants from his greenhouses. Gerald ambitiously set out some two hundred vegetable and flower plants and told Mater her gardens too had a child in the Rocky Mountains.

"We do not get in the least 'thick' with the Bells," he wrote; "we are always most formal and polite, and avoid them as much as possible. Consequently they think the more of us." They certainly did. Within a few weeks they had come almost to take for granted the inclusion of Jenny and Gerald in their nonstop social life. "I don't think they ever sit down to a meal without someone extra at table," said Gerald.

They invited the Webbs to go with them to teas at the homes of their friends in Colorado Springs and to concerts and dinners at the Broadmoor Casino, a large white "palace of refined pleasure in the grand European manner" built on the shore of Cheyenne Lake southwest of Colorado Springs by a German nobleman, Count James Pourtales. No one seemed to mind the young couple's invio-late rule of departure for home at nine o'clock; the regimen of the health-seeker was commonplace thereabouts.

"Mrs. Webb is the smartest woman I know" became Cara Bell's

habitual introduction, and it was hard to tell whether she was referring to Jenny's clothes or her brains, she admired both so much.

Jenny worked for hours over her skirts and frocks, adding or subtracting ribbons, collars, flounces, "so that my few dresses will seem to be many." She even remodeled her wedding dress of thick ivory silk into an elegant dinner gown. And she fussed endlessly with her hair, which was coming out by the combfuls daily. Gerald tried to reassure her that it would grow back in but she knew it would never again be so thick or so strong. "Illness is such an un-beautifier," she lamented.

But she had a lively intelligence and read a great deal too, so that Gerald was as proud as their new friends were impressed to hear her discuss with wit and spirit the latest books and "the deepest problems of humanity."

Gerald's reading included the weekly packet of newspapers and magazines that Mater sent on from Cheltenham, among them always the *Daily Telegraph, Graphic,* and *Punch,* so that no reference to events at home among the transplanted Englanders in the Bells' circle found him without information and opinion. But his chief asset next to his charming manners was his excellence at tennis. "The best tennis player in Colorado," Dr. Bell called him, and though he commented privately "Poor Colorado!" he enjoyed the compliment.

He played every afternoon on the Bells' court, and almost every day Jenny would cross the lawn at five to join the party for tea. Often they would be asked to return for dinner, and twice Jenny, at Dr. Bell's request, took over the role of hostess in the Briarhurst dining room—"as big as a banquet hall" Gerald called it—when Cara, off on a picnic at Glen Eyrie or calling on the parson in Colorado Springs, forgot she had invited guests for dinner.

Gerald did not much like Mrs. Bell. He thought her "snobby" and irritatingly affected. "Would not trust her a yard with a shilling," he told Mater. The daughters he considered dowdy and feckless. "They are great walkers but cannot do anything else. All the women are a careless set, one time serve you tea that has stood *an hour* and the next time forget to serve you at all." He did not know that stories of Cara Bell's scatterbrained behavior were legion in Little London.

But she was well liked just the same, for she was kind and unfailingly cheerful. She came often now to chat with Jenny while the

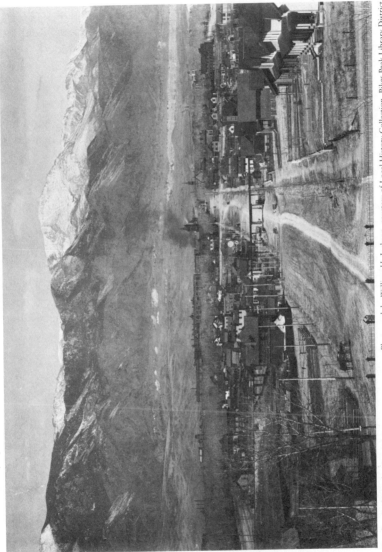

Early Colorado Springs

Photograph by William H. Jackson, courtesy of Local History Collection, Pikes Peak Library District girl was putting in her hours of rest on the verandah and reminisced of early days in Manitou.

She told Jenny of Queen Mellen, the winsome young hothouse flower whom General Palmer wished to transplant from eastern high society to the Colorado mountains as his wife. The town he planned for her was to be no rough and noisy assemblage of saloons and brothels like others roundabout; it was to be a colony of people of wealth and refinement, a "Saratoga of the West," a "Newport in the Rockies." So the sale of liquor within the town was forbidden by the Colorado Springs charter and the plat for Manitou included only a few lots of ordinary size in the center of town; the surrounding hillsides were divided into much larger sites for beautiful villas like the one General Palmer built for Queen at Glen Eyrie.

Alas, sighed Cara, lovely little Queen could not share her husband's dream or endure the discomforts of its beginnings. She had tried living at Glen Eyrie a few times but had eventually established herself and her three daughters permanently in London, where she held court for young artists and writers.

Queen had died suddenly last winter, and this summer General Palmer, after only infrequent visits to the seven springs for two decades, had brought his daughters with their English governess and housekeeper to make a home again at Glen Eyrie. What would he do, Cara wondered, about the upstart promoters who were stirring up such an unseemly commotion in the leisurely, refined life of Colorado Springs?

Dr. Bell had fared little better than the General in his plans for Manitou, said his wife. The hard times of the mid-70s had slowed development of the town almost to a standstill. What few of the villa lots were sold had soon been cut up and resold as little plots for unsightly stores and cottages, so distressingly different from the handsome castles the doctor had imagined in his dreams. Still, Cara shrugged, Manitou had become the most fashionable watering-place in the West and many people worth knowing had come there.

One of the social assets of the young Webbs was that they knew in one way or another so many of these people worth knowing. The connections that kept turning up astonished Gerald. Cara Bell herself turned out to be a cousin of one of Mater's friends in Cheltenham. And when Jenny was seated beside General Palmer at dinner one night, she discovered that he and Uncle Homer Bates had begun their business lives as colleagues on the staff of the Pennsylvania Railroad and that she and the General had many friends in common in Philadelphia.

At another dinner party the Webbs met Theodore Whyte, the partner of Lord Dunraven in the development of Estes Park. Whyte had a sister living in Cheltenham and knew all about the spa. His wife and children having stayed at their home in Scotland while he was looking after his Colorado investments, he was a lonely man and took to calling on the Webbs to confide his woes with the playboy lord who was wont to go yachting in far waters instead of tending to business in Estes Park.

Whyte knew the Bells well, indeed had occupied the Webbs' cottage the previous summer, and talked so admiringly about the doctor's many enterprises and the enormous extent of his grounds and staff at Pendell Court that Gerald dropped for good his irreverent private nickname for his landlord, "old ding-dong."

There were also the Pearces, frequent visitors at Briarhurst because the eldest son, Harold, was engaged to the eldest Bell daughter, Cara Rowena. Mr. Pearce, the British consul in Denver, was one of the great smelting barons of Colorado and also the discoverer in the state's mountains of a new metal for which no use was yet known; it was called uranium.

Stanley Pearce, the second son, greeted Jenny with cries of pleasure when they met; they had come to know each other at Old Point Comfort, Virginia, when both were visiting cousins there. He too came calling often at the cottage thereafter. His mother, stone deaf but a true *grande dame*, lorgnette and all, took a fancy to Jenny and to Gerry the poodle.

But the most pleasing surprise was the fruitful connection with Dr. S. Edwin Solly. Within a week of meeting Gerald, William Bell took him to play tennis at the doctor's house in Colorado Springs. Not only did Solly know Cheltenham well from having sought the cure there, but his two daughters, Lily and Alma, had finished their education at the Women's College in that city and Lily remembered vividly the sprightly Mrs. Webb who had come often to visit with the headmistress.

Another guest that afternoon, James J. Hagerman, also remembered Cheltenham because, like Solly, he had sought health there when consumption forced him to give up his partnership in steel with Andrew Carnegie. A feisty little man who felt good only when he was angry about something, Hagerman had put his millions to work at Aspen and at Colorado Springs; it was he who began the "commotion" that roused the Springs from its genteel doldrums in the 1880s. Edwin Solly, his physician and friend, had often smoothed the way for Hagerman's aggressive undertakings.

Dr. Solly, aged forty-eight now and showing streaks of gray in his thick dark hair but suave and handsome and richly baritone of voice as ever, did not drop his air of soothing assurance even on the tennis court. Graciously he offered to examine Jenny and, if he found her a suitable case, accept her as a patient.

Gerald returned home brimming with excitement about their incredible good luck. Dr. Solly had the best and biggest practice in Colorado Springs, he told Jenny. According to Dr. Bell, he was the foremost authority on consumption in all of Colorado, knew all the doctors thereabouts, even in Denver, and was often called in consultation on their cases. And he would be her doctor!

They went to see Dr. Solly in his office the very next day. He judged Jenny to be no worse than when she had left England, perhaps even somewhat improved. The Colorado air would without doubt make her wholly well again if she took care not to tire herself. She must go to bed no later than ten o'clock each night and rest for several hours each day, but she must also get plenty of exercise outdoors in the sun. And she should plan to remain in Colorado for some time, to give the altitude time to work its magic.

When Gerald protested that he must get back to England and his studies at Guy's the coming autumn, Dr. Solly advised strongly against it. Why not plan to spend the winter in Denver taking a medical degree at the university there and return to London next summer if Jenny was able? He himself had added the Denver degree to his English diploma and found it useful. He promised to introduce Gerald to the Denver doctors himself and to take him to observe operations at the Denver hospitals.

The Webbs returned to Manitou subdued by the need to rethink their plans but much encouraged in their hopes for Jenny. Gerald wrote Mater:

"It is nice to get such a satisfactory opinion from one who knows. In consequence of the great number of consumptives here, Solly is an authority on the disease, so we can take for certain all he says.

"And look at all the cures the air here has effected—Bell, Solly himself, Nichols the proprietor of the Cliff House, who says he came here 20 years ago from the East when the doctors gave him only 3 months to live but is now a hale old fellow of 55 with a grown-up family, two old Guy's men who got consumption before they completed their course and are now in business at Colorado Springs, a good many army men whose lungs gave out. One of them came here nine months ago from India, could not stand up when he came but is now driving around as well as anyone.

"I am so thankful we got here in time and did not dally. Don't forget, if ever you hear of weak lungs, pack them off to Colorado *at once*. Don't delay trying one place and then another, come direct here. Consumptives seem to add 20 or more years to their lives by coming here. What do you think of Solly's proposal about Denver?"

He did not act immediately even after a second visit to Dr. Solly's office for the express purpose of discussing the Denver degree. The fact was he was not certain at the moment that he wanted to go on with medicine; he thought he might prefer to tend one of Dr. Bell's irons in the fire.* The man's wealth and power dazzled him. He had never been close to the likes of it before; the Bates and Myers fortunes were in no way comparable.

The wonder of Bell's private railway car, for instance. It stood always ready on the short siding of the Denver and Rio Grande that ran alongside Briarhurst, and whenever Dr. Bell wanted to go some-where at a distance, such as the five hundred miles southwest to look over his coal mines at Telluride, he bundled family and ser-vants into the car, had it hooked onto a passing train, and went off to live in luxurious comfort in the roughest of mining camps.

Gerald watched guests arrive at Briarhurst in their own similar private cars, which stood shining on the siding until they were ready to leave. And Cara Bell told him General Palmer had spent his years alone mostly rolling from coast to coast in his private car named *Nomad*.

A life of that free and opulent style would be exciting, and no doctor, not even Dr. Solly, could hope to earn it. Gerald knew Dr. Bell thought well of him and kept hoping he would be offered a post somewhere in the Bell empire. He made sure the Bells knew

---

*Perhaps it was at this time that Gerald impulsively applied for American citi-zenship. He did not pursue it for some fifteen years. In his request to have the ap-plication reinstated in 1912 he gave the date of the original request as 5 June 1894. But at that date he was still in London, with no thought of living in America. His memory for dates was never reliable.

he needed money and even was bold enough one day to hint that the busy man could use a private secretary. But after a while he realized that his announced intention of returning to England as soon as Jenny was well had put him out of the running; neither Dr. Bell nor any of his lieutenants wanted transient help.

Gerald's thoughts then turned back to medicine and he made arrangements to enter the University of Denver medical school in September. He could receive his degree the following April and the work would help prepare him to pass his English examinations quickly when he returned to London.

Once again he dusted off his medical textbooks and began reviewing the clinical and surgical lectures published in back issues of *Guy's Gazette*, which he received regularly and always read from cover to cover. To prod him back onto the track Trixie Finch sent him a gift of an especially fine binaural stethoscope; he thought it "a beautiful piece" and was delighted to have it.

But his former dedication and concentration were lacking. There were too many pleasant distractions at hand and, feeling better than ever before in his life, he was so alive with energy that sitting quiet over books was intolerable. Jenny teased him that he was "getting positively fat." His appetite was enormous. A typical menu for his breakfast at nine, Jenny said, was "Blackberries. Hominy and cream. Corned beef hashed on toast. Fried tomatoes with muffins. Griddle cakes and maple syrup. Coffee with cream. And of course milk for Gerald."

Not content with daily tennis, gardening, and long rambles among the rocks with Jenny, he chose an out-of-the-way stretch of land beyond the railroad tracks, roughed out a small golf course, and began teaching Dr. Bell the game. He practiced there often himself, taking Jenny along to get the exercise Dr. Solly had prescribed by retrieving his lost balls or trotting Gerry the poodle around the course.

In mid-August Gerald whooped with joy when Mater wrote that Wilfred, Sophie, and Amy were on the way to visit them. He had been urging Mater herself to come but she thought she was too old to cross the ocean.

In a hurried letter Gerald arranged for Cousin Homer Bates to meet the travelers at the dock and put them up for a night or two in Monmouth Beach, where the Bateses had a summer home. To the travelers themselves he sent urgent instructions about where to go and what to see. Surely echoing Jenny, he warned them not to waste time and money now in New York and Washington because it was out of season in such cities; they would be empty of people and all their great houses would be shut up. The places to see this time of year were the resorts along the Jersey Shore, Newport, and Bar Harbor.

When the "trippers" blithely disobeyed and spent ten days happily sightseeing in New York and Washington, Gerald was exasperated. He washed his hands of the silly trio, he told Mater.

But his temper was sunny again when Wilfred and the girls finally arrived, and they all had a lively week together, highlighted by attendance at the Briarhurst wedding of Rowena Bell to Harold Pearce, an afternoon of tennis and tea at Dr. Solly's, and a farewell fling of dining and dancing at the Broadmoor Casino, which Jenny recklessly insisted on sharing. Her pleasure in dancing again was so good to see that Gerald had not the heart to restrain her.

As soon as the English three had departed westward—Sophie and Amy to turn back for home after seeing the Grand Canyon and Salt Lake, Wilfred to proceed on around the world—Gerald hied himself quickly to Denver to begin his courses at the medical school and find a place for them to live.

The heat in the capital was scorching, climbing day after day to high readings in the 90s, and after a week of it Gerald pled the need to help Jenny pack up as an excuse for escaping back to the cooler heights of Manitou.

Taking advantage of these last days at Briarhurst, he went with a friend of the Bells on his postponed hike to the top of Pikes Peak. They got back just in time, for Gerald was astonished to wake the next morning to a deep chill in the air and two inches of snow on the ground. In Denver the sudden storm had felled hundreds of trees and left a foot of snow; it would have been perilously worse on the trail to the summit.

The snow at Manitou having melted by midday as usual, the Webbs spent the afternoon entertaining callers come to wish them godspeed: the Bells, who were "terribly cut up at our leaving," the Sollys and James Hagerman, and Theodore Whyte. All promised to see them soon in Denver.

Gerald called it propitious that it was on September twenty-fourth and his twenty-fourth birthday that he and Jenny moved into the house he had chosen at 950 Corona Street, east of Capitol

Hill "in the healthiest and smartest part" of Denver. The house was small but well furnished and its modern conveniences delighted them both: electric lights and bells, hot-air vents in every room, bathrooms off the bedrooms, and each fireplace fitted with an ash disposal chute into the cellar.

In the yard patches of deep snow still lingered amid the litter of leaves and branches left by the storm. After clearing away the worst of this debris and having found "an Irish biddy" to help Jenny, Gerald returned at last to intensive study of medicine.

III

Unsettled

"No, Mater, of course I shall not use this Denver degree. I do not care a snap for it. You know it has always been my ambition to get the London MD, the best medical degree in the English-speaking countries. And I still mean to have it. But I must fill my time here this winter and it is easier to study hard if you have a goal, so I shall get this American degree in April, then return to Guy's in May, take my MRCS and LRCP in June and my MB in July. A pretty big order, I know, but I mean to do it."

That was the attitude with which Gerald began his studies at the University of Denver. But within two weeks he was confessing his pleasant surprise at the excellence of his American teachers and teaching: "In many ways they are better than at Guy's."

They were certainly different. Guy's being a hospital school, its emphasis was on teaching and learning at the bedside and the complementary lectures were loosely grouped into only three subjects: medicine, surgery, and obstetrics.

At Denver the university medical school offices, classrooms, laboratories, and free dispensary—all located in the Haish Building at Fourteenth and Arapahoe streets—were independent of any hospital, and the curriculum was divided into more than a score of courses extending through four years of seven months each.

First- and second-year students never approached a patient, being drilled wholly in the basic sciences, including such developing fields as histology, osteology, embryology, and microscopy. In the third year the classroom lectures shifted to assorted phases of the practice of medicine and the students were introduced to clinical training by observing at the bedside and in dispensary clinics.

All these preliminaries Gerald Webb was assumed to have completed at Guy's, so that he was enrolled with the fourth-year students, who attended classes in sixteen subjects, including pediatrics, dermatology, ophthalmology, otolaryngology, nervous and mental diseases, hematology, bacteriology, medical jurisprudence, medical ethics, history of medicine, and a fad of the times, electrotherapeutics. At the end of the term the student was required to pass an examination in each course in order to receive the degree.

But such didactic training was less than half the work. American medical educators had quite lately come to recognize that without having felt a pulse, assuaged actual bleeding, or examined a sick person to discover the source of his ailment, a graduate was poorly equipped to practice medicine no matter how many good lectures he had heard or how many textbooks he had memorized.

The University of Denver was not far behind the nation's best in the amount of bedside experience it provided. Its fourth-year students mingled with those of the University of Colorado and the Gross Medical College in the wards of six Denver hospitals. Three of these were public institutions staffed by the University of Denver faculty: the Arapahoe County Hospital, the Steele Contagious Hospital, and the Infirmary of the State Home for Dependent Children.

Most important for University of Denver students was the County Hospital, which served also as the city's general hospital. Begun in 1873 as a simple frame building fitted with a few cots and using water carried in barrels from the Platte River, it was now a two-hundred-bed institution with all the latest arrangements: a surgical amphitheater, separate medical and surgical wards, a special children's ward, and a lying-in department. Its patients were attended by the fourth-year students under the supervision of faculty physicians. So too were all patients who came to the medical school's free dispensary.

Perhaps because of these clinical services, Denver's seniors paid no tuition fees providing they had taken their first three years' work at the school. Since Gerald Webb had not done so he paid £20, about a hundred dollars, for the year of instruction and was delighted that it cost no more.

His class numbered eleven students. Among them were one woman, a rarity in English medical schools, and four men who were more than fifty years of age. Gerald being the youngest member of the class, he wryly called himself its "beardless boy."

He thought his classmates a rather rough, casual lot, not at all "polished" like his fellows at Guy's, and he felt himself to be conspicuous among them in the high-buttoned cutaway coat and striped trousers that had been a required uniform for a medical student in London. But he would not change costume: "I am an Englishman still, and always will be."

Each morning at eight o'clock he took the streetcar down Capitol Hill to the Haish Building for lectures that lasted till noon. After a hasty lunch brought from home he took another streetcar to an assigned hospital for two or three hours of work in the outpatient clinics or the wards. Then he rode back to the Haish Building for additional classes or work in the laboratories until the school's dispensary opened at five o'clock.

The last patient there was seldom taken care of until seven o'clock, after which came weekly quizzes on some nights and on others a second trip to a hospital for rounds on assigned patients. Free at nine o'clock as a rule, he caught the streetcar home for a late dinner with Jenny and, after she had gone to bed, a session of study at the diningroom table until midnight or after.

It was a grueling schedule but Gerald enjoyed it. "I quite revel in being back at hard work again," he told Mater. Three courses he singled out for comment: special pathology, because it stressed diagnosis, skill in which Gerald had already decided was the most valuable asset of a physician; nervous and mental diseases; and bacteriology.

Gerald had been nudged into heightened awareness of "nerves" since coming to Colorado, perhaps by experiences of his own, more probably by Jenny's fits of weeping and irritability, and he had come to think the altitude might be responsible. Cara Bell assured him he was right; she and Dr. Bell fought much more often at Briarhurst than at Pendell Court, she said, "for no reason at all except the air."

He now devoured the treatises of S. Weir Mitchell, the American physician (and novelist) who was pioneering in the application of psychology to medicine, and decided to take a competitive examination in the subject which was open to all medical students in Denver.

He won second place, losing the gold medal to a student from the University of Colorado. "Woe is me," he said, "but I beat all the women up for the prize anyway, and I learned more about nervous diseases than I should have by not competing."

The course in bacteriology was an afterthought, added late to the Denver curriculum that year, and Gerald was permitted to take it without extra fee. This was a lucky bit of timing for him, because in it he seems for the first time to have learned anything of substance about bacteria as a cause of disease. He must have heard something at Guy's about the work Louis Pasteur and Joseph Lister had done some three decades earlier, but here he first saw the organisms under the microscope and was introduced to contemporary methods of isolating, culturing, staining, and identifying some of them.

He could have got no more than an introduction to the subject, for the teacher was Dr. William C. Mitchell, a hospital pathologist at the time, and Gerald was to learn that he was neither skilled nor outstandingly bright. But he may well have been the one who first showed Gerald Webb the tubercle bacillus that produced tuberculosis.

Such tardiness is puzzling.

It was in 1882 that the great German bacteriologist Robert Koch announced his discovery of the tubercle bacillus, and in 1890 and 1891 that he proclaimed the tuberculin he had prepared from dead bacilli to be an effective vaccine against tuberculosis. But the inevitable cultural lag in medicine was prolonged in those days because the diffusion of scientific and medical discoveries was much slower than today.

When Edward Trudeau in 1890 tried to show his physician, the venerated Dr. Alfred Loomis of New York, the tubercle bacillus on a microscope slide, Dr. Loomis smilingly waved it aside, saying "I don't believe in these newfangled germs," and it took Trudeau ten more years to convince the man that tuberculosis was of bacterial origin. Indeed, the infectious nature of consumption was not officially accepted, after a long and bitter battle, in New York City until 1907.

Still, one would expect knowledge of Koch's work to have been current in London and at Guy's Hospital when Gerald was a student there.

And Gerald, writing some forty years later about Koch's claims for tuberculin in 1891, did say: "I was a medical student at the time and can well recall the excitement produced in the world and the hopes aroused in consumptive patients."

Yet nowhere until this year of 1895–96 in Denver had Gerald

shown any sign of ever having heard of a bacterial agent in consumption. He reported nothing of the kind from Dr. Shaw, dean of the College at Guy's, or from Dr. Goodhart, "the best chest man in London," or from Dr. Solly, "the foremost authority on consumption in Colorado." Quite the reverse. Until now all Gerald's scores of references to consumption had implied a constitutional cause: "weak chest," "weak lungs," "worn-out lungs," "fallen into consumption," "gone into consumption," "declined into consumption." Now for the first time he began to write of "contracting consumption" and "the consumption bug."

He was of course hyperreactive now to any fact or theory about consumption, and, far from avoiding tuberculous patients as he had at Guy's, he sought assignments to work with them, mostly at St. Anthony's Hospital, Denver's newest. Its three-year-old building accommodated two hundred and fifty patients, many of whom were consumptives segregated in special wards in accordance with the latest practice.

As Gerald worked in those wards, he began to think he might prefer to specialize in the treatment of consumption rather than in his early love, surgery. "I want to do some original work someday," he said, "trying to discover something that will kill the consumptive 'bug' or bacilli."

Gerald left no record of what he was being taught in his other courses or which of them he especially enjoyed. How advanced and how truly aseptic were the operations he observed or assisted in? He did not say. Nor did he comment on the course in hematology, although examinations of the blood were to preoccupy him later, or on the teaching in medical history, which was to become an absorbing and productive avocation for him.

His most influential teacher by far was Dr. Henry A. Sewall, professor of physiology. Just past thirty years of age, Sewall already had a great record, though he did not insist upon it and few recognized it. From studies at the newly established Johns Hopkins University in Baltimore, before it had a medical school and when pre-med courses in science were called "the stinks," and in Europe at Cambridge, Leipzig, and Heidelberg, he had acquired what Thomas Huxley called "the divine dipsomania of research."

With a Ph.D. but not an M.D. from Johns Hopkins, Sewall moved to a chair in physiology at the University of Michigan, and there turned a few small, cramped rooms in a cellar under the amphitheater into a laboratory and began acquiring "the little snakes," two-foot rattlesnakes, which he milked of their venom. This toxin he injected in repeated small doses into pigeons until he proved that in time the process made the birds immune to the venom.

His work was interrupted by an attack of the pulmonary disease that had killed his father and an older brother. He went south to Asheville, North Carolina, for a month or two "to escape the northern blasts." When he returned to Ann Arbor he finished his experiments and wrote a report of them which was published in the British *Journal of Physiology* in 1887.

He called the report "Experiments on the Preventive Inoculation of Snake Venom," but he went well beyond the facts to point out their implications: "I assume an analogy between the venom of the poisonous serpent and the ptomaines [toxins] produced by bacterial organisms. If immunity from the fatal effects of snake-bite can be secured by repeated inoculations of doses too small to produce ill effects, we may suspect that the same sort of resistance against germ disease might follow the inoculation of the appropriate ptomaine."

He wrote that suggestion three years before Von Behring in Germany and Roux in France began their work on diphtheria antitoxin and before Koch announced tuberculin. Sewall thought all three men must be readers of the *Journal of Physiology* and since none of them even mentioned his article, he wondered whether he was the victim of a nationalistic "conspiracy of silence."

That experience of Sewall's became of enormous importance to Gerald Webb a few years later.

During a summer back at Johns Hopkins, in the new hospital this time, Henry Sewall examined his own blood under the microscope and diagnosed his "pulmonary disease" as tuberculosis. He did not take this seriously until the Hopkins doctors became concerned about his look of ill health and his favorite teacher, Newell Martin, got stern with him. "Go to the Rockies, and go at once! Stay here in Baltimore or at Michigan and you will be dead in a year," Martin thundered at him.

Henry obediently resigned his post at Michigan but he did not go to the Rocky Mountains. He had to earn a living and so took the post of resident physician at the Adirondack Cottage Sanatorium* which Edward Trudeau had established at Saranac Lake, New York. This was in 1889.

He stayed there only one year. He and Dr. Trudeau did not get along. Both men had explosive tempers and Trudeau did not like to have a rival near his throne. But both were great talkers too, and Gerald Webb never could believe that Henry Sewall did not tell Trudeau about his antitoxin theory or demonstrate the methods in bacteriology he had learned. The following year Dr. Trudeau published the account of experiments in inducing immunity with tuberculin that made him forever famous. He made no mention of Henry Sewall, then or thereafter.

Meanwhile Dr. Samuel Fisk, a medical graduate of Harvard who had gone to the Rockies to cure his tuberculosis and had become dean of medicine at the University of Denver, asked young Sewall to come west to practice in Denver and teach physiology at the university. Glad to escape from Saranac Lake, Henry accepted and began his long professorial career at the University of Denver. By taking courses as well as teaching them the first year or two, he acquired the doctor of medicine degree he had not bothered to take earlier.

The obviously English Gerald Webb and his superior performance in class caught Dr. Sewall's attention, and when in late October the doctor's teaching began to strain his infected throat, he asked young Webb to take over the lectures in physiology for a while.

Gerald did so, but with butterflies in his stomach at first. He gave credit to the childhood theatricals at Heimat for enabling him to mount the platform at all, but he was soon relishing his own performances and enjoying the students' response; they all came to the class every time now as few of them had before—because, they told him, his descriptions were more "lucid" than Dr. Sewall's. He supposed that being young and fresh in teaching he took more pains with his lectures than had Sewall.

After coming "to peek in the door" and listen to Webb's lecture a few times, Dr. Sewall told him the course was his to teach for the

*The word was spelled *sanitarium* at that time. The two spellings were used interchangeably and haphazardly in those years, but I have chosen to use throughout the spelling that became standard for tuberculosis hospitals.

remainder of the term and Gerald rejoiced — because of the honor but also because he liked having the run of the physiology laboratory for extra experiments.

He went often to Sewall's home to report and consult and soon was like a younger brother in the house, helping Mrs. Sewall tend her garden and listening to her endless tales about the many heirlooms among the furniture. She was a devoted and forbearing wife. She always traveled to medical society meetings with her husband, "to make sure he wore clean collars," she said, but Gerald was sure she went along to look after his health, about which he was exasperatingly careless.

Most of all, Isabel Sewall grimly endured the nuisances of Henry's research. He carried it on in a small third-floor garret of their house and there was no way to get his materials and his guinea pigs in and out except through the downstairs living room and out the front door. Gerald sometimes helped with the carrying and was aware of the compressed lips with which Mrs. Sewall watched the procedure.

Like all the medical school faculty members, Dr. Sewall really earned his living by conducting a private practice. His office was on the first floor of his house and Gerald frequently arrived to find it full of waiting patients, whereupon he ran upstairs to help Mrs. Sewall rout Henry from his absorption in some laboratory experiment.

Soon the young Webbs were being invited to the "simple but charming parties" Mrs. Sewall liked to give. "I met many eminent physicians from the East at those parties," Gerald said.

Each Tuesday evening the senior classes of the three medical schools and some of their professors assembled at the County Hospital to hear Dean Fisk present a case. With the patient present he would describe the symptoms and history of the illness, demonstrate the physical findings, and discuss alternative diagnoses and modes of treatment. Wanting to introduce some variety into these weekly clinics, Dean Fisk in December decided to risk the experiment of having a student work up a case and present it. He chose Gerald Webb to make the try.

"I was bound I would make it a success," said Gerald, "and spent a lot of time on it. It was something of an ordeal, about 100 being present, but my experience with the physiological lectures helped me out wonderfully and I was well rewarded with applause and

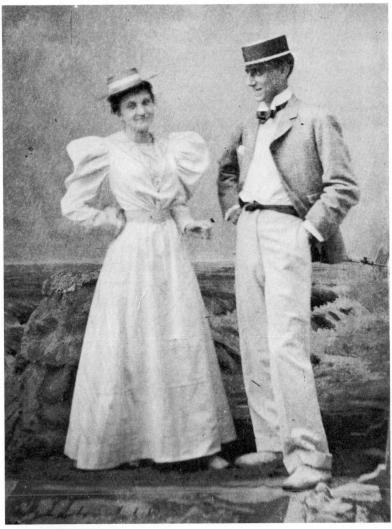

Jenny and Gerald in Denver, 1896

congratulations." Dean Fisk was so pleased that he embarrassed Gerald with his praise.

All this while the Webbs were continuing their active social life and their days of play. They were introduced to Denver high society by the Pearces, who gave a splendid dinner party in their honor soon after they arrived. The table was of banquet size; dozens of American Beauty roses "at $1 apiece" complemented the elegant settings of crystal and silver; the menu featured a special delicacy called "Reed birds" sent out from Philadelphia plus half a dozen wines and liqueurs. The Webbs were awed, and grateful.

When Rowena and Harold Pearce returned from their wedding trip, Gerald and Jenny were included in the extended round of teas, dinners, and receptions given for the newlyweds, becoming always such centers of interest that they had to take care not to outshine the guests of honor.

Jenny struggled to return the social favors showered upon them by entertaining callers at tea. She considered it a wife's duty to help her husband get ahead by winning friends for him among people who counted, and she fretted that her limited strength and budget permitted her to do so little. She was happy when Nell Holbrook, her best friend from childhood, came to spend several weeks with them because she knew "Nelly" would win them added cachet among their new friends in "the swagger set."

Nell was a chic beauty, spoiled by her inherited millions, but she knew everybody in Society, even in Denver, and quickly dominated any gathering at which she appeared, as Gerald unhappily discovered when he escorted her to a charity ball that Jenny was too "down" to attend. Nell's self-assured independence repelled him; he was glad Jenny was not so "hard and shiny."

Dr. and Cara Bell came to see them, bringing armloads of asters and hampers of vegetables from Gerald's gardens. The Sollys invited them back to Colorado Springs for a weekend. Theodore Whyte took them to dinner and the theater, secured a membership for Gerald in the Overland Park Country Club, and when he left to return to his family, made a gift to Gerald of his fine Scottish golf clubs.

The Overland Park club became virtually the Webbs' home on weekends. Gerald could not get enough of golf; some days he went round the three-mile course five times. He inched up steadily in tournament play, won enough prizes to keep him well supplied with new balls, and finally captured first place in an exciting playoff.

"You can't imagine what good all that sun and fresh air do me," he told Mater. "I come home with the blood just boiling through me, I feel so good."

Jenny still walked round the course and occasionally played a few holes with him, but she said her main pleasure at the club came from seeing Gerald mingle happily with the other men. "I like him to gather ideas from the opinions of many. I think it broadens him and makes him more manly. Sometimes we have a jolly time with twenty or thirty nice young men — all refined and sporty and genuine-hearted. It makes his laughter ring and his face glow."

Robert Kenney and his wife came from Wahoo to spend the Christmas holidays, for which Gerald had a fortnight free from the medical school. He was astonished to find Jenny's father so young — "only 44 and looks no older than Harold. I have to call them by their Christian names." Robert, who had been elected justice of the peace in Wahoo, turned out to be a merry guest, tender with Jenny and sympathetic with Gerald about his daughter's illness.

That illness was a nagging worry for Gerald. He could not help seeing that Jenny was increasingly less well than she had been during the summer at Briarhurst; her relapses were more frequent and lasted longer. Yet Dr. Solly, examining her on one of his visits to Denver, had pronounced her improved and ready for more exercise; he suggested bicycling, along with singing to stretch her lungs.

Gerald vetoed the "wheeling" as too much for her but was willing to try the singing. He set aside an hour on Sunday mornings for accompanying her on his violin, his piano being still in storage at Heimat.

When it quickly became clear that the singing did Jenny harm rather than good, Gerald began to question Dr. Solly's opinions. She should have a doctor in Denver anyway, he decided, and took her to consult Dr. Karl Ruedi, a newcomer to Denver whom he had met at Dr. Sewall's home. Ruedi had been an attending physician at Davos in Switzerland, where he took care of Robert Louis Stevenson and became the hero in a bestselling English novel, *Ships that Pass in the Night*.

Shaking his head gravely over Jenny's condition, Dr. Ruedi advised her to take much less exercise and much more rest, in the open air if possible. He suggested that she go south to Santa Fe in New Mexico when the weather turned bad in Denver, so that she could spend eight or more hours each day in hot sunshine. In the meantime she should have eggs and whole milk daily, take an ounce of whiskey each day, and drink all the ale or stout she could swallow.

It was no help to Gerald at this juncture to receive a letter from Mater recounting a recent conversation with two of his friends at Guy's. They thought Gerald had made a serious mistake; he had sacrificed what was sure to be a great career to no purpose; he should have sent Jenny to America to seek her cure in the care of her family while he stayed on in England to complete his education at Guy's. Obviously Mater thought his friends were right.

"I do not at all agree," Gerald replied. "Do they not understand that I love the girl, and that being separated from her would have been a far greater sacrifice?" Besides, he did not think he was damaging his career. Did Mater not remember how poor health had hampered him at Guy's? Here in Colorado *he* at least had grown strong and well.

"Therefore, Mater, do not waste time worrying over things that only in imagination might have been. Your boy is doing supremely well and has only one thing against him, that he is always wishing he were in England—but he is wise enough not to be discontented in his present surroundings."

The weather remaining mild, Jenny stayed on in Denver until early March. Word came from Uncle Homer in late February that the Reverend Myers had died and Beade was inconsolable. Gerald immediately suggested that she might find distraction in going to Santa Fe with Jenny. But the ladies preferred southern California to New Mexico and were soon established at a luxury hotel in Coronado Beach not far from Pasadena.

Gerald disliked letting Jenny go off without him but he was too near his degree to give it up now. His final examinations began in mid-March and stretched on for almost a month. He thought it "a big grind to get up so many special subjects and be examined by specialists in each. The most you can do is get a good smartening for each exam."

With seven tests still to be taken, he got a letter from Beade saying that Jenny was terribly ill again; she had forbidden Beade to write him but the doctor had begged that he be told. Gerald stayed to finish his examinations, then, without waiting for the results to be posted, took the train west.

He found Jenny just past the crisis. She had been in bed three weeks, near death again from pneumonia. When she was able to sit up at the end of another week, Gerald decided it would be best to try to take her back to Colorado.

With Beade's help he packed her trunks, got her by carriage to Pasadena, and after two days' rest there carried her onto the Overland Limited for Denver, far from sure that she would survive the journey. He had to leave Beade, "still half dazed with grieving," to look after herself.

Jenny's gain in strength once she was at home again confounded him, but Dr. Ruedi confirmed the fear that had been growing in him: the disease had spread to Jenny's right lung and into her throat and was so far advanced that there could be no hope of cure for her. The Colorado air could prolong her life but not save it. In any other climate, the doctor thought, she would be dead within a month.

And there was a complication now, added the doctor: Jenny was three months pregnant—but she could not possibly carry the baby to term.

Numbly accepting the inevitable, Gerald a few days later sat waiting outside the operating room of St. Joseph's Hospital while Dr. Thomas Bagot, a surgeon lately come from Dublin chasing the cure, performed the necessary abortion.

Gerald marveled at Jenny's uncomplaining attitude going into the operation. She seemed to have no fear of anything. She had fought valiantly against the disease that consumed her. All for nothing it seemed. Well, as long as there was an inch of lung left in her he would do his best to see that she had every comfort.

He could not return to Guy's this summer as planned; instead he would take Jenny back to the cottage at Briarhurst where she had felt so well last summer, and he would open an office in Manitou. At least Jenny had lived long enough to see him become a doctor.

The American doctorate in medicine had been conferred upon Gerald Bertram Webb during his absence on 16 April 1896. He had ranked first in twelve of the examinations and had won the only honor the University of Denver medical school conferred, a first prize in the practice of medicine.

When he showed his diploma to Jenny, saying it was as much hers as his, she teasingly commented that it meant he was now "duly qualified—to kill." No further hospital internship or residency was then required.

Gerald wrote to Heimat of all that had happened and of the consequent change in his plans:

"Jenny cannot live so very long, Mater. Of all the awful things, consumption of the throat is the worst. I want to be with her as long as she lives, could not bear to come over for my London exams and have something happen while I was away. Sometimes she suffers so much she longs for death to relieve her, and unless there is some change for the good, I shall too, for there is no pleasure for her in dragging on like this. I sometimes think Jenny might be well now if we had come directly here. Georgia was a great mistake.

"No, Mater, the Denver MD is by no means a London MD, but it is equivalent to the MRCS–LRCP, which is the general practitioner's qualification as a rule in England. I'll get the London someday, but meanwhile this is quite good enough to begin practice with and it took me some hard work to get it. I shall do all right with it in Manitou."

Jenny was not happy at the prospect of returning to last summer's cottage. In comparison with their Denver house it seemed to have been dirty and barren. But the Bells had it all refloored, repainted, and repapered for them, and Gerald arranged with Mater to ship over their household goods, including Jenny's knickknacks and his piano. "It will make things more homey for her to have her lovely things around her, and I should like the Bells to see what good things we have."

Expectantly Gerald opened a modest office above the post office in Manitou, had a quantity of letterheads printed with the new rubric Gerald B. Webb, M.D., and hung out a sign by the roadside in front of the cottage.

But few patients appeared. Gerald had underestimated the strength of the competition from the established doctors in Colorado Springs. The friends of last year were friends still, but not to the point of calling or recommending an untried physician. He had plenty of time to play tennis and plant his gardens again and begin raising baby chickens. But not so joyously now. What was he to do?

Dr. Bell was having trouble at Manitou Park, a beautiful property of his twenty miles up Ute Pass where he had added a huge hotel to his operation in lumbering and ranching. He could not get the resort project off the ground and Gerald thought of proposing himself as its manager. He was sure that the obstacle was "lack of posh," and if he were there to lay out a golf course, put in a tennis court, and in general "make things go," the resort would soon be a success.

But the idea was not so compelling as it would have been the summer before; he was sure now that he wanted only to practice medicine.

There was a constant tug from Heimat; old Mater, not having seen him for almost two years, wanted him to come home. And he wanted to go. Jenny, with her amazing resilience, had got well enough again to make her death seem much less imminent than it had in the spring, so there was no telling when he would be going back to live in England. Could he get in a quick trip now, when he had no practice to speak of? Dare he leave Jenny alone for a month?

A letter from Cousin Homer Bates saying he was coming for a visit at the end of August gave Gerald his chance. Homer was a gay blade, full of fun, devoted to Jenny; she would not be lonely with him around.

Gerald sailed on 22 August, spent ten satisfying days with Mater and the family, had some new suits made for him by Thomas the Tailor in Cheltenham, paid a flying visit to his old friends and haunts at Guy's, and was back in Colorado Springs, much refreshed, on 17 September.

In his trunk were gifts for Jenny, a "fine and full set of blood instruments" that his brothers had given him, and some of his favorite books from the library at Heimat. His mind was full of exciting stories from "the sweetest-looking old maid imaginable," Clara Barton, the Red Cross heroine, with whom he had talked for hours on the boat coming back. He had a new game to teach Jenny too, for a trio of young Englishmen on board had introduced him to poker.

He was reassured to find Jenny feeling and looking better than when he left. But he would have been annoyed if he could have read Cousin Homer's letter to Mater, which must have confused her:

"Although Gerald seems to take a decidedly serious view of Jenny's condition, personally I think she will get well if she only remains in Manitou. Her trip to Coronado Beach was exceedingly unfortunate. She looks well but her body is severely thin. She coughs badly and her throat rattles at night and when she stoops, but I know of many people in a much worse state than Jane who have entirely recovered. I understand that before my visit she was quite downhearted, cried, and said there was no use in living any longer, but when her mind is kept employed with other matters, she doesn't have time to think of her sickness and picks up immediately."

Probably so, but Gerald was not an insouciant visitor with nothing to do except keep Jenny's mind on other things; he had a living to earn. He wanted to be rid of the need for Uncle Homer's largesse as quickly as possible and still give Jenny the creature comforts she wanted.

A letter was awaiting him in Manitou from Dr. Henry Sewall offering him the position of assistant professor in physiology at the University of Denver for the following year. Gerald was sure this was his big opportunity. He would have to risk taking Jenny away from Manitou. Denver, with its booming growth, all its hospitals, three medical schools, and a lively medical society, was surely the best place for him to practice, and he would be starting off with the prestige of a university position.

He accepted Sewall's offer immediately and in late September moved Jenny and their possessions into a house at 950 Pearl Street in Denver. He had chosen a place farther toward the outskirts this time and bought Jenny a pony and light carriage so she could go daily into the fresh air of the open country.

But in mid-December he was packing to move again. He was getting nowhere in Denver. The university position, for all its honor, paid little in cash, and patients just did not come to the office he had opened in downtown Denver.

He put out feelers everywhere, sometimes with letters of introduction from Dr. Sewall, but all he got was dashes of cold water. One doctor told him, "There are 600 doctors in Denver already. There seem to be more doctors here than anything else. Every other house is a doctor's home, and they're all extremely discouraging about the prospect of making a living."

Another was blunter: "There are too many God-damned doctors here now. Go some other place, for God's sake!"

Dr. Sewall would not listen to such views. He shook his finger at Gerald and shouted, "There's always room at the top. Go and get to the top!"

Subduing his pride, Gerald went canvassing from office to office offering himself as an assistant trained and willing to take over the doctor's laboratory work. But he found only one man who felt enough need for such work to want help with it. Dr. Charles W. Powers, a surgeon whom Gerald had assisted in a few operations, was hoping to expand his laboratory services but could not afford to do so immediately. In a few months perhaps.

Gerald's idea was ahead of the times. The day of laboratory medicine, of scientific aids to diagnosis, was barely beginning. Its dawn would create his opportunity later but at the moment urinal-ysis and use of the stethoscope were as far as most practicing phy-sicians went beyond use of their own senses.

Gerald could not afford to wait for Dr. Powers' uncertain prop-osition. Besides, Jenny was failing again. In his frustration and dis-couragement Gerald for the first time expressed exasperation:

"She knows too many people here, there are too many amuse-ments, and worst of all, too many nice stores. Instead of driving her pony into the country—which is not inviting anyway—she goes into town and spends her time in shops like so many others of her sex. She is so run down that if we stay in Denver I don't think she will survive Xmas."

On 16 December he wrote from "The House at Austin Bluffs" in Colorado Springs—"a kind of farm house four miles east of town where Jane can get the best of milk and cream and town life can be avoided." And on 23 December he sent off almost a prayer with his Christmas greeting from his new office in the Hagerman Block: "After being so wretchedly unsettled for so long, now at last I think we are stationary for good."

IV

Building a Practice

GERALD WEBB and Colorado Springs were both twenty-five years old when their fortunes came together in mutual benefit.

General Palmer's dream town now numbered some twenty thousand inhabitants and covered about ten square miles, encircled on the north by the Rampart Range, on the west by Pikes Peak, on the south by Mt. Rosa and Cheyenne Mountain. To the east, beyond Austin Bluffs, gray-green prairie rolled gently to the horizon.*

The little city was an attractive place of wide graded streets bordered by walkways of packed gravel and shaded by the arching branches of tall trees. Under a lacing of wooden bridges and paralleled by the railroad tracks on which the trains of five companies traversed the city, Monument Creek flowed south through town to its junction with Fountain Creek just southwest of the low mesa on which the townsite had been platted. The shops, livery stables, "lounges," hotels, and office "blocks" of the business district, which centered on the intersection of Cascade and Pikes Peak avenues, were multiplying northward along Tejon Street and Nevada Avenue.

In and around this downtown section clustered a mixture of old houses. Unpretentious cottages like the one in which Helen Hunt Jackson had lived before she fled to California to write *Ramona* and the shabby shack that was home still to recluse William Stratton, erstwhile carpenter become the "Midas of the Rockies," stood comfortably cheek to cheek with the gracious larger dwellings of long-time community leaders like Dr. Edwin Solly.

A mile or so north of the elegant Antlers Hotel on Pikes Peak

---

*This name appears in the records variously as Austin's Bluff, Austin's Bluffs, etc. I have used Austin Bluffs because that is what Gerald and Jenny called it and they lived there.

Avenue sprawled the Colorado College campus, and beyond its heavily wooded acres newcomers who were making quick fortunes in one way or another from the gold fields were building conspicuously splendid houses along North Cascade and Wood avenues. North and east of this affluent section the prairie was checkered with new houses of more modest size and cost.

Gold made the mare run now in the Springs. Tourists and health-seekers still came in droves but the business of attracting and caring for them had fallen to second place. Most of the Cripple Creek mines and the attendant financial, milling, smelting, and transportation facilities were owned or controlled by Colorado Springs residents, and city affairs were dominated by an interlocking group of half a hundred wealthy mining and milling engineers, financiers, investment brokers, bankers, and lawyers.

In varying combinations these entrepreneurs ran the banks, held the seats on the Mining Exchange, built the newer business buildings, organized the companies that provided electricity, gas and coal, and streetcar transportation throughout the city. They gathered at the exclusive El Paso Club to drink, dine, and deal with associates from the East and Europe and at the Cheyenne Mountain Country Club to play hard at sports of all kinds and sometimes indulge in less respectable merriments.

They also built churches, created parks, financed charities, and as trustees supported and guided the growth of the city's principal cultural asset, Colorado College.

As a speculative venture one of this group, William A. Otis, had bought up a large acreage of ranch land around Austin Bluffs, intending to develop it into a suburb of sumptuous estates. He began by building on one of the choicer sites his own luxurious mansion with capacious stables nearby. But his project fell flat; the Bluffs were too far east, too far outside the northward stretch of the city at that time. By late 1896 Mr. Otis had given up his scheme, decided to move his family back into Colorado Springs, and was trying to sell his property.

Dr. Solly had built himself a second house on the western slope of Austin Bluffs, relished living there, and thought the pure air, unsullied by the smoke and dust of town, was beneficial to his health. At his suggestion, the Webbs rented one of the old ranch houses on Mr. Otis's land.

The house stood alone, more than a mile from its nearest neighbor, but Jenny, lonely as she often was, came quickly to love it. Its wide front windows faced west and from her place of rest on the long windowseat she could look across the prairie and watch the shifting lights and colors along the whole front range of the Rockies. Even the Spanish Peaks, one hundred and thirty miles away, were clearly discernible. "A lordly scene" she called it.

When she felt equal to exercise she could ride her pony and take her dog (Gerry the poodle had died of intestinal tuberculosis and been replaced by a female counterpart called Clorinda) to the bluffs and wander through their fringe of pines looking for birds and wildflowers.

Gerald was preoccupied with getting started in practice. His expectations and determination ran high: "I may be the youngest doctor in this town, but I expect to be its most famous."

He felt lucky to have got an office at the most prestigious business address in town, the Hagerman Block, recently built at the corner of Tejon and Kiowa streets by the current dean of Colorado Springs entrepreneurs, James J. Hagerman, the testy little millionaire with whom the Webbs had become acquainted during their first summer at Briarhurst. With the help of his son Percy, Mr. Hagerman conducted his ramifying affairs from headquarters in rooms 4 through 8 of his new building, and Gerald was delighted to secure room 11 down the hall.

Exuberantly he placed his furniture, shelved his medical books and journals, and adorned the walls with his two framed diplomas, two engravings of Guy's Hospital, and a portrait of Robespierre clipped from the *Graphic*. On his desk and an adjoining table he laid out some brass ornaments Mater had sent him, a leather writing pad from Ida, the cases of blood instruments Harold and Roly had bought for him, his precious microscope acquired in Denver, and the handsome stethoscope Trixie Finch had sent him. Thinking it all looked very professional, he had a picture taken of the office to be sent home to Heimat.

But within a month he was feeling inconveniently cramped, moved everything down the hall into the larger room 9, and added the small adjoining number 10 to serve as a waiting room. Knowing he really could not afford such expense, he began looking around for a suitable doctor to occupy room 11 and share the cost of the waiting room in 10.

Having bought himself a pony and secondhand yellow trap, he

set up a regular schedule for himself. He drove off at 8:30 each morning to reach his office by nine, saw patients there till noon, took a light lunch in town, made sick calls until four, then drove home to have dinner with Jenny. After she went to bed at 7:30 he drove back to the office to see more patients and study and write up his cases until ten.

This he meant to make the pattern of his life seven days a week, except for some tennis on Saturday afternoons "to shake up my liver" and a few extra hours of rest on Sundays.

But of course patients were too few at first to fill the hours allotted to them and while seeking ways to increase their number Gerald decided, after watching Jenny fight through a bad spell of coughing and fever, to give some time to "original experiments on guinea pigs to see if I can find something to kill the beastly bug of consumption. There is so much clinical material in this town in the way of consumptives but so far no original work has been attempted here."

How or on what project he began I do not know, except that he kept his guinea pigs at Austin Bluffs and wished he had a "bacteriological outfit" for better handling of his bacillus cultures.

He had expected to draw patients from among the friends he and Jenny had made during their two summers in Manitou but he was soon disillusioned; those friends remained cordial but they ventured nothing to give him a boost.

The one exception was the Hagerman brothers, Bert and Percy, and Percy's wife, a wealthy woman in her own right and a good friend of Jenny's. Gerald had barely opened his office when Mrs. Hagerman engaged him to deliver the baby she was expecting in early spring and a few days later she sent him her ailing maid, whom he found to have a badly diseased kidney. Judging removal of the organ to be imperative, he took the woman to Dr. Bagot, Jenny's Irish surgeon in Denver, and stayed with her through the operation and the first days of recovery. Mrs. Hagerman was as grateful as the maid and paid him well for his trouble.

The Hagerman brothers had little need of his services themselves but they talked him up at every opportunity among their friends. Bert, a practicing lawyer, was especially helpful, on one early occasion diverting to Gerald a fellow lawyer from Michigan who was Solly-bound with his tuberculous wife, the daughter of Professor Demmon of the University of Michigan.

Gerald said at once there could be no hope for Mrs. Ninde be-

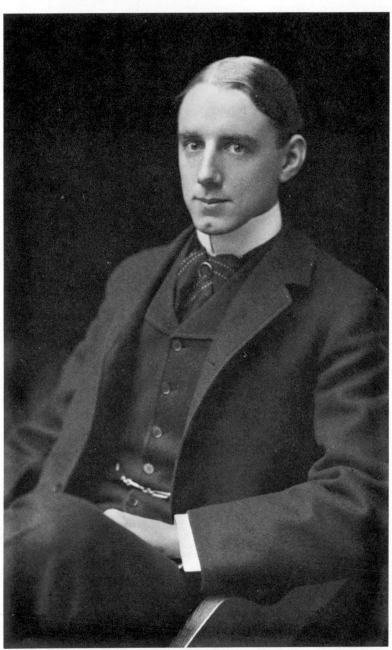

New young doctor—awaiting patients

cause her heart was not strong enough to sustain the kind of fight Jenny was waging, but for six months the Nindes and the Demmons were among his most lucrative patients. And the care and comfort he gave them so won their devotion that when Mrs. Ninde died the Demmons impulsively offered to secure for him any post he wanted at the University of Michigan if he would move to Ann Arbor. But he knew he must not take Jenny away from Colorado.

In those early months it was mostly the poor who sought his services. His letters to Mater were full of such items as "An old woman with Bright's disease gave me 25¢ in gratitude for relieving her. Can't do more and she can't live long so maybe I can collar her heart, kidneys, and brain in a postmortem as recompense." And "A colored girl up at the College needs an operation but can't pay much, so shall operate on her for $10 and experience."

Callous as such private comments seem, face to face with a patient Gerald forgot whether he would be paid or not. He was absorbed by the challenge to his skill. He could not stop himself from probing deeply into the history and circumstances of every symptom or making an exhaustive physical examination, noting his findings on an anatomical chart he devised and had printed for the purpose. When puzzled he combed through his textbooks and back issues of medical journals, especially the clinical sections of *Guy's Gazette*, until, he confessed wearily, "I know them almost by heart."

In what he came to call an "anxious case," if the family could not afford to hire a nurse he would take over the intensive care himself, sometimes spending two or three successive days and nights at the bedside and worrying himself, said Jenny, "to the verge of nervous prostration" until he had got the patient out of danger.

Gardeners and ranch hands, cooks, waitresses, and maids, barbers, butchers, and carpenters responded with a vocal devotion to "my doctor" that spread his reputation among high and low in the community. Looking back, Gerald came eventually to say, "The best thing I ever did for myself was to look after all those poor people when I began. They brought me some of my best patients."

They also brought him his first tastes of a special kind of pleasure. "I really think I was cut out to be a doctor," he exulted to Mater, "because diagnosis is so easy for me. I make brilliant diagnoses but I always am careful to confirm them by all medical means. I do enjoy it so when achieving success where others fail—am jolly glad they do too, for success in making a correct diagnosis means success in medical life, for patients go around saying 'Those other d———d doctors didn't even find out what was the matter with me, but Dr. Webb did right away.'"

This experience came to him most often with what he called "itinerant patients," the chronically ill or complaining who had been making the rounds of doctors' offices for months or years without benefit and now came to see what this newcomer could do for them.

Among the first was a young waitress whom three different doctors had been treating for asthma, the ailment for which she had been ordered to move to Colorado. In a careful examination of her throat, Gerald found an inflamed soft palate protruding an inch and a half at the back of her tongue. "I promptly whacked it off— and no more 'asthma.'" She paid him three dollars.

He got the same fee from a man whose little boy had been crippled for five months with what several physicians had treated as "rheumatism of the hip." Gerald found the trouble to stem from a dislocation and had the youngster running about normally in a few weeks.

Gerald called such instances of corrected diagnosis his "reputation-building cases." The most dramatic group of them began when he was summoned to see a woman who had been ill for eighteen months and bedridden for the last eight. The trouble was in her left leg; varicose veins a succession of doctors had called it, and several of them recently had advised her to have the leg amputated. But she would not submit. She was a widow, aged 48, and had been supporting her seven children by working as a restaurant cook.

Her leg was in shocking condition, swollen to twice its normal size and covered from knee to ankle with ulcers, abscesses, sinuses, and scars, with a few patches of hard skin in between. It looked hopeless to Gerald but he raised the foot of her bed with bricks and prescribed the application of hot boracic bandages every two hours. Since she also complained of constipation, he gave her a dozen two-grain calomel tablets with instructions to take one occasionally.

For several weeks the condition of the leg slowly improved. Then it grew gradually worse again "and she despaired and so did I." But on his next visit he found a new ulcer that unlike the previous lesions looked typical of tertiary syphilis. He suddenly remembered the improvement that had occurred while the woman was taking calomel "and I told her at once that I could get her leg well."

He immediately began treatment with mercury and iodide of potassium (Paul Ehrlich's 606 being still a decade in the future), and in six weeks the woman was able to return to her job as cook. When she appeared in church, her jolly old self again, the entire congregation joined the pastor in thanks to the Lord for her marvelous recovery "at the hands of Dr. Webb."

"A gain of forty new patients for me," exulted Gerald.

He took the experience very much to heart. It drove home the admonition he had heard at Guy's, that fledgling doctors were likely to overlook the ramifying effects of syphilis, and the extravagant dictum of William Osler that syphilis was the only disease medical students needed to know thoroughly in all its manifestations. And he could hear again Henry Sewall's thunderous preachment: "Always consider the possibility of syphilis even in the Holy Family."

Alerted now, he found this venereal disease in one or more of its three stages to be the cause of an astonishing variety of complaints that patients brought to him, ranging from shortness of breath and headache to spasms of vomiting and swollen knees. Often, with nothing like a Wassermann test as yet available to help, the diagnosis was difficult and Gerald was certain of his verdict only when the mercury and iodide treatment cleared up the symptoms.

In other cases the signs were so unmistakable that he could not imagine how previous doctors had missed them. One case he diagnosed as the patient walked into his office. Although a young woman, she was a pitiable sight. Her body was thin and wasted; spots on her scalp were wholly bare; her arms and face were covered with dark patches of hard scaly skin; the glands of her neck were enlarged into thick cords; on her lower lip lay a square of adhesive plaster.

Into Gerald's mind flashed the picture of a woman of like appearance he had examined in Guy's Hospital three years before. He had not seen a similar patient since but he remembered the diagnosis: simultaneous first and second stages of syphilis.

This Colorado Springs woman had been under treatment for three months for a supposed cold sore, actually a chancre, on her lip. Now she had also a sore throat and constant fever, her hair was falling out, and she was steadily losing weight. Gerald administered his mercury-iodide treatment and "within a few weeks all symptoms had vanished." He called in the woman's husband, found the expected signs, and dosed him too.

Gerald needed such dramatic successes because he was up against formidable competition. By his count, confirmed by the city directory for 1896, there were already sixty doctors in practice in Colorado Springs. Remembering Henry Sewall's "There's always room at the top," Gerald concerned himself primarily with the six or eight men who had large, well-established, well-paying practices of the kind to which he aspired.

Of these Dr. Solly was the leader. He seemed to have a virtual monopoly of medical practice among the transplanted British in the town and also among consumptives sent to Colorado Springs by eastern physicians; his writings were still serving him well in that respect. Gerald counted heavily on his friendship with Solly, expecting to acquire quite a few good patients by referral from the older man. It augured well, Gerald thought, when Dr. Solly made a point of taking him to the January meeting of the El Paso County Medical Society and introducing him all around as a protégé.

Of about equal standing with Solly was Dr. Boswell P. Anderson, a courtly graduate of the University of Virginia Medical School who had sought the cure for consumption at Manitou when the resort was just beginning. After a year or two as attending physician at Dr. Bell's bathhouse, he had opened the first doctor's office in Colorado Springs in 1872.

Named physician and surgeon to the Midland railroad when James J. Hagerman was pushing its tracks through Manitou, up Ute Pass, and down through Cripple Creek in a frantic race to reach Aspen ahead of the Denver and Rio Grande, Dr. Anderson attended to the cuts, bruises, and breaks of the workers in a barn alongside the tracks. When a major accident brought him a score of wounded on stretchers that could not be got through the barn door, he persuaded the Sisters of St. Francis that the best thing they could do for Colorado Springs was to build it a hospital. The consequent St. Francis Hospital on east Pikes Peak Avenue was still the city's only real hospital and Dr. Anderson was still the chief consulting surgeon on its staff.

He was also the medical director of Glockner Home, the nearest thing to a sanatorium for consumptives in the Springs. When one of his patients, Albert Glockner of Pennsylvania, died of consumption, he had used his southerner's arts of suasion on the grieving widow so successfully that Marie Glockner bought a block of land between North Cascade Avenue and North Tejon Street and built there a hospital for victims of throat and lung diseases. It opened in 1890.

So many of the patients admitted were charity cases that within three years the deficits were beyond Mrs. Glockner's resources. This time Dr. Anderson turned to the Sisters of Charity, who agreed to accept the Home as a gift and take over its management and all the nursing. Most of the several hundred consumptives they took care of annually were Dr. Anderson's patients.

Gerald Webb wanted very much to establish friendly relations with Dr. Anderson but to his dismay the Virginia gentleman remained uncharacteristically aloof, almost hostile. So did a number of the other doctors, including Charles Fox Gardiner, with whom, however, the initial antipathy was mutual.

Dr. Gardiner, a descendant of the Lion Gardiner for whom Gardiner's Island in Long Island Sound was named, was an unpolished diamond whose bluff ways and fanatical advocacy of pet theories in medicine affronted Gerald.

Afflicted with a puny body and devastatingly severe migraine headaches, the young Gardiner fifteen years before, after graduating from Bellevue Hospital Medical College, had headed for the West, determined to harden himself into strong muscle and good health by fighting raw nature and rough men in the wilderness. He had found what he sought in Colorado, first alone in the isolated mining camps at timberline around Crested Butte and later with his wife in the somewhat gentler cattle country near Meeker. To ensure a good education for his children he had moved in 1886 to Colorado Springs.

However uncouth Gardiner seemed to Gerald, he was a popular doctor in the Pikes Peak region and was currently president of the El Paso County Medical Society.

In contrast to the inexplicably cool reception Gerald got from Anderson, Gardiner, and several others, the cordial friendliness of Dr. James A. Hart was all the more encouraging. He was another of the many Colorado physicians whom tuberculosis had driven west, in his case from a good practice in Albany, New York, to Colorado Springs in 1876. He was now the most beloved family doctor in the city, was known widely as "Uncle Jimmie," and was president of the staff at St. Francis Hospital. He took an immediate liking to the young newcomer and began at once to send him patients and to telephone him almost daily to make sure all was going well with him.

At the February meeting of the county medical society Gerald planned to make a bit of a splash. The paper of the evening was to be on "The Value of an Examination of the Blood in Diagnosis" and he was willing to bet, he told Jenny confidently, that he knew more about that subject than the speaker did, so he would make himself known in the discussion.

He got a chastening surprise. The speaker was the secretary-treasurer of the society, Dr. W. B. Fenn, a "lunger" who had been practicing in Colorado Springs for eight years. He knew quite enough about the blood to win Gerald's wholehearted respect.

The two men quickly became friends and in a few weeks Dr. Fenn agreed to take room 11 in the Hagerman Block and share the waiting room in number 10. Gerald was jubilant. Now he had a proper suite of offices and he and Dr. Fenn could assist each other in operations and as consultants.

More important, Dr. Fenn believed as strongly as Gerald did in the importance of the new scientific aids to diagnosis and was disturbed that they were so unavailable in the Colorado Springs vicinity. He was certain that no other member of the county medical society had a set of blood instruments like Gerald's—or would know how to use them. He did not think any of them even had a microscope.

Would the other doctors make use of hematological and bacteriological tests if they were offered laboratory service? Gerald wondered. Some of them might, Dr. Fenn thought.

That was all the encouragement Gerald needed. He immediately bought the "bacteriological outfit" he had been wanting, including an incubator in which to maintain bacterial cultures at the proper temperature, and had printed a circular announcing a long list of determinations on blood, sputum, gastric contents, urine, and feces that Drs. Fenn and Webb would be pleased to make for their colleagues at a modest fee of ten dollars per analysis. He mailed out several hundred of these circulars to doctors in Colorado Springs and several nearby towns.

The response came slowly but increased steadily. It was gratifying to Gerald to have the great Solly himself be among the first to bring in specimens for analysis, and even more so to see one after another of the doctors who had greeted him so skeptically come to seek his assistance. Even Dr. Gardiner appeared. Only Dr. Anderson kept away. "He just won't have anything to do with me — I can't imagine why," Gerald confessed to Mater.

Meanwhile he was pursuing another course toward public favor. Dr. Henry Sewall had wanted him to continue as assistant professor of physiology at the University of Denver, but since doing so would have meant three days a week away from his office and the university could pay no more than his expenses, he refused the honor. Instead the big news of the day in Colorado Springs turned his thoughts toward Colorado College.

"THE BIG CHECK HAS COME!" blared a banner headline in the *Gazette* in early January 1897, and the Springs community breathed a collective sigh of relief at the success of its sustained effort on behalf of the college.

When the eloquent President Edward F. Tenney allowed his enthusiasm for acquiring beautiful acres for the campus to lead him beyond the bounds of fiscal responsibility and was forced to resign, he left the college in financial straits. The new president, William Frederick Slocum, another clergyman from the East, being determined to expand curriculum and enrollment and assemble a first-rate faculty, had first to raise adequate funds. He returned from a solicitation trip through the Midwest with a pledge from D. H. Pearson of Chicago to give the college $50,000 when and if it had raised an additional $150,000.

The Colorado Springs millionaires must have been somewhat less than generous because it took three years of persistent drumming to accumulate the required sum. The campaign reached its successful end just after the Webbs moved to the Springs and it was the arrival of Mr. Pearson's promised check that occasioned the January headline.

To the eager Gerald the story meant that Colorado College now had enough money to pay well for a professor of physiology. James J. Hagerman was a trustee of the college and had built its dormitory for men, Hagerman Hall. Why not ask Bert and Percy to persuade their father to use his influence on Gerald's behalf?

The first fruit of this scheming was a public lecture at Colorado College on January 21 by Gerald B. Webb M.D. on "The Anatomy of the Brain," for which the young speaker worked long hours preparing a set of large drawings as illustrations. Whether or not his effort attracted much of a public audience, it must have proved his worth to the college officials because he soon thereafter told Mater that he had been granted the faculty appointment he sought—"at what pay I don't know yet."

Nothing much in the way of teaching or salary can have come from this appointment because the name of Gerald Webb does not appear on the college faculty lists for those years. But Gerald had gained the friendship of President Slocum and the Swiss-born Florian Cajori, professor of mathematics and physics; he acquired patients among faculty and students; and most important, he was given the run of the college laboratories for his own analyses and experiments.

Professor Cajori, an able and dedicated scholar, was engrossed that spring with efforts to produce satisfactory "skiagraphs" by means of the new X rays, the discovery of which had been announced the previous year by the German physicist, William Conrad Roentgen. The rays were still mostly the subject of silly commercial exploitation in the staging of demonstrations for amusement, the production of X-ray-proof underwear and X-ray opera glasses, and the like. But Cajori's interest was strictly scientific. He had assembled his own apparatus for using the Crooke's tube to produce the rays and was achieving respectable results in making X-ray pictures.

Gerald Webb was fascinated by the procedure, and when Cajori suggested that he experiment with its usefulness in medical diagnosis he seized the chance.

One of his new "itinerant patients" was a woman who had been hobbling around town with a crutch for some four years. She had taken her painful leg to half the doctors in town, always being told she had an incurable disease of the ankle joint. Gerald decided to see whether Cajori's apparatus could tell him anything helpful about that ankle.

He got a clear picture which showed the trouble to be not with the joint at all but with the flange of bone just above it. He operated the next day, removed the difficulty easily, and soon had another conversation piece in town.

One thing was discouraging. It had taken him an entire day to set up the apparatus and prepare the patient for one hour and fifteen minutes of unmoving exposure to the X rays. Hardly a practicable procedure. But the Knox Apparatus Company of Boston was offering for sale the Tesla Oil Coil, a small X-ray machine that required a much shorter exposure time, and Gerald at once ordered one sent to him.

When the Tesla arrived in July and Gerald had assembled its components on a table behind his desk, word of the novelty spread fast and in only a few weeks as many as five doctors a day were bringing him patients to be X-rayed.

His pictures located all sorts of objects for them — bullets, pieces of glass, swallowed carpet tacks and safety pins — and revealed many kinds of abnormalities, including breaks and fractures, in the bony structures of the body.

Making clear pictures of the internal organs, especially the lungs, and interpreting the shadowy outlines the rays produced were arts not so quickly gained, but Gerald kept practicing.

One success pleased him mightily. He had been puzzling over the case of a teamster who complained of excessive weakness and fatigue. After a couple of hemorrhages the man had been sent from Chicago to Colorado as a consumptive but the prescribed open-air exercise was doing him no good. Twice after a hard day's work he had suffered another hemorrhage. He had no other symptoms of tuberculosis and Gerald could find no trace of the tubercle bacillus.

What he did find was a pronounced bulge in the upper sternum and feeble heart sounds and a weak pulse. Under questioning the patient remembered having occasional dull pains over the heart and dizziness on exertion. Gerald turned to his new X-ray machine for help, and the nature and location of an abnormal shadow on the skiagraph clinched his verdict: an aneurysm of the aorta.

He was so excited by reaching this diagnosis of "a very rare disease" that he failed to record what treatment he prescribed or how the patient fared thereafter.

It was the X-ray machine that at last brought Dr. Boswell P. Anderson to Gerald, not once but repeatedly.

By this time Gerald had learned from Dr. Fenn what had caused his cool reception by Anderson and the others. He had been introduced to them as a protégé of Dr. Solly and they had no respect for that gentleman as a doctor. They were willing to give him credit for promoting Colorado Springs as a health resort but they considered him little more than a charlatan in the practice of medicine, and they were bound to look askance at anyone he sponsored, especially another charming, cultured Britisher like himself.

When Gerald first learned of this attitude he was inclined to discount it as professional jealousy, but as the weeks passed he began to hear from patients and see for himself the evidence of Dr. Solly's incompetence.

His first lesson came from Mrs. J. S. Luckraft via Jenny. Mr. Luckraft, an English mining engineer and "the most popular Britisher in town," was Gerald's next-door neighbor in the Hagerman Block. His wife, a cousin of the Allen brothers of Somerset, tennis stars who had been Gerald's heroes in England, invited the Webbs to one of her formal receptions, took an instant liking to Jenny, and went often to visit her at Austin Bluffs.

One of Mrs. Luckraft's tales to Jenny was of grievance with Dr. Solly, who had been the Luckraft's physician since their arrival in Colorado Springs. They had little need of his services but he persisted in making a call each week and then sending them a big bill every few months. And now they could not even trust his medical advice; he had treated a friend of theirs for chronic rheumatism over a period of many months before sending him to take the baths at Glenwood Springs, and the doctor there had found the man to have a dislocated shoulder which he set right almost overnight.

Then came the Henry C. Halls. Mr. Hall, the distinguished head of the law firm in which Bert Hagerman was a junior associate, had been an attorney on the staff of the American Embassy in Paris for many years before bringing his diseased lungs to Colorado Springs and Dr. Solly.

Now it was Mrs. Hall who was the patient, with painful swellings and sores on both legs. Dr. Solly named the cause milk leg and kept changing her medicines and dressings with expensive regularity. But her condition only grew worse. Bert Hagerman persuaded her to try his friend, young Dr. Webb, and Gerald recognized the lesions as the gummata of tertiary syphilis. He was shaken to find upon analysis of Dr. Solly's latest prescription for Mrs. Hall that it was only a placebo.

Mr. Hall, understandably, was outraged by Gerald's diagnosis and would submit himself for examination and treatment only after Gerald's doses of mercury and iodide cleared up Mrs. Hall's ugly sores. Thereafter the Halls were among Gerald's most loyal and helpful patients.

As Gerald witnessed and heard of more such instances of Dr. Solly's gross errors, his disgust with Solly became as intense as Dr. Anderson's, and all the more bitter because he had been so duped. "The man is a fraud, an unprincipled scamp," he told Mater. "He will do the most despicable things just for money. His reputation is not in the least enviable now, and he is losing his patients fast."

Jenny Webb was one of the patients Dr. Solly lost. Gerald asked Dr. Hart to look after her instead.

Gerald's disillusionment spread to include his former benefactor, Solly's friend Dr. Bell. He too was a fraud, Gerald decided. "He is recognized as the meanest, closest cuss in town. There have been many times when he could have done something to help me, but he hasn't lifted a finger. So having got into the wrong crowd, for 'getting on' reasons we are getting out of it."

The "right crowd" they wanted to join was what Jenny called approvingly "the swagger carriage set"—the El Paso Club and Cheyenne Mountain Country Club circle in which the Hagerman brothers moved. There, Gerald thought, he would acquire more of the well-paying patients he needed. But he knew he was not a likely candidate for election to the El Paso Club, and the country club was too far away for him to get there often. Besides, it was in a turbulent state at the moment.

William Otis, as part of his effort to develop a suburb at Austin Bluffs, had offered to donate land to the nascent country club but its founders had chosen instead to locate their clubhouse in the rival suburb of Broadmoor, near Count Pourtales' Casino a mile south and west of town, where beautiful Cheyenne Mountain provided a scenic backdrop for club activities.

Among these was golf of a sort, played on a scrabbly nine-hole course that had what Percy Hagerman called "sand greens the size of dinner plates." A few of the more serious golfers, including Hagerman, grew restive not only with the makeshift course but with the irresponsible antics, financial and social, of some of their fellow members, a group of devil-may-care young bachelors who called themselves the Socialites.

Leaders in this group were Spencer "Spec" Penrose and Charles Leaming Tutt, both Philadelphia blue bloods, and Charles Mather

MacNeill who hailed from Chicago. All burning with desire to get rich as quick as possible, they spent their weeks at hard labor and harder deals in the mining camps at Cripple Creek, then came to Colorado Springs for drunken, roistering sprees at the country club on the weekends. Not even the furniture at the club was safe from destruction during their boisterous brawling when they were in their cups.

Penrose was "a bull of a man," spectacularly tall and good-looking, shrewd, profane, socially shy and inarticulate. Intimidated by the brilliance and impeccable respectability of his father, a physician of repute, and his older brothers—one of whom was Boies Penrose, the famous U.S. senator and political boss from Pennsylvania—Spec was determined to show the family he could make more money than any of them.

Which he did, fantastically. He and Tutt and MacNeill became wealthy pillars of the community in their maturity, but in these early days they were raucous and crude by Jenny Webb's standards, not at all the kind of men she judged suitable companions for Gerald.

Percy Hagerman wanted to avoid them too. He and his friends in May 1897 withdrew from the Cheyenne Mountain Country Club, organized the Colorado Springs Golf Club, and bought William Otis's mansion at Austin Bluffs to serve as their clubhouse.

Gerald Webb enthusiastically joined the group, paid fifty dollars for a charter membership, and was elected to the board of governors and named a member of the Greens Committee. He was also asked to design and supervise the construction of the new nine-hole course.

"The prettiest links in Colorado" he gloatingly called the course when it was finished.

The new club brought more to the Webbs than a nearby playground; it became a source of influential new patients.

Among the first was Ellen the clubhouse cook when one day in early summer she lost a battle with a crab and developed blood-poisoning in her arm. Gerald managed to save both life and arm for her and thereupon acquired the entire staff of the club as a chorus of fans. By summer's end their audience included most of the people who counted socially in Colorado Springs, since membership in the new club quickly became fashionable.

Gerald's loyal patient, Henry C. Hall, was secretary-treasurer of the club and his word carried weight with his friend the president, Joel Addison Hayes.

Quite a power in the town was the quiet but popular Mr. Hayes, called Addison by all his friends and associates. He was president of the First National Bank and a director of a number of companies doing business in the gold fields as well as utility companies in Colorado Springs. He had been a banker in Memphis when he married the belle of the South, Margaret Howell Davis, daughter of Jefferson Davis, president of the Confederacy. But debilitating attacks of asthma forced young Hayes to leave the humid air of Tennessee and he and Margaret had moved to Colorado Springs in 1885.

Mr. and Mrs. Hayes liked what they saw of the young doctor of whom many were now saying much good, and before the year was out they had made Gerald Webb their family physician.

So had the Scudders and the Jewetts. William H. Scudder, a fellow member with Gerald of the club's Greens Committee, was a tuberculosis victim from St. Louis and the son-in-law of Samuel Cupples, one of the Missouri city's foremost philanthropists. Mr. Cupples came often to stay with his daughter and being old and frail had frequent need of a physician. He and the Scudders came to depend on young Dr. Webb, called him to one bedside or another often, and paid him well for the services they demanded.

W. K. Jewett and his wife Patty were newcomers to Colorado Springs, referred to Dr. Solly by Mrs. Jewett's doctor in the East. Ardent golfers, they joined the new club at once and there met Dr. Webb. Mrs. Jewett, disturbed by the tales she was hearing about Dr. Solly, appeared in Gerald's office one day and asked him point-blank: Could she trust Dr. Solly or should she change to another physician?

Gerald squirmed in his dilemma. He could not advise reliance on Solly but medical ethics forbade him to speak his mind about the man. So he told Mrs. Jewett that Edwin Solly had done much for Colorado Springs, that many of his patients liked him, but that she could change doctors if she wished providing she dismissed Dr. Solly in writing. He was pleased a short time later to receive Mrs. Jewett as a patient.

Clearly Gerald Webb had an asset working for him beyond his manifest ability, hard work, and advantageous connections. All his ingenuity in finding ways to extend his practice could hardly have paid off so quickly or so well had he not been handsome and personable, gifted beyond the average with a talent for winning friends and inspiring devotion. He must have possessed in extraordinary measure that indefinable quality of mind and manner variously called appeal, charm, charisma, magic.

Perhaps in him the charm came from, in addition to warmth and buoyancy, an unusual combination of diffidence and deference with assurance and authority. Whatever it was, patients found it easy to like and trust him; it somehow made them feel better just to talk with him.

Gerald was not unaware of this power in himself, nor wholly above some deliberate use of it. "I am becoming something of a courtier, I'm afraid," he wrote Mater. "I have adopted a new motto from Juvenal, wonderful in effect with most of the women here: 'Go persevere, and in most prudent strain / Praise wit in fools and features in the plain.'"

The "prudent strain" plus normal British reserve saved him from noxious blandishment, while his basic integrity and firm convictions kept him unswerving in medical matters. Two episodes will illustrate:

Among the young men who sometimes in late afternoon joined the Hagerman brothers in Gerald's office to watch him at work with his scientific "gadgets" were the Bonbrights, three bachelor brothers who constituted the William P. Bonbright Company, a brokerage firm in mining stocks.

William and Irving, the two older brothers, both of whom held seats on the Mining Exchange, shared a flat, though William was building himself a house at 1222 North Cascade Avenue. George lived at the El Paso Club and spent much of his time playing tennis. William, a consumptive, became Gerald's patient and George his occasional tennis partner.

One night during a Hagerman dinner party at which the Bonbrights and Webbs were guests George was stricken with dizziness and severe pain in his head. Gerald went to his aid and had reached a tentative diagnosis when George's own doctor, summoned by Irving, arrived. Gerald necessarily stood aside while the other doctor soothed and fussed, talked about overexertion, administered a bromide, and departed.

Tempted by galled pride and the canons of medical ethics to let it go at that, Gerald simply could not do so; if what he suspected was true, George's illness was too serious to be disregarded. As he bade George goodnight he casually suggested that it might be well to have the doctor make sure there was no possibility of a mastoid abscess.

Gerald said nothing when George heeded his suggestion and the abscess was found, but Bert Hagerman twitted George unmercifully about his poor judgment in choice of doctors. George soon joined William as Gerald's patient.

The second episode grew out of Gerald's conviction that every death of which the cause was in the least uncertain should be followed by a postmortem. How else could a doctor learn from his mistakes and improve his ability to correlate symptoms with an obscure origin? Gerald was therefore upset to learn that Dr. Fenn had failed to arrange for an autopsy after the death of a patient whose illness had baffled them both. When he protested, Dr. Fenn said it was too late now; the family was preparing for the funeral. Undaunted, with Fenn's permission Gerald went to see the family.

He found the body back from the undertaker's, all dressed and made up and laid out in a fine coffin surrounded with flowers. Relatives and friends were already arriving for the last rites. Nevertheless Gerald talked the family into postponing the services until the next day and letting the undertaker cart the coffin back to his parlors so that Gerald could do a postmortem on the body.

An incredible feat of persuasion! And behind it a will of steel.

The postmortem revealed a strangulated hernia which an operation could have repaired.

Another of Gerald's convictions, implanted by his father and Molière at Heimat and developed by his training, deepened rapidly as he gained experience in practice. He expressed it in reply to his sister Nell who, hysterically afraid of an operation her doctor had recommended for a retroflexed uterus, wrote to ask Gerald's opinion of two popular patent medicines that Roly's wife Lilian had suggested might relieve her pain. Advising Nell strongly against the nostrums, Gerald wrote:

"I am a great skeptic on most drugs, and I can almost count on my ten fingers the number I use. I prefer to rely on the '*vis medicatrix naturae*' and do not hinder it by dosing the system with gallons of drugs. Bowel openings regularly, fresh air, and good food are the most useful resources of my pharmacopeia. Doctors, I find, are the most deceitful and hypocritical of men, and the humbuggery that goes on is enormous. Ninety percent of patients will get well anyway, but the doctor who has been called in gets the credit instead of nature."

On another occasion he told Mater about one of his "anxious cases," a woman ill with puerperal fever with whom he had spent much time day and night for a week. When she recovered, her husband gave Gerald a pearl and diamond stickpin in gratitude for pulling her through, but "it was nature that pulled her through, not me," said Gerald.

The records provide only tantalizing glimpses of his methods in practice at this time. His penchant still was for surgery, and he described one week as "humdrum—several interesting cases but no operations." He seems to have done most of his minor surgery in his office or the patient's home, where effective antisepsis could hardly be achieved, but major operations he performed, through the kind auspices of "Uncle Jimmie" Hart, at St. Francis Hospital. Removals of a huge goiter, a brain tumor, a large ovarian tumor, and an inflamed appendix were the most advanced surgery of the day that he mentioned doing.

Chloroform was his preferred anesthetic, although he did on occasion use ether when he was assisting another surgeon who asked for it. Gerald shared the prevailing belief that ether was "tricky," unreliable, sometimes fatal, because the steady-drip cone method of administering it had not yet been developed.

A casual reference by Gerald to the application of "lint soaked in carbolic acid" is suggestive, but it seems unlikely that St. Francis Hospital was equipped for or its surgical authorities inclined to demand the use of Joseph Lister's carbolic acid spray for antiseptic surgery. The method was dramatic enough and the dripping spray unpleasant enough to have evoked comment from Gerald had he operated under it. The chances are that his antiseptic practices were as primitive as those of most surgeons at the time.

Yet he was able to say after seven months of practice that he had not yet had to write a death certificate, and when this depressing experience did come to him later, the instances he described to Mater were all from lung, kidney, or heart disease, not from surgery.

When Dr. Anderson, bowing to age, resigned from the surgical staff of St. Francis Hospital in October 1897, Gerald hoped to be appointed to the vacancy, since his good friend Dr. Hart was president of the staff. But the Sisters of St. Francis chose another man, because, Gerald surmised, "he has sent them more private patients than I have." It is equally possible that Dr. Hart thought young Webb had uncommon skills which the hospital needed more than his surgery, because the Sisters simultaneously named Dr. Webb "Pathologist to St. Francis Hospital."

Willy-nilly, Gerald was more physician than surgeon, treating whatever ills of the community were brought to him, from ingrown toenails and hives to diphtheria, pneumonia, and of course consumption.

For his consumptive patients Gerald on the whole followed the custom of the time and place, in which "Colorado, creosote, and whiskey" were considered the sovereign remedies. He put more emphasis than most on nourishing food and, remembering Jenny's experience in Georgia, always in severe cases prescribed an ounce of whiskey every two hours. Beyond that he believed with his contemporaries that fresh mountain air would cure any patient who could be cured, provided the patient cooperated by taking as much outdoor exercise as possible.

Looking back years later Gerald remembered how "feeble patients were allowed to rest the first week or two after coming to Colorado but then were told to throw away their thermometers and go for buggy rides. It was a matter of patching and breaking [the lesion in the lung]. Hence the idea that consumptives could never leave the Colorado climate. The complete rest regime was of slow birth."

He may well have been thinking of Jenny. None of her doctors, including Gerald and Dr. Hart, denied her exercise; rather they encouraged her to be as active as she could. Gerald allowed her to go alone to Denver to look for a suitable servant since a succession of local girls had frazzled her nerves—they were all either "drunk, crazy, saucy, or indolent." On a trip to the resort at Glenwood Springs with the Hagermans and George Bonbright in the Hagermans' private railroad car Gerald was delighted to have her swim with him in the hotel pool "though she could manage only a few yards." After a gala ball at the Antlers Hotel he marveled at "how much good it does her to dance—because it expands her lungs, I suppose."

It is curious that he did not find the reason in the good that dancing undoubtedly did for Jenny Kenney's soul, because, largely through his observation of her, he was beginning to emphasize attention to the consumptive's mind and spirits. "The whole art in successful treatment of consumption here," he told Mater, "is in administering to the mind. Keep that cheerful and your patient does well. The climate does the rest."

Later he would recognize that "for many, unfortunately, the clock was set back by those who, in their enthusiasm for climate, opposed the rest regime." But now he thought with Dryden that "the wise, for cure, on exercise depend" and with Ambroise Paré that the patient not too ill "must have viols and violins and a buffoon."

There is no evidence that in this first year of practice he offered more than reassuring words to cheer his consumptive patients, but to Jenny he brought books and magazines, news and gossip, and all the gaiety he could command at the end of a hard day. "I keep my problems and worries to myself." He encouraged visitors and was grateful when Cousin Homer Bates arrived in August to spend three months with them. "He is such a happy chap and does so much to cheer her up."

Perhaps what Jenny needed was more of Gerald's time, more of his company, to keep terror at bay, but he could see only the need to work harder and harder, climb faster and faster, to earn the money for her comforts and please her by his success.

By any objective standard Gerald was doing remarkably well. At midyear his practice alone was keeping him so busy that he turned over all the laboratory work to Dr. Fenn, who preferred it as less exhausting than coping with patients. And Gerald figured that with the major cost of equipment and instruments behind him he was now breaking even financially. Until he sent out semiannual bills for $450 and received only $85 in payment. It was a jolting lesson that "the doctor is the last to be paid, if at all."

He promptly made a precautionary switch in his accounting. He had been reckoning his income on what he earned, tabulating his fees day by day; now he began calculating it on what he took in each month. And by the end of the year he was receiving between three hundred and four hundred dollars a month, not at all a pittance in those days.

What to charge for his services was a constant problem for him. Fees of three dollars for a routine office visit, five dollars for a house call day or night, and ten to twenty-five dollars for a confinement were standard, but beyond those each doctor set his own. Wanting to avoid a reputation for exorbitant charges, Gerald was always afraid he was asking too much or too little.

One time he was really upset. Called to the scene when a visiting horseman was thrown from his mount and having to treat him for multiple dislocations and fractures over a period of several weeks, Gerald apologetically presented him with a bill for $188. The man, laughing as he wrote out his check, said he had expected to pay at least $350. For days Gerald berated himself for having been so timid.

Whatever his receipts he was always so near fiscal disaster that money became an obsession with him. When during one of Jenny's attacks of pleurisy the Hagermans and Bonbrights sent her florist's bouquets of roses and violets, Gerald calculated their total cost to have been twenty-eight dollars and fervently wished he had the money instead.

His difficulty came not just from the expenses of Jenny's illness but equally from his own impulsive extravagance. He spent the whole of his first sizable fee on a set of sterling silver orange spoons for Mater—and then had to explain their use to her, having forgot that oranges were not the staple at Heimat that they had become for him. He bought new instruments and equipment, always the best, with abandon. Telling himself repeatedly that he must not buy any more books, he always fell for the wares of the next itinerant book peddler just the same.

Hearing the Bonbrights discuss insurance, he at once insured his life for $10,000. And when Henry Hall, settling the estate of a deceased client, offered him a three-hundred-dollar phaeton for half its cost, he sold his pony and yellow trap and bought the fancier carriage and a team of cobs, justifying the indulgence on the grounds that "patients like to have their doctor drive up to their door in a handsome rig."

His offsetting economies were ludicrous. When he got too busy to continue the research he had started on the tubercle bacillus he threw away his cultures and in their place in his incubator set two dozen eggs to hatch so as to increase the flock of thirty chicks he was "raising naturally" at home.

And he bought not a stitch of new clothing, not even underwear, all year, though he complained that his professional suits, dating from his student days at Guy's, were getting threadbare and the two suits for "best wear" he had brought back from Thomas the

Tailor last year were too thick and hot for comfort in the Colorado summer.

It was a blow to Gerald when Dr. Fenn fell seriously ill in early August and after an operation in Denver decided to remain in that city doing laboratory work and teaching pathology. Now all the time-consuming tests and analyses were Gerald's to do.

His heavier duties made a burden of what had been a pleasure, the half-hour drive between home and office, and Gerald decided he and Jenny must move into town.

This was not the first time he had contemplated a change. Several other pastures had looked greener to his restless, impatient eyes, but Jenny had always "held him in line," she said. She had argued fiercely that he must not move again, that he was making good progress in Colorado Springs and would only lose everything if he tried to start over someplace else.

This time she could not counter his case. She "wept buckets of tears" at the idea of leaving the country, but Gerald would not be dissuaded. He must be nearer his office and in the midst of a potential supply of patients. All the other doctors were established in the older parts of town, leaving the rapidly developing area north of Colorado College without a physician near at hand. That was where he should be.

Hunting a house was discouraging. It must be furnished, since he and Jenny had acquired only accessories, nothing basic, and he thought the rents "absurdly high." The kind of house he wanted, "one like Roly's in Cheltenham," cost $150 a month, far beyond his means, and he had to settle for a lesser place, at 1423 North Tejon Street, which he could get for half that amount.

The move to Tejon Street in mid-September followed upon three simultaneous "anxious cases" that had allowed Gerald only catnaps for eight nights running. When with a little help from Cousin Homer and much direction from Jenny he had unpacked and stowed away their belongings, installed an electric bell for emergency calls at night, nailed a bird feeder to the windowsill in Jenny's bedroom, and bought her scrapbooks in which to paste their accumulation of photographs and clippings, he felt utterly fagged.

Usually after such a period of stress a good night's sleep and an afternoon of tennis or golf would make him fit again. But not this time. The fatigue was too deep. An unexpected opportunity to get off into the wilds for a while seemed heaven-sent.

Henry Hall's brother-in-law, Edmond Kelly, a New York and Paris lawyer, lecturer, writer, and sometime professor at Columbia University, had just arrived in Colorado Springs to recover from "nervous prostration." Mr. Hall brought him to Dr. Webb. When Gerald learned that Mr. Kelly owned a huge wilderness ranch across the Rockies, he told the man he could do nothing better for his nerves than to go there and live by his gun for a time. Mr. Kelly invited Gerald to go with him. And to bring Mrs. Webb and her cousin along.

So in early October the quartet set off by train on the journey of some three hundred miles through Glenwood Springs to the end of the tracks at Rifle and thence by wagon another hundred miles into "the heart of the hunting district."

Once arrived at the ranch they had no need to rough it. "Mr. Kelly has built a series of log cabins after the plan of the Trianon in Paris. Although so far from everywhere he has almost everything money can purchase and wagons can convey there—piano, good library, a chapel, French cook and English waitress, everything.

"[For more than two weeks] we all had the most delightful time hunting, shooting, fishing, in the saddle ten hours a day. We all lived on horseback, climbing over the most perilous places with sure-footed horses, sleeping in tents at times, eating venison and all kinds of game, and living as much with nature as is possible for a civilized animal. We are brown as Indians and my hair is bleached all shades by the sun. We have come back fit as fiddles."

Jenny was not strong enough to share much in such strenuous activities; she stayed behind in the cabins most of the time. Gerald thought she was better for the trip, but she said it had tired her and made her cough and fever worse.

Gerald himself quickly lost zest again. His load seemed only the heavier, his lot the less enviable, after the short spell of pure delight. He put his sense of letdown into words a few weeks later after the Twombley dinner party.

The Twombleys were Vanderbilt kin, "rotting with wealth," who had come recently to live in Colorado Springs. Having met the Webbs at the golf club and called Gerald to take care of a friend injured in an accident, they invited the doctor and his wife to their big November dinner.

It was sumptuous beyond belief, with plates of solid gold and everything to match. Jenny said it surpassed anything she had ever seen in Philadelphia and New York. And she was pleased to have done Gerald proud in such a company by winning the first prize at euchre after dinner. But Gerald was unwontedly sour about it: "To go to such dinners with such lavish expenditure and such displays of wealth makes one feel glum afterwards."

The contrast with his own financial plight was too great. The three weeks' holiday with Mr. Kelly had reduced his October receipts to eighty dollars and he was facing monthly expenses of more than three hundred. He listed them: rent $80, butcher $40, grocer $35, electric lights $10, coal $15, two maids $45, milk $12, boy to tend cobs and carriage $30. And if Jenny should have one of her bad attacks a trained nurse would cost $25 a week.

Plus, of course, the $100 rent for his offices. That was where he elected to cut back. Most doctors had their offices at home; why shouldn't he, now that he lived in town?

Deaf to Jenny's protests he turned a room of the Tejon Street house into a "surgery" and moved out of rooms 10 and 11 in the Hagerman Block, keeping only room 9 as his laboratory "and a place to see some of my poorer patients."

In hopes of increasing his income he sent round another circular offering his services in X-ray diagnosis, calling it wryly "my Xmas card." To make further hay with the doctors roundabout he wrote a paper about his syphilis cases to be read to the El Paso County Medical Society and then published in the *Colorado Medical Journal.* For that journal too he made a teasing little puzzle of the case in which he had found an aneurysm of the aorta, setting down under the title "Wanted: A Diagnosis" all the confusing symptoms and all his examination findings but, whether from modesty or conceit, withholding the conclusion he had drawn.

Under the stimulus of composition his ambition flared. He would send his articles to *Guy's Gazette* to keep his name alive at the hospital until he could get back to complete his degrees. He would write some articles for English medical journals. He would take a leaf from Dr. Solly's book:

"Solly derives all his practise from patients sent him by Eastern doctors, and I intend to know these Easterners myself. I am starting original work in X-ray examination of the lungs and also in blood work that I can make a paper out of and read before these learned Eastern doctors next spring. I have just joined the American Medical Association for that purpose. If I could come to Eng-

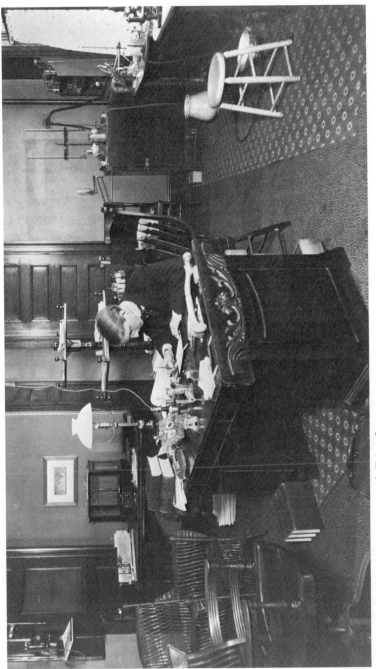

Gerald in his office at home on North Tejon Street

land I would canvass London chest specialists and get them to send their lung cases to me."

But the flare was momentary. When Henry Sewall sent Gerald's way the opportunity to collaborate with Dr. Louis E. Livingood of Johns Hopkins University on original experiments with guinea pigs and rabbits to determine what difference there might be in the germ-killing power of the blood at sea level and at the altitude of Colorado Springs, Gerald undertook the research with uncharacteristic lack of enthusiasm. "Original work is like buying gold mines," he commented; "there is usually nothing comes out of it."

The fact is that Gerald was ending his first year of practice with a clouding sense of failure, in what was for him severe depression.

Jenny thought him in good health, strong and vigorous, sleeping well. Out of her own many nights made sleepless by pain and coughing, she said enviously, "Oh, how he sleeps! Like a top. On and on. No matter what." She forgot the nights when, called out for a confinement or staying at the bedside in a worrisome case, he hardly slept at all. And she did not know that he was in a fret about his own mental state.

This concern grew out of Mater's letters about his brother Harold, who had suffered what his doctor called a nervous breakdown. From the symptoms Gerald judged the diagnosis correct and urged, in accordance with the regimen recommended in such cases by S. Weir Mitchell, that Harold immediately be isolated from all members of the family, even his wife. Recovery would be difficult and might take years, Gerald warned. "I would sooner have consumption, if it did not kill," he told Mater.

When he learned that Harold was taking his wife Enid, and brother Wilfred too, to a hotel in Cairo for a change of scene he was exasperated. Cairo was not at all what Harold needed; it would be too much like Cheltenham. He should go on a camping trip, live alone with nature, get away from people. "It is this d———d civilization that causes these nervous diseases," said Gerald.

But he soon found another explanation, at least for the Webb family. Reminded of Ida's recurrent spells of nervous exhaustion, Nell's tendency to hysteria, and Frank's continuing struggle against melancholia, he concluded they had all inherited "weak nerves" from their father. "Heredity is a wonderful thing," he wrote Mater, "and an alcoholic parent almost inevitably hands down delicate nervous tissue."

Naturally he began to find signs of incipient trouble in himself. "Harold started his symptoms with absent-mindedness and I am getting as bad as he was. But I am working to alter it and now am answering questions in two minutes instead of half an hour and try to get rid of thinking of other things than what I am doing, as for example at the piano."

More serious symptoms he seems not to have recognized, clinging instead to the notion that his cheerful disposition could banish all shadows. "If I were not blessed with a buoyant nature I should have terrible blues," he wrote to Mater. And to Sophie, "I never lose my spirits and just keep joyous and happy, crushing any gloomy feelings out of existence."

He was protesting too much. The blue funk came through in bursts: "How I would like to leave this place forever!" After reporting receipts of $400 in November, his highest for the year: "Being British, I'll never make it to the top here." In closing a letter, "Your good for nothing boy."

He grew increasingly self-centered, pouring out to Mater page after page about numbers of patients gained and lost, fees, unpaid bills, expenses, fancied slights, uncertainties about Jenny. Occasionally he would pull up and apologize for his preoccupation with "self" and "ego," only to return in the next sentence to his litany of worries.

He revealed intemperate judgments and loss of perspective. His dislike of Dr. Solly became a vindictive passion. Would the family please buy him subscriptions to the *Lancet* and the *British Medical Journal* so he could refuse the loan of that man's copies? It was disgusting the way Solly "namby-pambies his patients, calling on them twice a day and then charging them $250 a month," and the way Solly tried to steal patients from other doctors. Seeing how well Gerald was getting on with members of the golf club, Solly had applied for membership, and as a member of the board of governors Gerald longed to blackball him but knew he must not. So now Solly was coming often to play golf and "it is sickening to see how he toadies up to all the richest people there."

Brooding over what he considered his failure to get ahead, Gerald decided that "my three crimes are youth, poverty, and being a Britisher." At twenty-six he was calling himself thirty to offset the first, but he could only be bitter about the other two.

He made a little table for Mater, listing the five doctors he judged to have the largest practices in Colorado Springs—Anderson, Hart, H. B. Moore, Solly, and Gardiner. Alongside he guessed at their ages, all in their fifties and sixties except Gardiner whom he thought to be about forty, and in a third column he set down the supposed sources of their independent incomes—wealthy wives, brothers, or daughters. Below the tabulation he commented: "Hence these men, with gross ignorance of their profession, are able to live in swell houses and drive fine turnouts, and giving the impression of prosperity they get good practices. Then too, they are older and bar Solly are Americans."

No one in a normal state of mind could have accused all those five doctors of "gross ignorance" of medicine or could have expected in one year to equal the prosperity of men who had been developing their practices for decades.

The idea that it was a disadvantage to be British took root in Gerald's mind when he heard someone say that Colorado was a dumping ground for Great Britain's "bad eggs." He remembered being told at school in Cheltenham that this or that delinquent of the community had been banished to America, and thinking he had met a few of this kind in Colorado Springs he was sure they had so prejudiced the entire town against Britishers that being from England was a barrier to his success.

Jenny poohpoohed this notion, pointing out that half the most successful men in town were British and that Gerald himself was well liked by his associates and the members of the golf club. But Gerald was not to be argued out of his fixed idea and grew increasingly self-conscious about his "Queen's English" and "bobtailed British suits."

There is ample explanation for Gerald's depression in these closing months of the year. He had been working too long hours at too many things, without enough time to spend in the vigorous exercise to which he was accustomed. He had been losing too much sleep and worrying too much about his critically ill patients ("someday I may become as free from fuss about them as other doctors are").

He was spending beyond his income, partly for Jenny's sake but equally in a vain effort to keep up appearances among his wealthy friends and patients. He was living perforce a celibate life. He saw the prospect receding of his ever acquiring the "eight more letters after my name" that he desperately wanted from Guy's Hospital.

Trying to keep Jenny cheerful left him no outlet for his anxieties except his letters to Mater.

And over all his doings hung the threat and intermittent turmoil of Jenny's ups and downs. Early in December she was busy making herself a new dress "since we are too poor to buy one," but by the middle of the month she was "lying up after an attack of pleurisy."

"She is terribly weak and there seems to be nothing left of her. Her constant spitting up so nauseates her that she cannot eat, so her main food is whiskey. Every little thing upsets her and she cannot keep from crying. She feels she is only a terrible burden, and therefore begs to die. I often wonder if it is a kindness to keep her alive. Perhaps I am selfish in trying to do so. But I do so want her to see me a success. She has been so plucky, and entirely through her I have gained so many of my best patients."

On Christmas Eve Gerald sat on in his downtown office until after nine o'clock ("two in the morning in Cheltenham") writing a homesick letter to Mater. It would be such fun to be with them all at Heimat. He was sorry he could not afford to send them any presents this year. Maybe someday he would be rich enough to make his family and friends happy at Christmas. "Now I must rush home to Jenny. She is feeling better again."

V

Good Times and Bad

SEVEN MONTHS LATER the depression was gone and Gerald was singing. "You can't imagine how happy I am at making ends meet and not owing a cent. It makes me light-hearted again." Two years later he could claim to have the "biggest and best" practice in Colorado Springs and felt "exceptionally lucky" to have outstripped his older competitors. He had even made peace of a sort with Dr. Solly. And four years later his waiting room was always packed with patients and he was earning some $15,000 a year while contributing handsomely to the incomes of four other doctors who carried his overload of cases and assisted him in operations.

The turnaround in mood began with the advent simultaneously of Messrs. Blackman and Sanger.

W. H. Blackman was a retired businessman aged thirty-five who wanted to become a doctor and asked Gerald to take him on as a "pupil." Gerald agreed to supervise his studies and give him an hour of instruction each morning for a fee of thirty dollars per month.

When Mater observed with asperity that one dollar an hour was not a princely recompense, Gerald said yes, he supposed he should be charging twice as much but the teaching forced him into a valuable review of fundamentals and besides, even thirty dollars of certain income each month was a blessing in "this hand-to-mouth profession of uncertain payment."

The arrangement continued for a year, and when Mr. Blackman decided to continue his studies formally in Denver, Gerald was relieved to see him go, because "being so busy now I find him a little in the way."

John F. Sanger, whom Gerald always identified as John Pullman Sanger, the Webbs had first met while they were living in Denver. A cousin of Jenny's old beau, John Sanger Pullman, this John was the "favorite nephew" of the widow of the sleeping-car magnate and the stepson of W. S. Cheesman, a director along with Addison Hayes of the International Trust Company of Denver. Young Sanger, just Gerald's age, was assistant secretary of the company and manager of its branch office in Colorado Springs.

John had become a good friend and companion whom Gerald much admired because although John's salary was only $1800 a year he was finding ways to earn an additional $6000 a year on the side. In early 1898 he came to live with the Webbs in the Tejon Street house, paying them eighty dollars a month for his room and board.

Here was more certain income, enough to pay the entire rent for the house. And the way Jenny managed, it would cost no more to feed three than two. Gerald thought his financial load lighter by half.

The upward spurt in the number and wealth of his patients began with two dramatic reputation-building cases.

The first was the "Bennett babe." Born prematurely it was reluctant to take firm hold of life. But it was heir to an estate left in trust for it and its parents wanted desperately to keep it alive. A large segment of gossipy Colorado Springs watched avidly while the mother and father called in the doctors of the town one after another. All said the baby could not live.

At last Dr. Webb was summoned, but in consultation with two others whose recommendations for the care and feeding of the infant he could not agree with. So he withdrew while their plan was tried. It failed and the baby was barely alive when the parents asked Dr. Webb to return.

Gerald shed his coat, donned an apron, and took over the kitchen to carry out his plan "based entirely on physiology." With his own hands he prepared "the milk, etc. till I had nothing but peptones." Then he fed and hovered.

"From the very first the results were magnificent and I was soon able to put the babe with a good wet nurse and watch it gain and grow."

The advertisement of his skill proved to be far more remunerative than the "whopping fee" the parents paid him. They were so devoted to him that when they had a second son two years later they named him Gerald Webb Bennett. He grew up to marry the doctor's daughter.

The second tale is best told by Gerald himself:

"Dr. Gardiner has a rich patient a few blocks away from us whom he and Dr. Hart have been treating for months for stomach trouble. Having a sick headache Saturday, Gardiner asked me to run in and see the man. I did, and casually examining his chest I felt sure there was fluid on the left side. I put in a hypodermic needle and sure enough there it was. Yesterday I operated and taking out a piece of rib drew off over 4 quarts of pus!! Of course the tremendous pressure had upset the stomach and the man was rapidly dying. The sac of fluid might have burst any second. It was what we call an empyema.

"My name already is in everyone's mouth, as this patient is probably the most popular society man in town. His name is Godfrey Kissel.

"Last night was the first sleep I have had for nights, I have been so excited over this. As I was lying tossing in bed, Mater, I looked up at yours and the Pater's photographs and felt so grateful for the brains you had given me. Today I am going to try and rest. The strain has been so heavy my hand actually trembles."

Had Gerald been choosing a promoter of his name he could hardly have picked one more influential socially than Godfrey Kissel. A member of a family in New York City's "400," Kissel had journeyed westward for health and settled in Colorado Springs. Although he had no need to earn money he maintained a downtown office from which to dabble in assorted ventures, but he was primarily a sportsman and bon vivant, everyone's convivial friend. He had been a founder of the Cheyenne Mountain Country Club and continued to spark its activities.

But this was not his year. While he was still recuperating from the empyema his twelve-year-old daughter Bettye was stricken with acute appendicitis. Recognition of this disorder was little more than a decade old and the whether, when, and how of surgery for it were still matters of heated controversy. Gerald Webb operated without hesitation but then was torn with anxiety for days lest failure with the daughter undo the benefit of success with the father.

When Bettye was well along toward recovery Mr. Kissel decided he wanted to see his relatives and old friends in New York and arranged for a private car to transport him and his family thither. He insisted that Dr. Webb go along to take care of them, offering to pay all expenses to New York and back plus one hundred dollars a day. Mrs. Webb would be welcome to accompany him.

To go or not to go, and if he went whether to go on across the Atlantic to Cheltenham? Gerald agonized over the decision, trying to figure gain and loss both ways. If he went away his patients would scatter to other doctors and he might not be able to reassemble them when he returned. He could pay Heimat only a short visit at best. But Dr. Hart thought Jenny's nerves were now as bad as her lungs and it might do her good to see her people again.

In the end they went, but only to New York. Gerald decided to postpone his visit to Heimat until his practice was secure and he could stay away long enough to take the examinations for his degrees.

After delivering the Kissels safely to the country estate of Godfrey's brother Gustav near Morristown, New Jersey, Gerald took Jenny to the Bates home on West End Avenue in New York and left her to rest there while he made the rounds of the city's hospitals observing operations, "learning the latest," and making the acquaintance of the surgeons. What hospitals, what procedures, and what surgeons he did not say.

The Bates home was a deeply troubled place at the moment. The Tradesman's National Bank, of which Uncle Homer was vice-president, because of malfeasance, perhaps embezzlement, by its president, had been forced to close its doors and probably could never reopen. Uncle Homer, determined to make sure that no creditor or depositor lost a penny, was in the process of liquidating all his own and all Beade Myers's assets in order to assemble the required two million dollars. He thought he would have to sell their beautiful house.

"These people who when I first came here had so much of everything," mused Gerald, "now have to give up even their horses and carriages. Fortunes seem even more cruel in their departure than the loss of health. Thank goodness my star seems ascendant now, and long may it continue so."

Gerald's star was ascendant now not only because of the Bennett and Kissel cases but also owing to the misfortunes of Dr. Hart. He sent Gerald a specimen of urine one day and when Gerald reported back that analysis revealed incipient Bright's disease, Hart confessed that the specimen was his own. Soon thereafter he went off to Texas for a rest, leaving his many patients in Gerald's care. Quite a few of them liked Dr. Webb well enough to remain his patients after Dr. Hart returned.

But Hart did not mind; he was too worried about his wife of eight years, a consumptive patient with whom he had fallen in love. She was so ill now that she could no longer breathe well at the high altitude of Colorado Springs and after two months of indecision Dr. Hart concluded that she and he would both be better off in California. So he again surrendered his practice to Gerald, saying he might be gone for months or perhaps for years, he did not know.

He was away only five months, but when he returned to Colorado Springs he was too ill and dispirited to resume much of his practice.

The mantle of "Uncle Jimmie" was a tremendous boon. Gerald tried to show his gratitude by frequent letters full of news and by unswerving loyalty to his benefactor when Dr. Hart even in absentia was involved in the factional fights that kept things lively in the county medical society and at St. Francis Hospital.

"You don't know what a relief it is to be away from these brawls," Dr. Hart wrote from Pasadena, "but I want to hear about them. Do send me all the gossip." So Gerald wrote him the details of such goings-on as Dr. Anderson's week-long drunken spree and Dr. W. F. Martin's vamoosing to Denver in a huff after an argument with the Sisters of St. Francis.

The latter episode caused Gerald to make a decisive change. He considered Dr. Martin the ablest doctor next to himself in Colorado Springs and called him often in consultation or to assist in operations. So Gerald was outraged when he thought the Sisters of St. Francis had publicly "insulted" Doctors Hart and Martin in announcing a reorganization of the hospital staff.

It only added fuel to his anger when the Sisters invited him to join the new group as surgeon. Much as he had coveted such an appointment he now refused it and gave the Sisters "a piece of my mind" about the injustice they had done to two fine doctors. And he immediately transferred his surgical patients, eight of them at the time, from St. Francis Hospital to Glockner Sanatorium, as the former Home had been renamed.

This move may have assuaged Gerald's indignation but it did his surgery no good; the Sisters of Charity could provide excellent nursing service but they had only a primitive operating room. Gerald guided them in making some essential improvements in it and made do with these until a few years later he was able to secure from Mr. Cupples of St. Louis a donation of $1200 for installing a new and up-to-date operating room at Glockner.

As a rule Gerald managed to stay out of the professional quarrels, getting on well with most of his fellow doctors. He had been elected secretary of the county medical society for 1898 and optimistically expected to become vice-president and then president in successive years. But he encountered some spiteful jealousy.

A well-meaning friend told him of the rumors being spread around town by a fellow physician: that Webb was not a doctor at all, only a dentist, and had spent but a few months at the Guy's Hospital he made so much of.

The friend must have been astonished by the stiff anger that descended upon *him*. Gerald demanded an apology and insisted that the man immediately write to Guy's Hospital, the University of Denver, Dr. Henry Sewall, and Dr. Hart for authoritative confirmation of Webb's medical credentials. Gerald himself wrote to Mr. Dunn, his surgical mentor at Guy's, to prepare him for the questions he could expect. Mr. Dunn replied cordially and soothingly: No inquiry had been received and if one should arrive the writer would be told that Gerald Webb had indeed been an outstanding and most worthy medical student at the hospital.

As far as Gerald could tell, his action effectively squelched the rumors, which he thought had been started by Dr. Gardiner in pique over the Kissel case.

Mr. Cupples' gift for the operating room at Glockner was an expression of gratitude for Gerald's attention to his son-in-law, William Scudder. When William's consumptive lungs grew steadily worse in spite of Gerald's best efforts, Mr. Cupples proposed taking the sick man to Europe, along with his wife, their three children, two French maids, Mr. Cupples' St. Louis doctor, and Gerald and Jenny Webb.

Gerald longed to go but he advised strongly against the undertaking nonetheless, feeling certain that Mr. Scudder would die on the way. Then he had to wonder whether that might not have been better when a few months later Mr. Scudder suffered severe hemorrhages, developed a kidney stone, and contracted pneumonia.

Gerald was distraught. "The Scudders are people who demand

a great deal of attention because they can afford it, so for weeks I slept in William's room, being up and down all night. Jenny was gravely ill at the same time—I did not think she could pull through and had trained nurses with her around the clock, with Beade Myers too, who was visiting us. She surprised me again and is getting better but Scudder died."

Amelia Scudder, blind to all but her own plight, begged Gerald to go with her and the children in the private car carrying her husband's body to St. Louis. He could bring Jenny, for whom she would provide a good nurse, "the one who gives me massage." And upon arrival in St. Louis she sent the Webbs a telegram, "Am expecting you Friday without fail. Wire what train you will arrive."

They did not go. Not then. But Gerald was feeling tired and stale and they had a standing invitation through John Sanger to visit his aunt, Mrs. George Pullman, in Chicago. A month later, consequently, when Jenny was up and around again and Doctors Hart and Martin were on hand to look after Gerald's practice, they went with Sanger to Chicago for a week and on their way home stopped for a few days in St. Louis to see Mrs. Scudder and Mr. Cupples. Amelia having recovered some rational perspective, friendship was restored.

In Chicago Gerald had again spent his time observing "the big guns" at work in their operating rooms. There were indeed great surgeons there to learn from: the incomparable Christian Fenger, the surly but brilliant Nicholas Senn, the flamboyant innovator John B. Murphy.

Gerald Webb's preference was still for surgery, though he found it a strain. "These operations do knock me out so," he once admitted. Experience was making him more cautious, more aware of his limitations in this art. He was trying no more brash invasions of the brain to remove suspected tumors and after losing the patient in his first attempt to remove a gallbladder was risking only limited incursions into the internal cavities of the body. He was doing more ovariotomies and appendectomies but with a proportionate increase in the number of death certificates he must write.

It was a golden age in surgery, those decades when Joseph Lister's antisepsis and William Halsted's asepsis were permitting surgeons for the first time to operate inside the body with minimal risk of infection. But Gerald Webb was living in the wrong place and the wrong circumstances to participate in the excitement.

He was too far from the centers in Europe and the East where the bubbling invention and improvement of surgical techniques were taking place, he could not go often enough to those centers to learn and be stimulated by the ferment, and Colorado Springs did not provide enough surgical patients for the requisite experiment and experience. People did not journey to the Springs for surgical repair; they came to be cured of consumption.

Gerald did his best to keep up through constant reading of his medical journals and tried new methods both surgical and medical when he could understand them enough from written descriptions. He was elated to learn from the *British Medical Journal* a new and reliable method for the removal of hemorrhoids, with which he had been having indifferent success. He tried the injection of cocaine into the spinal column for anesthesia, and he knew from his reading the latest method of treating stricture of the esophagus.

The patient in the case was Donald Gregg, a Colorado Springs youth just out of high school who wanted to enter Harvard University but seemed more likely to reach an early grave. He was puny and frail, having lived since childhood on a diet of milk because he could swallow nothing solid. Gerald easily recognized the symptoms of esophageal stricture, which was usually the result of scar tissue formed in the healing process after the accidental swallowing of lye, a staple in most households of the day.

The obstruction could be cut through surgically by an ingenious "string-saw" method, but Gerald, having read of a less drastic procedure developed by Dr. Henry Plummer, the brilliant clinician who was a partner of the Mayo brothers in Minnesota, ordered a set of Plummer's instruments and showed Donald how to use them.

They were slender cylindrical probes fitted at the ends with soft rubber bulbs of graduated sizes. The patient began with the smallest, forcing it repeatedly through the stricture until he had made an opening large enough to admit the next size bulb, and so on through the set.

Donald Gregg had progressed to the third bulb and was eating small pieces of bread and meat when he left for Harvard. Gerald referred him there to Dr. Reginald Fitz, the physician-pathologist who had named appendicitis, and Donald reported back that Fitz had congratulated him on having found a doctor who knew what to do for him and had told him just to keep on with the bulbs. Except for "this vile climate" Donald was enjoying very much his first year away from home.

The youngest Gregg boy, Alan, nine years old at the time, watched with intense curiosity his brother's manipulation of the probes. Who knows but that here was planted the seed that grew into Alan Gregg's distinguished career as medical director of the Rockefeller Foundation? Whether that or not, Alan later worked and studied with Gerald Webb before following Donald to Harvard and its medical school.

Gerald Webb was wholly a clinician in these years. Under the pressures and excitements of his growing practice he had no time or inclination to cultivate his interest in research. The project he had undertaken in collaboration with Louis Livingood of Johns Hopkins came to an abrupt halt when Dr. Livingood, on his way to study in Germany during the summer of 1898, went down with the ship *La Burgogne* in a storm at sea. Although William Osler suggested that Dr. John B. MacCallum, an assistant in pathology at the Hopkins, might take up Livingood's end of the experiments, Gerald left the matter in abeyance.

Even his plans to write for publication remained mostly good intentions. The few papers he did turn out were all reports of cases, except one that described and pictured a wire contraption he had devised for the correction of ingrown toenails.

He did continue to mull over his major or unusual cases, trying to fathom the ways of disease and possible modes of cure. Once, excited by an idea about appendicitis, he wrote about it to Henry Sewall, who said in reply, "It is comforting and stimulating to find someone who *thinks* about his cases. I do wish you would give up practice and take over half the physiology here. Think of the glory you might win."

Gerald was not tempted. He was winning "glory" enough in Colorado Springs to satisfy him for the moment. And he was reveling in his freedom from the earlier "push, push, push."

With his office at home he could linger over breakfast or afternoon tea if he wished and relax after evening office hours, usually with a book since Jenny was in bed by then and his playing the piano disturbed her. She had turned one room of the house into a library, lining its walls with shelves and gathering upon them from all over the house hers and Gerald's many books. To their astonishment these totaled more than a thousand volumes. This room became the favored place for their hours together.

Jenny, refusing to surrender to her frailty and too full, Gerald said, of the *spes consumptiva* — usually called *spes phthisica* and described as "a feeling of being tinglingly alive," which tempted the tuberculous into activities disastrously beyond their strength — joined "a Shakespeare class" to which the members said they came "only to hear Mrs. Webb read." Gerald could believe it "for she reads very well, interprets *Hamlet* beautifully." He studied *Hamlet* line by line with her, and then *Macbeth*, reminded all the while of similar hours with Pater at 19 Tivoli Place.

Gerald could no longer read without spectacles but was glad he could do without them in public, since he thought the small round lenses in thin steel rims most unbecoming to him. He preferred to read history, biography, and poetry but could get absorbed in almost anything. Through one winter he read "Kipling's *Kim*, Roberts on the Boer War, Carlyle's biography of Schiller, Schiller's plays, and Lorell's *Ars Vivendi*." The Lorell he thought so wise that he ordered copies sent to Harold and Frank, both of whom were still beset by "nerves."

Gerald practiced the *ars vivendi* himself. "Last night I fixed my telephone so it could not ring and had nine hours sound sleep. I told some patients I would not go out again even if Queen Victoria sent for me! I can't burn the candle at both ends and feel when I have done $50 worth of work in a day I am entitled to a good sleep."

He had fallen into the engaging custom of marking his own birthday by sending a note to Mater and in 1899 he wrote her: "Knowing how you must remember 28 years ago today I want to let you know that I have yet the perfect health you gave me on that day and that I am very grateful for having been born. Health is indeed the grandest prize to be endowed with, and seeing so much illness as I do I appreciate my own health all the day long."

It was a problem, though, to find time for the exercise that meant true health for him. He was playing little or no tennis now, though the *Gazette* identified him as one of the best players in the city when it published an essay he had written at the editor's request.

"On the Tennis Court" revealed Gerald's un-American approach to the sport. Winning was not the sole purpose of the game, he said; good form, grace, and observing the etiquette of the court were equally important. The game showed up a player's character, whether mean or generous, and "one notes with disgust the player who tips the ball just over the net when his opponent is in the back court or in a doubles match plays always to his weaker opponent." Gerald advised choosing a better player as one's opponent in order to improve one's skills.

He was no longer playing much golf either. Returning home with a check for $1000 in his pocket in payment for escorting a mental patient to an asylum near Boston, he impulsively accepted membership in the El Paso Club and in the Cheyenne Mountain Country Club, but since the former was of little use to him except to provide him with prestigious stationery, in a fit of economy a short while later he resigned from it—and from the Austin Bluffs golf club too.

He got his exercise now by practicing his latest enthusiasm, polo, to which he had been introduced by John Sanger.

"Polo is to riding what golf is to walking" he said, and three or four times a week he and Sanger would rise at five in the morning to get in a couple of hours of practice before beginning the day's work. At first Gerald borrowed one of John's ponies but soon he paid $125 for a "beautiful animal" of his own so he would be equipped for the matches at the country club when he had gained skill enough.

Gerald was spending handsomely now. When Mrs. Cheesman, John Sanger's mother, took a notion to change carriages Gerald bought her Victoria, had it reconditioned, and presented it to Jenny as a surprise birthday gift. He replaced her pony with a "beauty of a saddle horse" and since she must spend so much time in her bed he spent $110 to buy her an elegant new one.

He also bought a houseful of furniture. A Philadelphia physician who had come to Colorado Springs to practice and brought along "$2000 worth of very good household chattels" went bankrupt and offered Gerald the whole lot "for a little more than $500." Gerald paid him $135 and the balance in small monthly installments.

Then he wanted a proper house to go with the furniture. He had come to look upon the Tejon Street house as "just a wooden shanty on a cheap street" and thought his position now demanded a residence in a better neighborhood. The place that took his fancy was the house of the late Dr. Jacob Reed at 831 North Cascade

Avenue, just across the street from the home of Gerald's friend and patient Addison Hayes. A further attraction was the separate office Dr. Reed had built adjoining the house.

Gerald offered Mrs. Reed $100 a month for the place but she stubbornly refused to rent it for less than $130. That was too much. The Webbs would have to stay on Tejon Street.

When Mater commented that things seemed to cost a dreadful lot in Colorado Springs, Gerald explained why: The town was booming. New mines were opening almost monthly at Cripple Creek and everybody was getting enormously rich. Wealthy health-seekers were arriving daily. All these moneyed people kept prices high and the invalids with families snapped up all the available dwellings. There was hardly a vacant house in town and hundreds of new ones were under construction.

When the Webbs' Tejon Street landlord moved his furnishings out to make room for the limed-oak pieces Gerald had bought, Gerald vowed he would insist that their rent be reduced. But he could not bring himself to do it. Instead Jenny coaxed the man into building another room onto the house to expand Gerald's office space, and then Gerald persuaded him to add on top of it an "outdoor room" so that Jenny could sleep in the open air all year round.

This was in step with the latest theory about the management of consumption. Long gone from Colorado was the fear of miasmic night air and the sight of invalids huddled always under shawls and blankets to keep warm. If pure mountain air was curative for the consumptive why not make him take it twenty-four hours a day?

All over Colorado Springs open-air sleeping porches and balconies began sprouting from the upper stories of houses and outside the windows of hospitals.

Gerald Webb did not go overboard about the idea as did some of his fellow doctors, especially Dr. Gardiner, but he wanted to try it for Jenny. And when he slept in the new room himself on a few chill winter nights he said he woke in the morning "feeling wonderfully fit." That the cold air was equally restorative for a woman reduced to 92 pounds and often sleepless with headache and coughing may be questioned.

Gerald's new affluence was sporadic, not in earned income but in money on hand. Almost as often as in his first year of practice he was without funds to pay his bills, and only then would he force himself to a Sunday afternoon of "working up my books" and sending out bills. "I hate the business side of my profession," he said, "although I have become as grasping as the Americans after the almighty dollar."

When John Sanger could no longer endure his friend's financial ups and downs, he took over the keeping of Gerald's books and set up a methodical system of quarterly billing. His first effort produced bills for $6000, of which one half were paid more or less promptly.

But Gerald's habits proved too much even for Sanger. Gerald did agree to increase his fees — to $50 per confinement, for instance — but half the time he made no record of them or jotted them down on scraps of paper that kept turning up in odd places if at all. And when Sanger by jogging his memory and hunting through the miscellany on his desk and tables had collected enough data to prepare bills, Gerald would on a third of them either reduce the amounts by half or write "Payment received in full" because he thought the charges too high or the patients too poor to pay.

The Webbs in England could have sympathized with John Sanger. Gerald was no more tidy in his letter writing. He seldom finished a letter at one sitting but kept adding bits to it sometimes for weeks before sending it off, with one or two last-minute postscripts scribbled hastily on prescription blanks. He was quite likely to use a half-finished letter as a bookmark and when he came across it as much as a month or two later mail it with no updating. He once kept a letter of Jenny's to Mater by him for six weeks, adding notes on the backs of Jenny's sheets from time to time, and when he did finally mail it he enclosed a partial letter he had written to Amy months before. The family must sometimes have got a weird impression of the sequence of events in his life.

No matter. Gerald was riding high. He had become *the* doctor in Colorado Springs and newcomers to town just naturally sought his office, "because I am so prominent now, I suppose."

Some of them were poor, like "the boy Arthur" from England who had Pott's disease (tuberculosis of the spine). Gerald bought him the brace he needed and gave him work looking after the Webb horses and carriages. And the English waiter who had to earn enough to support his family while Colorado cured his consumption. Gerald persuaded him to open a small shop for pressing, cleaning, and repairing clothes and was gratified when the man a year later was grossing $300 a month, half of it profit.

But most of the newcomers were persons of wealth, some of eminence. Benjamin C. and Maria McKean Allen, newly come from Philadelphia to become prominent leaders of the affluent in Colorado Springs, not only brought their own ills to Dr. Webb but summoned him when a visiting friend, a nationally known cricketer, suffered a serious accident. Mr. Paterson was so badly smashed up that Gerald was relieved when the young man's father arrived with his own doctor to take his son in a private car back to Philadelphia.

Other private cars brought Miss Helen Long from Massachusetts and her father, John Davis Long, former governor of Massachusetts and currently Secretary of the Navy, from Washington twice to visit her. When Miss Long's improvement was slight in Colorado, Dr. Gerald Webb escorted her in another private car back east to a sanatorium in Framingham, as all the eastern newspapers duly reported.

Of longer duration as a patient was the lovely Myra, wife of the handsome and dashing international playboy, Chester Alan Arthur II. The thirty-six-year-old son of the late President settled down in Colorado Springs in 1899 to add élan to the life of the city for the rest of his days. His bride presently engaged Dr. Webb to attend her in confinement and thereafter he was the Arthurs' family physician.

But Gerald Webb's biggest brush with eminence came to him not primarily as a physician but as a sportsman, through his friend and patient, Phillip B. Stewart, called Phil by one and all.

Mr. Stewart, seven years older than Gerald, had come to live in Colorado Springs the same year as the Webbs and was making his way rapidly to the forefront in various mining and public utility enterprises. Born in Middlebury, Vermont, the son of a Republican governor and congressman in that state, he had taken both bachelor and master degrees at Yale, where he was also an outstanding athlete. Between his junior and senior years he and a group of classmates had spent the summer on a horseback tour of Colorado and he had decided then that Colorado Springs was to be his home.

Phil cared little for the society life of the town; his interests lay in the out-of-doors—hiking, riding, hunting, nature study—and in education. He was elected a trustee of Colorado College in 1900 and became the volunteer coach of its baseball team. It may have been at the college that Gerald Webb first met him.

Perhaps through his father, perhaps during the campaign of

1900, Phil Stewart had made the acquaintance of Theodore Roosevelt and invited him to try big-game hunting in the wilderness of Colorado. Roosevelt accepted the invitation for a two-weeks' trip in January 1901, when he was vice-president-elect of the United States.

Stewart intended to take Roosevelt into an area on the Western Slope in the general vicinity of the Edmond Kelly ranch. Knowing that Gerald had hunted there and feeling concern for the safety and wellbeing of his distinguished guest, Stewart asked Dr. Webb to go with them.

Gerald was excited by "this chance of a lifetime. It is because I am a good sport! decent chap! and surgeon that I am asked. I am getting copies of Roosevelt's books so I can become familiar with what he has written and therefore be a better companion for his mind."

Jenny urged Gerald to go but John Sanger laughed at his eagerness and said he would not think of going if he "had not that beastly English instinct for worshipping anybody 'big.'" Gerald pondered the jibe but concluded Roosevelt really was worth knowing for his bravery and his brains "and being a literary wonder too."

Roosevelt having just resigned as governor of New York after a vigorous and bitter campaign for McKinley's election, wanted a rest from politics and reporters. Stewart and Webb therefore carefully concealed the date of their departure and tried to sneak their guest and guides away early in the morning of 10 January, but they could not avoid people and festivities until they had left the railroad behind at Rifle.

Thereafter the frustrated newsmen, deprived of any word about the doings of the celebrity, simply let their imaginations loose and sent throughout the country all sorts of fabricated stories about wild adventures and narrow escapes. In some tales Roosevelt was clawed by a bear and Dr. Webb saved his life; in others Dr. Webb was the victim of a mountain lion and Roosevelt was the hero to the rescue.

Jenny Webb and John Sanger must have been worried witless until Gerald, back in Rifle and reading the papers, wrote to say it was all nonsense, that the three had had a glorious time and excellent hunting and that nothing at all untoward had happened except that Stewart had been laid up a few days with tonsillitis.

Gerald added his impressions of Roosevelt: "I'm afraid my

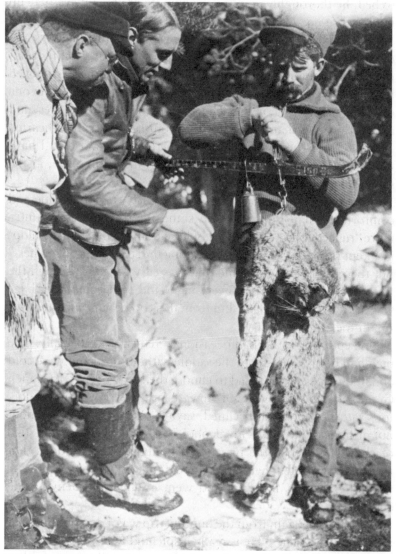

Hunting with Theodore Roosevelt, who looks over Dr. Webb's shoulder as the guide weighs the kill

literary ability is not equal to the task of describing him. He is a man of indomitable energy both mental and physical. What he has not read and studied is nil. He seems equally at home with the names and habits of the birds of the air and with the beasts of the earth including mankind. The first up in the morning and the last to bed, he thoroughly enjoys every minute of life, always 'way up in G' to use one of his own expressions.

"Thorough seems his watchword — exact too in all he says and does. He is strong in his likes and dislikes and unhesitatingly expresses his opinions of prominent men. He is not in the least spoiled by his success and dislikes any attempt to make him more than one of the party, waiting on himself, chopping wood for the fires, and always doing his share of whatever is required. Very simple-hearted — democratic — perfectly genuine. A better all-round man I have never met. I feel immensely strengthened in his presence, at the same time ignominiously small."

Gerald found the ranch at which the party stayed less fine and comfortable than Edmond Kelly's and the surrounding country more "rugged, bleak, bare. We could seldom get much of a gallop, just kept riding up and down and along the steep sides of gulches." But there was plenty of game that was easy to track through the fresh snow that fell almost every night and their combined "bag" was a good one. A cougar skin from this trip became an attractive rug in the Webbs' library.

One episode Gerald had occasion to remember especially. The men had been ten hours in the saddle without food and were cold and hungry. As they paused to choose their way back to the ranch Gerald offered Roosevelt and Stewart some whiskey from his doctor's satchel. Roosevelt declined, saying "A good sportsman does not profane the woods with alcohol," and accepted instead a stick of chocolate. When the papers later published accusations that Roosevelt stocked up with liquor and drank heavily on his hunting trips, Gerald was incensed and went about hotly denying the charge.

An additional gain from the hunting trip was a deeper appreciation of Phil Stewart. "He is really a splendid fellow," Gerald told Jenny, "so thoughtful and gentle. He is physically powerful but constitutionally delicate. I said this to Roosevelt and felt confirmed by the tonsillitis."

Vice-President Roosevelt returned to Colorado later in the year to participate in the state's Quarto-Centennial celebration and during his visit to Colorado Springs Gerald felt honored to ride beside him in the parade and to play opposite him the next day in a polo match at the Cheyenne Mountain Country Club. Roosevelt was an aggressive competitor but a good sport when his team lost.

When the following month Roosevelt succeeded to the presidency after the assassination of McKinley, Gerald thought he could without presumption send him a note of congratulations.

The hunting trip in January initiated a year of much traveling for Gerald. Every month or so he accompanied a patient somewhere — to San Antonio in Texas, Coronado Beach in California, Boston again, Philadelphia again, with Mr. Cupples to St. Louis again after the old gentleman had spent the winter with Amelia Scudder, who had brought her children back to live in Colorado Springs.

Gerald's fee of $100 a day plus expenses for the round trip had become standard for these journeys and he relished the big checks for a thousand or more dollars each one produced. But he kept hoping for one that would take him home to England. And it came in October.

Just across Tejon Street from the Webbs lived Verner Z. Reed and his family. The thirty-four-year-old Reed, having come to Colorado Springs as a youth "with bare feet," had made a fortune dealing in mining property, educated himself, and written several "sparkling" books for children. He and his wife took no part in the social whirl of the town, but Gerald had got to know and like them as patients.

Jenny, though, did not care for Mrs. Reed, thought her "ordinary," perhaps because Mrs. Reed spent more time in good works among the poor than in reading or keeping her house up to Jenny's standards.

Mr. Reed's business took him often to London and he had solved Gerald's clothes problem by serving occasionally as courier from Thomas the Tailor in Cheltenham. Gerald had once bought a ready-made American suit for twenty dollars but felt "so funny" in it that he would do anything to get back to his English cut. So Jenny sent Thomas the Tailor instructions to make his suits a trifle bigger and the coats an inch or so longer, Mater took them when finished to London, and Mr. Reed brought them home as his own to avoid duty.

In September 1901 Mr. Reed went to London as William Stratton's agent to conclude the sale of the famous Independence Mine for $10,000,000. Since his commission was to be half a million dollars, he took Mrs. Reed along for a holiday, leaving their infant daughter Margery with a nurse under Dr. Webb's care. The baby got sick and went into convulsions. Her condition was not at all alarming but Gerald thought he ought to let the parents know, and Mr. Reed by return cable asked him to bring the baby and her nurse to London.

Gerald took Jenny with him to New York City. She had been having an especially bad time, her headaches so severe that she had twice tried to kill herself with morphine, and Gerald, fearing for her sanity, had put her under the care of a specialist in mental diseases in Denver for a few weeks. She was still distraught and Gerald hoped another visit with her family would calm her.

The Bateses were continuing to live in their West End Avenue house, their financial affairs having turned out better than they had expected. The bank had reopened with Uncle Homer as its president but the period of stress had affected his health and seeking rest he and Aunt Sally had twice visited Jenny and Gerald in Colorado Springs. They now welcomed Jenny so warmly that Gerald felt it was safe to leave her with them.

The long-awaited return to England did not give Gerald the pleasure he had expected because he had complicated matters by permitting Henry Hall to cross the Atlantic with him. Mrs. Hall, to Gerald's great distress, had died with her baby in childbirth the year before and Mr. Hall, growing more and more ill and lonely, wanted to see Paris again. But the Paris climate was no better for him than before and Gerald had been in Cheltenham only a few days after delivering the Reed baby to its parents when he received an urgent summons to come take care of Mr. Hall.

He never got back to England. He had to agree with the French physician that Mr. Hall must go south immediately and Mr. Hall would not go without Dr. Webb. So they went to Biarritz and thence to Italy, sailing for home finally from Naples.

Having picked up a more relaxed Jenny in New York, Gerald arrived back in Colorado Springs feeling tired and disappointed. All that traveling and so little time with the family! One good thing, he had brought more books from the library at Heimat, among them biographies of Jenner and Pasteur, Carlyle's *Life of Cromwell*, and a volume of Browning's poems, and these kept him in good company during the winter nights that followed when he sat alone by the fire in the library after Jenny and John Sanger had gone to bed.

The Webbs' landlord, having enlarged the house to suit his tenants, found a buyer for it and gave them notice to move out in

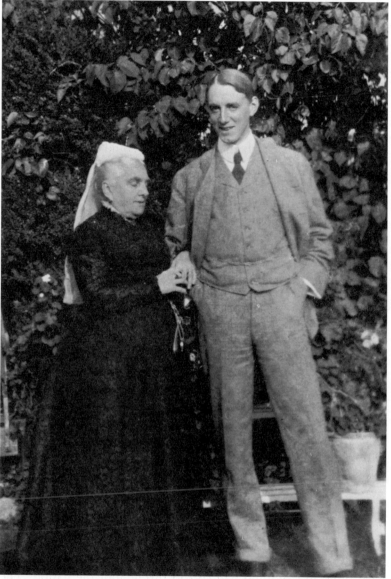

Gerald with Mater at Heimat, 1901

sixty days. It was their good luck that coincidentally William Bonbright decided to return to New York and was willing to rent them
his four-year-old house at 1222 North Cascade Avenue.

It was a large and splendid house of many rooms, with an exterior of brown siding and white shutters. Across its front stretched

a long pillared porch with an open balcony above. There was a big barn in the rear, the grounds were spacious, and the whole was enclosed by a high board fence.

No house and no location could have pleased Jenny more and Gerald rejoicingly signed a two-year lease and moved Jenny and the household into their new quarters in September 1902. Never mind the high rent of $135 a month; it was worth it just to see Jenny so happy living at last in the fine house of her dreams at Briarhurst.

But the timing of such an upward move could hardly have been worse.

There were ample signs of the coming slump for Gerald to read if he had not been blind to them. Why was William Bonbright going back to New York? Why were "To Let" and "For Sale" signs appearing all over town? Why did the Johnson Dry Goods Store close its doors and Mr. Johnson declare himself bankrupt, leaving Gerald with an uncollectable bill for $700? Why, indeed, were so many of Dr. Webb's "sure-pay" patients not paying?

The bonanza of Cripple Creek was running out. Many of the mines were shutting down for lack of ore and labor troubles were reducing production in the others. The diminishing flow of income was bringing business in Colorado Springs to a standstill. The boom was over.

By the end of 1902 three hundred carpenters and probably an equal number of other workmen had left the town to look for jobs elsewhere and nearly a thousand houses stood vacant, so many that the real estate dealers agreed to take down all for-rent and for-sale signs so as not to discourage tourists.

When Gerald became aware of what was happening he at first consoled himself that he would feel the pinch less than others because so many of his patients were easterners whose fortunes did not derive from the gold fields. But a hurtful number of these left and few others arrived, because, Gerald falsely assumed, the hard times in Colorado had spread throughout the nation. The fact was that Colorado Springs had become a depressing place to be.

Gerald's income dropped by two thirds and he could not pay his monthly bills. Determined that Jenny should not know how bad things were and should not be deprived of her luxuries, he began borrowing, first at the banks, where John Sanger co-signed his notes, then from John Sanger himself, and finally from his brothers in England, especially Wilfred.

Worried sick by his mounting debt, he once again donned his mask of cheer with Jenny. She could seldom be out of bed now and he coaxed her to fill the time by copying poems and quotations she liked into a scrapbook, but she wrote only three entries in it, one from John Keats:

Oh what a misery it is, to have an intellect in splints!

One from Omar Khayyam:

The bird of time has but a little way
To flutter—and the bird is on the wing.

And one from Owen Meredith:

And we are punished for our purest deeds
And chasten'd for our holiest thoughts, alas!
There is no reason found in all the creeds
Why these things are, nor whence they come to pass.

She had lost interest in reading; her one delight was to watch the many birds that came to feed at her windowsill tray. So Gerald brought her books about ornithology and on the rare days when she was strong enough he took her on short drives to see birds in the woods. When the prairie bloomed in the spring he brought her wildflowers and studied them with her.

Friends helped. Patty Jewett drove by often to bring her armfuls of flowers; Addison and Margaret Hayes placed their brougham and coachman at her disposal when she wanted a drive while Gerald was busy; their daughter Varina, who had become her closest friend, came daily to chat and run errands for her. Varina had often scolded her for not resting more, for squandering her meager strength on social amenities and housekeeping trifles. But it was too late to change her now.

Jenny's nine-year struggle ended at 3:45 in the morning of 16 July 1903. She had been unconscious all the day before but she rallied for an hour just after midnight and talked with Gerald about their life together. She regretted only that her body had been so frail when her love was so strong. She was tired of suffering now. Would he let her go to sleep and make sure she did not wake again?

When, knowing nature was about to take care of that, Gerald did not answer, she told him what she wanted done with some of her trinkets and asked for a quick and simple funeral. All she wanted was lots and lots of roses on her grave.

Gerald sat in reverie beside the bed until dawn.

How could such spirit, such intelligence as Jenny's be gone with a breath? He remembered how pretty she was, how pert and lively, when they were married. Should he have kept her in England and let her go quickly instead of subjecting her to this long ordeal?

No, they had had many hours of joy together despite her torment. How they had laughed and joked and teased each other when she rode with him on his rounds and sat reading in the carriage while he called on his patients. And all that partying. She had loved it. He had grown tired of it but he knew he had gained social ease and poise from it. She had taught him so much, not least the ways of getting ahead in this alien land. With her he had grown from an inexperienced youth to a capable, responsible man. Without her illness to make him see and feel he could not have become so understanding a doctor.

But he had given her much too. For her sake he had surrendered his dream of a career at Guy's Hospital and had worked hard in America to win the success she admired. He had endured the ups and downs and strains of her illness without complaint. He had forsworn sexual intercourse and the hope of a family of his own. In a few months he would be thirty-two. What, where, was to be his future?

Gerald had sent word the day before to Alice Evans, the cousin at whose house he and Jenny had been married and who was now living at Rocky Ford in Colorado, asking her to come at once. She arrived the day after Jenny died and the funeral was held the next morning, with the Reverend Benjamin Brewster of the Episcopal Church officiating at a short service of poetry and music.

Gerald was willing to admit his and Jenny's many friends to these rites but he did not want them at the interment in Evergreen Cemetery. He took only Alice Evans and John Sanger with him to the graveside, along with Jenny's saddle horse and the poodle Clorinda. He thought Jenny had loved these animals more than people.

Jenny had her roses; her grave was lined with them and they blanketed the ground around. Patty Jewett alone had sent one hundred and fifty of them.

The next day John Sanger and Godfrey Kissel took Gerald out into the mountains for two weeks. Before leaving he wrote a hasty note to Mater: "Poor little Jenny is at rest. You can have no idea how much she meant to me and how I worshipped her. Soon you will see me, but I must arrange matters here. I am in debt and must work hard to clear myself, but I have not the heart to try. Troubles have come so thickly of late that I feel just about crushed."

VI

Enter the Varinae

RUNNING AWAY to the mountains did Gerald Webb no good this time. It merely quickened his slide into a paralyzing lassitude.

Not that he was crushed by Jenny's death. The long years of her dying, the many recurrent crises in which he had thought her life at its end, had inevitably diminished grief to sadness. But the effort to meet her needs had kept him on the stretch in mind and body too long; with release the spring snapped. He felt listless, drained, "constantly tired," without strength or will to face his problems.

"There is no health in me anymore," he told Mater. "I know now how Harold must have felt when he had his nervous breakdown."

If only...if only he could dust his hands of everything and go back to Heimat...

But he had a huge debt to repay and his lease on the house had fourteen months still to run. He offered the place for sublet and his horses and carriages and polo ponies for sale, but there were no takers. The best he could do was rent the barn and his equipages to a patient and put the ponies to pasture on a nearby ranch. The one horse and runabout he needed for making calls he transferred to a livery stable.

He dismissed the servants, all but one part-time maid to keep his office clean and admit his patients, and he tried to cash in his life insurance, but some bit of fine print in the policy prevented immediate surrender; instead he had to scrape up the dollars for another premium payment. He could not bring himself to ask John Sanger for more money. In desperation he cabled his brother Wilfred for a further loan.

He said he felt no loss of caste in all his "climbing down"; everybody in Colorado Springs was "scraping the can" as strikes rippled out from the gold fields to engulf thousands of coal miners, carpenters, plumbers. Departures from the Springs swelled to an exodus, and when John Sanger decided to join it and move to New York, Gerald felt wholly alone.

Slowly he assembled Jenny's clothes and bibelots, packed them into a couple of trunks, and dispatched them to her cousin Alice Evans, asking Alice to distribute them according to Jenny's instructions. He bought some black-edged stationery and tried to acknowledge the stacks of letters and telegrams he had received, but he made little progress. A "brief but lovely note" was all he could manage to Uncle Homer, and a short apology for his silence even to Mater. To her he added, "I have been having terrible blues today but must work up some cheer now to go out and make my calls."

Those calls on patients became almost more than he could endure. "If I cannot soon get out of these sickroom atmospheres, I think I shall go to pieces," he said. He passed more and more of the calls along to other doctors until by year's end he was doing little beyond seeing the patients who came to his office in the mornings. Even these grew steadily fewer because in the hard times people were "economizing on their ills by doctoring themselves." His practice was reduced to "influenza, measles, pneumonia, and drunks."

He was sleeping badly and having strange dreams. One nightmare that kept recurring was of Pater in bathrobe and slippers hunched forward in his old chair by the fire glowering at a frightened little Gerald in the corner.

A waking nightmare ended when "Tiny" Alvord, a neighbor across Cascade Avenue, died of alcoholism. He had been a cherubic, lovable drunkard, "a fine person in every other way," and Jenny and Gerald had been fond of him. When his wife buried him in the lot next to Gerald's in Evergreen Cemetery, Gerald was relieved. "I know it is foolish," he said, "but I have had a horror of someone being laid next to Jenny whom she did not like. Now I know she lies between two good friends."

On her other side was buried Frederick Hitchcock Morley the financier, whose widow Helen was keeping fresh flowers on Jenny's grave as well as on her husband's. The Morleys had long been both patients and friends.

For the most part Gerald was able to keep his troubles to himself, so that even his closest friends assumed he was preparing to return permanently to England. On his birthday in September, at dinner with Helen Morley, Godfrey and Josie Kissel, and Frank

Gilpin, the manager of the Broadmoor Casino, and his wife Emma and daughter Laura, Gerald was given a leather writing pad with a verse expressing the hope of these friends that he would write them often from his new home in London.

Patients and friends showered invitations upon him. Social chit-chat was a black demand upon him now, yet he could not always find a graceful excuse for refusing and sometimes felt he must accept lest he antagonize. "A professional man cannot please himself in these things as a layman could."

But when Christmas came he no longer cared. Pleading a bad cold, he said no to everyone and, leaving his gifts unopened, spent the Eve and the Day alone in bed.

He diagnosed his illness as "nervous prostration" and told himself he must fight this "neurasthenia" with activity and diversion. Shortly after the turn of the year he took in as a paying guest a new patient from New York, Chaloner B. Schley, a scion of the well-known family of Wall Street brokers. An excellent violin-player, young Schley often wheedled Gerald into accompanying him on the piano, but Gerald was of two minds about the companionship: "I suppose it is good for me to have him around, but I would prefer to be alone."

Again, encountering a Colorado College student of German birth and rearing, Gerald asked him to come to the house at seven-thirty each morning and converse in German for an hour over breakfast. "It leaves me less time for thinking—and who knows, I may want to make my way around the Fatherland someday."

Thinking "to rest my head by wearying my legs" he sometimes sought out a partner who could give him a hard game of tennis in the evening; "it makes me tired so I can sleep better." And recalling the dictum that "the outside of a horse is the best thing for the inside of a man," he occasionally went for long rides on horseback, one day as far as twenty miles. But at other times he had to say, "The horse needs exercise but it's too much trouble to put on my riding clothes."

He confessed to Mater that his eyes were troubling him so much he dared not use them for reading and so spent much of his afternoon and evening time "just sitting by the fire dozing, as Pater used to do."

By mid-March he could take no more. "I am off to the mountains for a month," he wrote, "ostensibly to hunt bear but really for a rest away from everything. I am a nervous wreck and can work no longer."

Chaloner Schley and his brother Kenneth went with him to a ranch northwest of Glenwood Springs. Neither the hunting nor the weather was good and the ailing Chaloner soon returned to Colorado Springs but Gerald and Kenneth stayed on as supernumerary ranch hands, "ploughing, riding the range, roping and branding cattle," and in general living a hard outdoor life.

The good effects did not long survive his return to Colorado Springs, which was dictated by the approaching birth of Mrs. Chester Alan Arthur's second child. Soon his head was whirling dizzily again and he could not concentrate for more than a few minutes on anything.

All the while Mater was urging upon him an ambitious program of travel and study. The burdensome house lease would soon expire and the family would somehow take care of his debts. He should plan a long journey, perhaps westward around the world, and then settle in England to resume his work at Guy's Hospital. With all the experience he had now, she was sure, he would quickly reach the top of his profession in London.

No, Gerald replied, he must pay off his own debts, and only in Colorado Springs could he earn enough to do so. Besides, "I do not believe I have the physical strength to compete with the top-notchers in medicine. I do not doubt that I could get to the top and probably at race-horse speed, but I lack the staying qualities. At least I feel so now — when I admit I am no competent judge."

He was in despair about his future. He knew, as Mater did not, that it was futile to dream any longer of those English examinations and degrees and a staff position at Guy's; the best he could expect in England now was a mediocre practice in some provincial town. And did he really want to go back to live in the damp and overcast of England when he so much enjoyed the clear air and sunshine of Colorado?

He did not know what he wanted. "A doctor's life is a dog's life anywhere. I can fight along each day but when I think of the emptiness of the future it is hideous and I long for something to destroy me."

One idea occasionally sparked his interest — "if I only had the energy to pursue it" — that of building a new sanatorium for consumptives in Colorado Springs.

The prolonged hard times had convinced the Springs community that it had made a grave mistake to let itself become so dependent on the Cripple Creek gold mines instead of continuing to build its reputation as a health resort, that it should now once again actively promote its mountain climate and mineral waters.

This change of heart was a welcome call to action for Dr. Solly, still the city's prime booster in the health business. He had long been urging that what Colorado Springs most needed was an up-to-date, deluxe tuberculosis sanatorium. Glockner Sanatorium would no longer do, he said; it was too old, too unpretentious, more than half a general hospital. And all the other places that claimed to care for consumptives were little more than custodial boardinghouses or clustered rows of Dr. Gardiner's tepee tents, which might give patients plenty of fresh air but hardly much comfort or serenity. A new institution elegantly accoutered and properly managed would restore the Springs' "somewhat faded prestige as a health resort."

The segregation of consumptives in sanatoriums, well established in Central Europe and France and to a lesser extent in England, was just beginning in the United States. Germany could count more than a hundred such institutions, France at least eighty, but the United States fewer than a score worthy of the name. Their purpose was twofold: to permit physicians and trained attendants to supervise the regimen of tuberculous patients and to isolate such patients from the community.

The initial impetus for the sanatorium movement had come from the first of these purposes but the second was emerging as medical and lay leaders awoke to the implications for public health of the infectious nature of tuberculosis. No wonder the disease was endemic in the nation, they said, when its victims mingled freely with the populace, breathing their germ-laden droplets into the common air and depositing their deadly sputum at will on public walks and streets and in whatever places of assemblage they chose to frequent.

Dr. Solly, whose faith in the curative properties of Colorado's air and sunshine was absolute, cared little about the public health aspects of the problem; his concern was with the attitude of prominent eastern and midwestern physicians upon whom depended the referral of affluent patients. In Colorado Springs, Dr. Solly pointed out to local newspapermen, such doctors not only found no suitable accommodations for their patients; they could readily see how badly the city was polluting its good air.

Just look, he instanced, the Antlers Hotel had frequently to remove guests from its south rooms because these were filled with smoke from the power company's chimneys, and the horse-drawn traffic, especially the narrow-wheeled coal wagons, ground the unpaved streets into clouds of choking dust because the city did not water or roll down its roadways often enough.

Even the social gaiety of the town had become a disadvantage because it "encourages the invalids to lead too exciting and careless a life." They should be directed to "new quiet resorts in the suburbs" — or better still, to a fine new sanatorium built well away from town. Otherwise doctors would stop sending tuberculous patients to Colorado Springs.

By 1903 Dr. Solly had secured resolutions of moral support for a new sanatorium from a variety of civic organizations, including the Chamber of Commerce, had persuaded General William Palmer to donate one hundred acres of land plus $50,000 toward the cost of a building, and had engaged the foremost local architect Thomas MacLaren to prepare elaborate plans.

The grand "Sun Palace" of Solly's dream was to stand on a plateau on the western slope of Austin Bluffs, five miles northeast of the smoke-plagued Antlers Hotel, and was to be surrounded by some ninety acres of woodland park in which the expected one hundred patients could take their exercise in the purest of air.

MacLaren designed a U-shaped building consisting of an impressive central block (to house administrative and communal activities) flanked by two wings sweeping north and south at a sixty-degree angle so as to provide each patient's room with full exposure to the sun and with the view of the mountains that Jenny Webb had called "a lordly scene."

Clusters of luxurious individual cottages were to dot the surrounding woodland. Of prime importance to Dr. Solly, each cottage and each room were to include a spacious open sleeping porch on which the patient could take his rest day and night in the invigorating open air.

The name of the sanatorium was to be Cragmor (shortened from Cragmoor, which the Englishman in exile coined to designate the site where the "crag" met the "moor") and Dr. Solly was to be its physician-director.

With only General Palmer's $50,000 Solly could not even begin to execute his plans, "owing to the high price of materials and the disturbed state of the labor market." He would need at least $300,000 more. So he launched a newspaper campaign for public subscriptions; in view of the benefit the sanatorium would confer upon the city he thought every citizen should contribute to its cost. He also sent out nationwide thousands of copies of a description of the Cragmor-to-be, hoping to secure additional donations and equally to prepare the way for an influx of referred patients.

These plans for Cragmor were "the sanitarium scheme" to which Gerald Webb fitfully alluded that spring of 1904.

His flickers of interest came from some vague hope that if he bestirred himself to collect money "the company" might send him to Europe to study sanatoriums there. He talked enough about the plan to win from Samuel Cupples a pledge of $10,000 in support of it, but he did nothing more; "I suppose I could get more contributions but I don't have the energy to try."

Gerald had gone to St. Louis at the invitation of Mr. Cupples and Mrs. Scudder to see the much-advertised Louisiana Purchase Exposition of that year, but if he found anything to interest him at the Fair he did not say so; his appreciation was for the quiet of the Cupples home and the leisurely carriage rides around the city, on one of which Mr. Cupples showed him the campus of Washington University, for whose new buildings the old gentleman had contributed more than two million dollars.

In Colorado Springs the one home Gerald enjoyed visiting was that of Addison and Margaret Hayes, four blocks south on Cascade Avenue. He had come to feel at ease there. He could wander out into the garden and "steal" fruit from their trees because "it tastes so much better when I pick it," and he liked teaching Jefferson Hayes-Davis, the elder son, how to play polo.

(Jefferson's name, with the consent of his parents, had been changed from Davis Hayes to Hayes-Davis by official vote of the Mississippi state legislature when at the death of the President of the Confederacy there was no male descendant left to carry on the revered name.)

Gerald spent relaxing hours working with little Billy Hayes in the woodshed carpenter shop. He entrusted Jenny's beloved Clorinda to the willowy blonde younger daughter Lucy, who welcomed the dog as a playmate for her own black poodle Marquise. And he found he could without effort discuss city affairs with Mr. Hayes, exchange teasing flatteries with Mrs. Hayes, and talk companionably about music, birds, and flowers with the older daughter Varina.

Gerald was now the object of undisguised pursuit by the community's unattached females. As the end of the conventional year of mourning approached, he was becoming an eligible male again — handsome, charming, a man of local repute and, as far as most knew, means. "As you can imagine," he wrote Mater, "women of all sorts are hurling themselves at my head, from widows with millions to debutantes without a cent."

The only one of them to whom he gave a second thought was Varina Howell Davis Hayes. "She was Jenny's best friend, and as you know, Jenny's taste was good," he wrote. "She told me much about this girl and I have found all she said to be true. Varina has been in love with me for a long time. I have known this and fought hard against it. But she has finally conquered my wretchedness and made me care for her."

But should he marry her?

Varina was twenty-six years old to his thirty-three and a petite five-feet-three-inches to his six-feet-two. He did not think her pretty but not plain either, with her dark hair brushed high above gray eyes set wide in an oval face of flawless complexion. He considered her "mentally brilliant" and loved her warmth and solicitude, her animated ways, quick wits, lively imagination. She shared many of his tastes. It was a tonic to go with her for rambles in the woods because she was so gay and alive with curiosity about everything they saw. And in spite of her social prominence — "she is the most popular and sought-after girl in town" — she did not really care for society life any more than he did.

When he told a few close friends — the Kissels, John Sanger, Chaloner Schley — what he was considering, they responded with unalloyed approval. Nothing could be better. Why on earth was he hesitating? They reminded him that with the backing of Joel Addison Hayes as his father-in-law there would be no limit to what he could achieve in Colorado Springs.

Gerald did not doubt that Mr. and Mrs. Hayes would bless his marriage to Varina. "They think the sun rises to shine upon your boy," he told Mater; "they treat me like a Tin God on Wheels."

Mrs. Hayes was unrestrained in her affection for him. "Like all

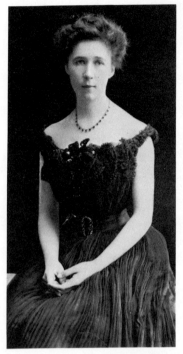

Varina Howell Davis Hayes
at age twenty

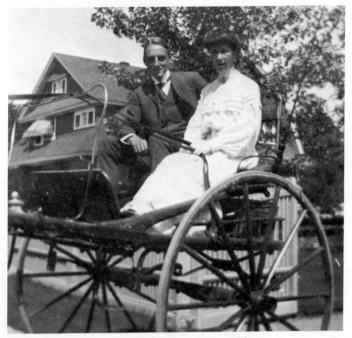

Varina and Gerald on the day before their wedding

his patients, I just worship him," she said. "He is like a beloved younger brother to me. I do not think he has a single fault; he is without a peer among men." For years she had been half admiring, half indignant as she watched him "forced to work so hard because of the extravagance of poor little Mrs. Webb." Since he had lived such "a self-forgetting, *clean* life" through all his tribulations, she dubbed him Sir Galahad.

Still, Gerald could not make up his mind. By marrying Varina he would be committing himself to a life in America and practice in Colorado Springs. Could he settle for that? After all his ambitious hopes and plans...

And could he honorably ask Varina, reared to financial security and genteel pursuits, to share his unstable fortunes and limited income? Surely he ought in any case to wait until times were better, until he had rid himself of debt and got himself somehow out of this neurasthenia.

He did not know his Varina. Once Gerald gave her the chance she resolved his questions without ado. If they were to be married it should be at once, she insisted, so that she could come and help him. He was feeling so ill because for years he had needed someone to take care of him. And their children would give him a future to work for.

As for his debt, he would be surprised how well she could economize; working together they would have him financially free in no time. After a word with her parents, she promised him immediate relief from one burden; he would have no more rent to pay. Mr. and Mrs. Hayes would buy the Cascade Avenue house for them as a wedding present.

Writing Mater on 26 July for the first time in six weeks, Gerald told her about his indecision. He had been in too unsettled a state to write, he said, trying to choose among three ways out of his terrible existence, "a gun, gin, and a girl. This new struggle took a great deal out of me, but now that I have succumbed to my love for the girl I feel well again and all my ambition has returned. The last few days I have actually enjoyed making calls again."

He concluded the letter with a request: "Do, dear mother, send Varina a little note addressed to her as my wife, for I hope to make her so on Saturday next."

The wedding took place on 30 July 1904 at the Hayes home with the Reverend Benjamin Brewster reading the vows. Only the

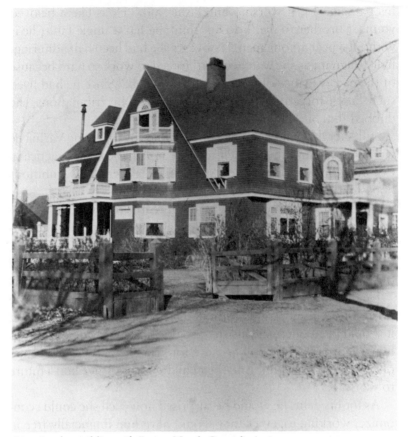

"A princely wedding gift," 1222 North Cascade Avenue

Hayes family were present. It had been a choice between no guests and inviting half the town, and Varina, to her bridegroom's immense relief, unhesitatingly elected the former.

But Margaret Davis Hayes had her innings. When Varina and Gerald had left after the ceremony for a week's stay at Woods Lake, she gave the *Gazette* enough information to produce a rapturous account of this "scintillating" union, including the "princely wedding gift of one of the finest houses in the city." Then Mrs. Hayes settled down to the pleasant task of sending out fifteen hundred announcements of the marriage, including, much to Gerald's amusement, one to King Edward VII, whom she had met once at a soirée in London, and dozens more to members of the British peerage.

She also wrote a long and gracious letter to Frances LePlastrier

Webb in which she included a mother's view of Gerald's new wife:

"Varina is not pretty but very stylish, clever, and talented. She is popular and witty, and adapts herself to any situation. She is a sensible girl, not extravagant, and cares little for fashion or society, is devoted to music and loves nature and animals. She is quite artistic, models well in clay and draws and paints cleverly. She loves to sew and does it well. She can also cook well. I am sure she will make it up to dear Gerald for all his years of sacrifice and will bring him the happiness he so much deserves."

Mrs. Hayes's letters suggest that Varina may well have developed her good sense and resourcefulness as a means of self-preservation. Her mother, a celebrated beauty as a maiden and still at forty-nine considered "a queenly and beautiful woman," was so often defensive about Varina's lack of prettiness that she must have given the girl from childhood the self-image of an ugly duckling. Yet Varina's photographs show her to have been a most comely young woman.

She was now a happy one, making it her first duty to nurse Gerald back to mental health. "I am allowed to be a nervous race horse no longer," he said in wonderment at her loving care. "I am made to lie down and rest at every opportunity. This Sunday afternoon is the first one in years that I have spent like the old ones at Heimat. After a heavy midday meal I went to sleep immediately and have had six hours of perfect rest."

But he continued to have trouble concentrating and complained of "brain fag after a few hours of work." Varina, though, watching quietly, saw him grow gradually less nervous and begin to gain weight. She drove him on his daily rounds, not only to save the expense of a coachman but to relax him between calls. She waited until September to send out their "At Home" cards and found excuses for postponing the parties their friends insisted on giving for them. And she coaxed Gerald into frequent truancy from his office. According to Mrs. Hayes:

"He and she go on long drives in the country and come back delighted with having had a glimpse of a rare bird and laden down with wild flowers, happy as two children. He has gone back ten years in looks and manner and seems about twenty-five years of age."

Varina also took over the handling of Gerald's accounts and was amazed to find him so unbusinesslike. With dismay she watched him throw away the bills that arrived, saying wearily that he had no money to pay them. And no wonder: *he* had sent out no bills for more than a year. When Varina had pieced together enough information to make out overdue accounts amounting to some five thousand dollars, she, like John Sanger before her, had to watch Gerald tear up half of them. She hardly knew whether to scold him for the waste or "kiss him for being so gentle-hearted and generous."

For his part Gerald was astonished at Varina's gift for saving money. "I never knew a woman could be so economical," he told his mother, whom he had always thought the thriftiest of women. "I tell Varina she is her father's daughter and has the hoarding habits of a banker. She seems to be able to make one dollar do the work of five. She does all her own sewing and even makes shirts for me, wonderful ones out of a fabric called Viyella."

Gerald was wrong. It was not the hoarding habits of her father he was seeing in Varina but the scrimping skills of her mother—that "Maggie Davis" who through ten years of her adolescence had to learn the arts and tricks of genteel poverty while her father was kept in prison by vindictive Union forces and struggled with meager means for years after his release—until well past the time, in fact, of Maggie's marriage to Addison Hayes. Margaret Hayes knew quite a few things to teach her daughter beyond the pretty manners of a southern belle.

When the parties could no longer be put off, Gerald submitted to them with good grace but was glad to see the last of them, a reception by Myra and Chester Alan Arthur. "I have been through all these social affairs so often I am tired of them and would prefer to spend the time quietly at home. Varina feels the same, I am glad to say."

In October Varina happily told Gerald she would be bearing him a child the following May. Gerald's neurasthenia seemed to vanish at her news. One day he told Mater she could expect an American grandchild and the next he wrote her: "Today I have done a full day's work and for a wonder my brain is not spinning round and my mind is in working order. I have just finished off a whole pile of letters without effort."

He was soon back at work in earnest, taking an active interest in everything once more. The continuing stagnation of the economy roused him to indignation now and when the mine-owner husband of one of his obstetrical patients from Cripple Creek was shot while making a speech in Colorado Springs, he joined the local chapter of the Citizens' Alliance against the strikers. Agreeing with Mr. Hayes that the reelection in 1904 of Theodore Roosevelt and of the Republican governor of Colorado was essential to economic recovery, Gerald, since as a British citizen he could not vote, made sure that Varina did so.

Gerald's primary task was to mend the medical fences he had let fall into disrepair. He got back into touch with former patients and medical colleagues by tending to the huge basketful of unopened letters that stood in a corner of his office and was soon rewarded by the appearance of new patients as well as old ones long unseen.

One of the former was the tuberculous niece of both Dr. Silas Weir Mitchell and Horace Howard Furness, the noted Philadelphia editor of the New Variorum editions of Shakespeare. Young Mrs. Mitchell was a charming and cultivated woman with whom Gerald enjoyed discussing her uncles' work, and she may have persuaded him to think again about the curative possibilities of rest.

For it was at this time that Dr. Webb first, as far as we know, tried a period of absolute rest in the treatment of a consumptive patient. When Henry Hall brought him a cousin who had tuberculosis, he put her to bed without activity of any kind for a period of six weeks—and, unbelieving, watched her emaciated frame take on thirty pounds of flesh in that time.

Somehow Gerald had acquired a firmly negative attitude toward "the rest cure," which he thought of as the regimen of isolation and bed rest developed by Dr. Mitchell for the treatment of nervous disorders. Gerald was at this time, in the winter of 1904–05, as a further part of his program for recovering lost ground professionally, preparing a paper to be read before the El Paso County Medical Society and published in the *New York Medical Journal* in which he proposed an alternative, "a recreation nerve cure."

"I have always felt the term 'rest cure,' to be a misnomer," he wrote, "for my best results in the cure of nervous patients have always been brought about by keeping them the busiest people in town. To use a quotation, the author of which I cannot recall:* 'Lack of occupation is not rest, / A mind unoccupied is a mind distressed.'"

The subject of the paper was the treatment of Graves' disease, otherwise known as exophthalmic goiter. Good physicians were

*He later remembered the author to be Dryden.

familiar with its symptoms—the goiter, protruding eyeballs, and in recurrent crises extreme nervousness, fast heartbeat, vomiting, diarrhea—but nothing was known of its cause; discovery of its connection with malfunction of the thyroid gland was still a decade or more ahead. In treatment of the disease there had been no advance since William Osler, writing in 1892, recommended the application of an ice bag over the heart. Gerald Webb had cured two cases of Graves' disease and was ready to propose a theory about the cause of the disorder.

The first case had occurred in 1900 when Dr. Webb was summoned to the bedside of a widowed boardinghouse-keeper aged forty-five. She had had the goiter and exophthalmos for nine months and was now in crisis, her pulse too fast to be counted, her body and limbs all atwitch and in constant motion.

"While observing the patient, I was struck by the great waste of nervous energy going on, due to the tremor and jactitation of the extremities. The thought came to me that could I stop this leak in the nervous energy reservoir, she might improve. Going further, I pondered the question, why could not the whole disease be due to a neurasthenic condition in one who had forced herself along with a determined will when the nervous system had been exhausted and should have relaxed."

He sat down beside the bed and with soothing authority talked the patient into control of her muscles and nerves. "Then realizing the too wide awake and active state of her brain, with her mind running in every direction, I selected some simple inspiring poems for her to memorize. Personal experience had taught me that it was far easier to relax the body than the mind, and that if the brain continued its unchecked riotous behavior, little good was gained by bodily relaxation."

He instructed the patient to repeat his prescribed poems with intense concentration at fixed intervals every day. "From the first, improvement was marked, and in a few weeks she was wonderfully changed, though it was nearly a year before she was wholly herself again."

The second case, occurring in the spring and summer of 1904, was strikingly similar, the patient again being a widowed landlady, this one aged forty. The treatment was the same: "Absolute relaxation for mind and body was to be methodically carried out." But rapid improvement did not occur until Dr. Webb separated the patient from her family and responsibilities by removing her to a ranch a few miles from town.

"There in a few weeks all the remaining symptoms entirely disappeared. Finding that piano playing and horseback riding absorbed the patient, and keeping in mind that 'The pleasures we delight in physic pain,' I allowed her these pursuits in moderation, the riding in spite of the fact that she had been warned by a previous physician that she might fall dead any minute if she took much exercise."

In summary, said Dr. Webb, "My theory in regard to the origin of Graves' disease in these women is that it resulted from nervous exhaustion, and that the escape of nervous energy needed blocking, as was proved in both cases by the result of the treatment practised."

Gerald hoped this paper would bring him national recognition, and it did receive substantial circulation in medical circles. But later discoveries proved his theory to be in error, and it must be left to a modern man of medicine to explain how Webb effected two cures of Graves' disease, one of four years' duration at the time he wrote, without administering iodine or resorting to surgery or irradiation.

The paper retains significance despite its mistaken theory. It shows Gerald Webb at work as an observant, thinking, innovative clinician, much more inclined to encourage the body than to drug it. It reveals the role of his personal experience in forming his medical ideas and practices. And it foreshadows dramatically his later approach to the rest cure for tuberculosis.

Varina had turned one of the upstairs bedrooms into a cozy sitting room with writing table and bookshelves along one wall so that Gerald could work on his paper and do his reading away from the office downstairs while she sat nearby making Christmas gifts for her family. She had decreed no buying of presents this year and compromised only by sending photographs of herself and Gerald to Mater, with an apology for Gerald's being so poor a likeness. "But then none of his pictures ever does him any sort of justice. His eyes don't come out right, and the important coloring is missing."

Mrs. Hayes was less economical. It delighted her to watch Varina's and Gerald's eyes open wide when she unveiled the lavish layette she had brought back from a visit to her mother in New York. The crib and baby carriage were to follow and she and Mr. Hayes insisted on paying for the redecoration of the room Varina had chosen for the nursery. Gerald called Mrs. Hayes Lady Bountiful but said firmly that she must stop her purchases lest she make the baby "a dude living beyond its means."

In April President Roosevelt came to Colorado for another hunting trip with Phil Stewart but Gerald refused the invitation to go with them this time and also said no to a similar expedition with the Schley brothers; he would not risk being away from Varina so near the time of her confinement.

At six in the morning on 13 May 1905 the baby was born, a six-pound-four-ounce girl with a fluff of dark hair. Naming her Varina Margaret for her great-grandmother Varina Davis and her grandmother Margaret Hayes, her parents intended to call her Margaret but in only a few months, for some unremembered reason, she was "Binks" to all the family. To Gerald, who liked Latinisms, she and her mother, whom he called Varina Mea, became "the Varinae."

Phil Stewart and Helen Morley were named little Margaret's godparents at her formal christening but "Mamie" and "Papa" Hayes conferred their personal blessing on her when she was two weeks old. They gave her, held in her father's arms, a twenty-dollar gold piece and helped her to carry it up the stairway "so that she may go up in the world from the start."

The first weeks of fatherhood were wearing for Gerald. Varina, rejecting her father's offer to pay for a wet nurse, breast-fed the baby but in accordance with the custom of the day was not allowed to do much else for a month, so the chores of baby-care fell on Gerald. They were made less onerous by his "doctor's orders" that the babe was not to be picked up and fondled except when she was being fed or changed. She was to be left alone, kept quiet, so that she would develop regular habits. He watched so carefully for misbehavior to be corrected that Varina told him to ask Mater whether he had been as good a baby as he expected Binks to be.

To Mrs. Hayes Gerald seemed puzzlingly aloof and reserved toward his new daughter. Could he be one of those strange men who do not like babies? Even Varina thought him a little too professional about the infant.

Gerald Webb was not one to cluck and coo over a baby. He had other ways of delighting in his firstborn. He made endless "kodaks" of her and enclosed some in a whimsical note to Mater:

"My dear English Grandmama—I do nothing but eat, sleep,

and play. I am getting my father's complexion and dimple. The other night I slept eleven hours without eating. I have not yet been away from house and garden. Father cannot do baby talk, so he whistles the 'Toreador Song' to me. When I know that one I am to learn another. Goodnight. Varina Margaret Webb."

"It does make a big difference in life having a youngster to raise," added Gerald.

During baby Margaret's first summer her father spent his leisure time playing polo.

This ancient game of kings and nobles, imported into the eastern United States in the late 1880s and making its appearance among the English ranch hands of Wyoming at about the same time, was now beginning its long vogue as *the* fashionable sport of the mountain states. Games and tournaments in Denver, Colorado Springs, and Glenwood Springs were already producing long columns of copy not only for the sports pages and the national polo magazine *Rider and Driver* but also for the Society pages, where the names, costumes, and equipages of the spectators were faithfully reported along with elaborate descriptions of the pregame luncheons and postgame dinner dances that made each contest a social event.

Gerald Webb had become an excellent polo player and was in this summer of 1905 the captain and mainstay of the Cheyenne Mountain Country Club team. Again and again the Denver and Colorado Springs sportswriters headlined their accounts "Dr. Webb the Star of the Game." They applauded his hard riding, accurate driving, and phenomenal backhand stroke. And they cautioned opponents to beware whenever he made a mistake or was penalized for a foul; his "grimace of disgust" might be "sidesplittingly funny" but an icy anger at himself was likely to make him invincible on the next drive.

Two visitors made the 1905 polo season memorable. President Roosevelt on the way back from his hunting trip with Phil Stewart stopped over long enough to participate in a game, in which, according to Gerald, he showed himself an able player and a good sport when his team lost.

Even more exciting was the summer-long presence of Foxhall Keene, the nation's foremost polo player. He had been chosen to captain the American team that was scheduled to play in Britain for the international trophy but in a fall during spring training had

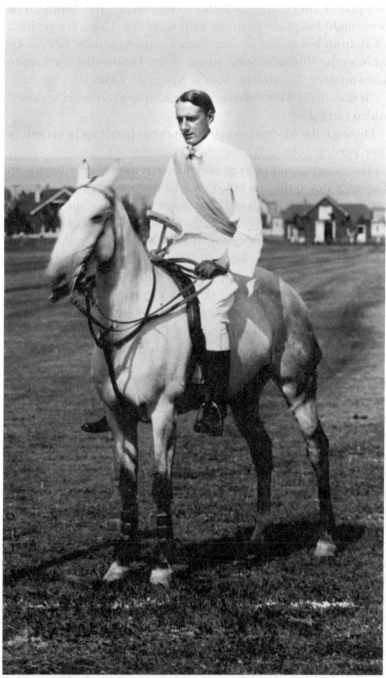

Captain of the polo team

broken his collarbone and so had come instead to spend the summer as the guest of Captain Ashton Potter and his wife, Grace Goodyear Potter, in Colorado Springs.

Keene confessed himself surprised by the skill of the players and ponies he saw on the country club grounds and as soon as he was able involved himself wholeheartedly in practice and play. It was a gala day when two local teams lined up for a joust, the Blues captained by Keene, the Reds by Webb. Keene, courteously given his choice of teammates, picked the best players available; he was out to win. So astonishment reigned when the Reds won, 5 to 4.

"The natural question is," said an account of the game in *Rider and Driver*, "how could Webb's team conquer four picked players headed by Keene. The answer lies in Webb. The mildest of men in his professional and social life, Dr. Webb in a game becomes the cold disciplinarian. He demands absolute control of his team, and he gets it. He knows every inch of the field, and even how to take advantage of the wind and the slight drop in level on the east of the grounds. He times precisely his commands to ride off the opponents."

Playing match after match against the Denver and Glenwood Springs teams, the Prairie Dogs and Ranch Hands of Sheridan, Wyoming, and the 10th Cavalry Division Team from Fort Robinson, Nebraska, the Colorado Springs team swept the western tournaments that summer, winning the Phipps Cup at Denver, the Devereux Cup at Glenwood Springs, and Colorado Springs' own new trophy, the Foxhall Keene Western Polo Cup, donated by the celebrated visitor.

When the triumphant season was over, Gerald said wearily, "I don't think I'll play polo any more except on special occasions; it takes too much out of me."

With the Varinae he went southward for ten days of rest on the Acorn Ranch in the mountains of northern New Mexico—"a heavenly life after the dog's life of a doctor"—and then settled in for what he expected to be a quiet winter of medical practice.

But the Furies were not yet done with Gerald Webb.

One of his first patients that autumn was a little friend, Laddie Armit, whose father, Captain John Lees Armit, a nephew of Mrs. Godfrey Kissel, had been a member of the Queen Victoria Guards and served under Lord Kitchener in Africa. He and Dr. Webb often indulged in discussions of politics and personalities in England.

Laddie had acquired a painful abscess on his leg and his father brought him to Dr. Webb to have it lanced. This was a minor procedure and the two men were probably talking while the doctor worked. The scalpel slipped and made a slight cut in Dr. Webb's finger.

Ten days later Gerald was near death from acute bloodpoisoning. Five local physicians, unable to control the raging fever that kept him in delirium, agreed that he could not live. Only at Varina's insistence did they summon in consultation Dr. Charles W. Powers of Denver, the surgeon with whom Gerald had wanted to work nine years before.

Dr. Powers too was pessimistic. All he could do was cleanse the seventeen suppurating sores on Gerald's left arm and wait, in the hope that the patient's own defenses would win their battle against the multiplying bacteria.

Varina had cabled the dire news to Mater, and Roland and his wife Lilian, hurrying to Gerald's bedside, were halfway across the Atlantic when the fever began to subside and Gerald returned to lucidity.

Now Dr. Powers could act. He excised the seventeen sores, placed the arm in a splint, and prescribed an extended rest. The prostration would be severe after so virulent an infection, he warned, and it would take months for Gerald to regain his health. He suggested a long sea voyage as a fine aid to convalescence — and a good diversion for Mrs. Webb, for whose "poise and strength" throughout the ordeal he expressed the highest admiration.

The only sea voyage Gerald wanted was the short one back to England. But he had not the wherewithal to finance it; he had only recently finished paying off his old debts and settling the bills for some necessary repairs to the house.

Addison Hayes solved the problem. He offered to defray all the expenses of a long holiday abroad for Gerald and the Varinae. Gerald refused to accept the offer unless it could be firmly understood that the money was a loan which he would be obligated to repay in full. With heightened respect for his son-in-law Mr. Hayes agreed and hurried preparations for the trip began. Hurried because Gerald, weak and one-armed, wanted to travel with Roland and Lilian so they could help Varina look after the baby.

When, after a brief stopover in New York City to let the aged

Varina Howell Davis see her infant great-granddaughter, they all sailed from Boston aboard the White Star liner *Cymric* on 9 November, Gerald was quietly thinking of more than convalescence in England. He had written his sister Sophie that early in the new year he would be coming to London to do postgraduate work at Guy's Hospital.

VII

Opsonins and Vaccines

GERALD was disappointed that he and the Varinae could not stay at Heimat. The old house was shuttered and sheeted for the winter and Mater, feeble and ailing at seventy-seven, had gone with her nurse-companion to spend the cold season with Nell at Stoneygate in Leicester. Nell, recently widowed, welcomed her brother and his family into her roomy house and she and Mater's nurse took care of the baby while Gerald and Varina devoted themselves to recuperation.

Doctor Gerald put the lustily growing Binks onto a bottle for two feedings a day "lest there soon be nothing left of her little mother" and also to free Varina for long walks and excursions with him. They had wondrous, healing days together, exploring the countryside on foot and going by boat and train to visit the museums and monuments of the district.

The reunions were restorative too, as the Webb brothers and sisters came one by one to see Gerald and meet Varina. She won unqualified approval from them all, especially from Mater, who was pleased to conclude that Gerald had a suitable wife at last.

By early January Gerald felt able to make his move to London. The splint was gone, the sores healed into the scars that would always remain, and he was exercising the arm into useful mobility again. So he and the Varinae became paying guests of his sister Sophie, who at the age of forty had courageously begun putting herself through the courses of study and apprenticeship necessary to qualify as a professional midwife and was now the owner-manager of a large and flourishing nursing home at 258 Elgin Avenue in Maida Vale.

But it was not to Guy's Hospital that Gerald went for his postgraduate study. He found that cherished place disconcertingly strange, much changed by a dozen years of rearrangements. Few remained of the staff members he had known, but one who did, now as a senior surgeon, was the kindly paternal confidant of his undergraduate days, L. A. "John" Dunn. It was probably Mr. Dunn who advised him that his major interest was not at the moment ascendant at Guy's.

The new surgery, still the medical world's wonder child, was maturing nicely, but general medicine was on the whole resting placidly in a mood of Oslerian nihilism. The exciting advances of the day were being made by the laboratory doctors, especially in medical bacteriology and its promising but puzzling infant, immunology. In this scientific ferment Guy's Hospital, somewhat tradition-bound and just beginning to emerge from a long period of financial stringency, was participating little.

During the two preceding decades, labeled by historians the golden age of bacteriology, the pathogenic organisms responsible for many infectious diseases had been identified and each new discovery had led to a frenzied competitive hunt for an immunizing vaccine or antitoxin. These efforts had been successful in, among others, diphtheria, tetanus, cholera, bubonic plague, and typhoid fever.

But a vast lot remained obscure about even these diseases. In some others, yellow fever for example, discovery of the agent of transmission had pointed the way to potential control but the causative organism itself had still to be identified.

The existence of filterable viruses — then called "filter passers" because they are so small they can pass through a porcelain filter as most bacteria cannot — had been demonstrated but none had as yet been isolated. And against many plagues upon man — typhus, leprosy, polio, encephalitis, a score of mysterious fevers — the attack had barely begun if at all.

Tuberculosis was a special frustration; though Koch had made known the offending bacillus, effective defense against it continued to elude the hunters.

Alongside the largely hit-or-miss groping for microbes and cures, some of the more science-minded of the laboratory men were beginning to probe into the underlying physiology and chemistry of parasite and host, trying to discover how microorganisms produce disease and by what processes the animal body resists and destroys them.

The current London star in this quest for the secrets of immunity,

Mr. Dunn would have had to tell Gerald Webb, was Almroth Edward Wright, who worked at St. Mary's Hospital, where at the moment he was trying to rehabilitate Koch's vaccine, tuberculin, as a cure for tuberculosis.

Sentiment yielded to sense. Turning away from his beloved Guy's, Gerald joined the group of American and Canadian doctors then doing postgraduate work with Wright, who was to be dubbed Sir Almroth and made a Fellow of the Royal Society in this year of 1906.

St. Mary's was a forbidding place. Though one of London's newest hospitals, established in 1854 to serve the people who flooded into the Paddington district after the building of the big railway terminus there, it was gloomy-looking, ugly outside and in, ill-lighted, badly furnished. Wright's laboratories were housed in just two small rooms fronting on the bleakness and dust of Praed Street. Both space and equipment were minimal, neither of them nearly enough to accommodate the work, the workers, their patients, their visitors.

But what went on in those jumbled, jampacked rooms set Gerald Webb afire. "It is not marble halls which make for intellectual grandeur; it is the spirit and brain of the worker."* It was the extraordinary brilliance, learning, eloquence, dedication, pigheadedness, and ferocious determination of Almroth Wright that made life in his laboratory an arousing experience. He was in all things, not least in his prejudices and foibles, a personality larger than life. A massive rumpled figure, looking slow and clumsy, he won the startled admiration of his acolytes as much by his nimble dexterity in delicate manipulations as by the quickness and soaring of his mind.

When Wright, with whoever was on hand of his half dozen assistants and equal number of students, broke work for tea, in late afternoon or just as likely at midnight, the conversation usually became a monologue by Wright, delivered from his armchair or his workbench stool while the others sat on the floor around him. His topic might be medical but it was more apt to be some matter of politics, literature, or philosophy, present or past—perhaps a sarcastic tirade against women, for whose minds and pursuits he felt only a lively contempt. Best of all for Gerald Webb, reminded of

*Statement by Sir Alexander Fleming.

dinnertimes with Pater at Heimat, it might be a dramatic recitation of some great chunk Wright knew by heart from Dante, Kant, Sophocles, Goethe, Thucydides, Shakespeare, Milton, the Bible. His memory was prodigious, and well, well stocked.

Almroth Wright, a decade older than Gerald Webb, was born of an Irish father and a Swedish mother who hired tutors to educate him, then sent him to Dublin University to become a master of languages. He thought briefly of taking up the literary life—"You handle the pen as well as I do," George Bernard Shaw told him— then read law awhile and traveled around the world for a year or two. Finally he settled upon a career in scientific research and trained for it at a succession of German universities, where he became expert in using the microscope and in contriving laboratory tools.

In his first post, as chief pathologist in the British army medical school at Netley Hospital, he devised an effective method of preventive vaccination against typhoid fever, always the dread enemy of soldiers at war. Stormily outraged by the way the skeptical and incompetent military men bungled the use of this vaccination in the Boer War, he resigned from Netley and in 1902 became professor of pathology at St. Mary's Hospital. There he speedily rid himself of all duties and concerns apart from immunization and in a single tiny room set up an Inoculation Department.

He shared the common puzzlement of the laboratory doctors about immunity. Why did some individuals appear to have a natural resistance to a specific kind of bacteria while others did not? Why among the latter did many acquire an artificial immunity from vaccination while some did not? What caused the differing responses?

Wright knew well the controversial theory of the rambunctious Russian Elie Metchnikoff, the man who watched wide-eyed while white corpuscles (white cells, leucocytes) in the transparent body of a starfish larva under his microscope floated toward the bits of red matter he had poked into the larva and engulfed them—as he said, "swallowed" them. He then stuck a thorn into a water flea and again watched the white cells move toward the intruding point, surround it, ingest it.

By a flashing leap of his amazing mind, Metchnikoff equated his bits of carmine and thorn with invading bacteria and triumphantly announced, before ever seeing a leucocyte attack a microbe, that he had discovered the process of immunity. Seizing upon the Greek word *phagein* meaning "to eat" he coined the words *phagocyte* for the white cell that "eats" bacteria and *phagocytosis* for the ingestion process.

The ensuing debate was long and raucous, and conspicuously unscientific. "It's the white cells that destroy bacteria," shouted Metchnikoff and his disciples in every medical journal and at every medical convention for years. "No! It's the blood serum that kills them," cried the enraged followers of Emil von Behring, whose work with immune serum had produced diphtheria antitoxin, and Richard Pfeiffer, who with his microscope had seen bacteria explode into bits in the blood with no white cells anywhere near them.

Almroth Wright, working quietly in his cramped laboratory with his assistant Captain Stuart Douglas, who had followed him to St. Mary's from Netley, bridged the gulf between the combatants by demonstrating that the cellular and humoral theories of immunity were each half right.

Wright and Douglas mixed bacteria and leucocytes in a salt solution and turned the microscope upon the result. Nothing happened. The white cells and microbes just lay passively side by side. Then the experimenters suspended their germs and white cells in blood serum — and saw the bacteria "swallowed" into the leucocytes at a rapid rate. They concluded there was some substance in the serum that made the bacteria appetizing to the leucocytes.

In naming this newfound substance Wright locked neatly and wittily into Metchnikoff's conceit. From the Greek *opsono* meaning "I prepare food" he formed the word *opsonin* to denote the "relish" or "sauce" that makes bacteria edible.

"Opsonin is what you butter the disease germs with to make your white corpuscles eat them.... The phagocytes won't eat the microbes unless the microbes are nicely buttered for them," explains Sir Colenso Ridgeon, the principal character in George Bernard Shaw's *The Doctor's Dilemma*, published this year of 1906. Sir Colenso in his medical persona is unmistakably Sir Almroth Wright.

(Shaw was a close friend of Wright's and got the idea for his play as he sat in the St. Mary's laboratory late one night drinking tea and listening to Wright argue opsonism with a poohpoohing Harley Street doctor of the old school.)

It was later learned that there are many opsonins, one for each kind of microbe, and they came to be called antibodies.

Sure now that the degree of an individual's immunity depended on the amount of opsonin in his blood, Wright set out to find a way of measuring this constituent. After countless experiments he arrived at the "opsonic index." It was based, to put it briefly, on the number of bacteria ingested by a given number of leucocytes in a suspension containing the patient's blood compared with the same numbers in an identical suspension containing normal blood.

Calculating the index was laborious and time-consuming; it required not only taking blood samples, making slides, and identifying the culprit microbes, but especially the careful counting of leucocytes and bacteria. Under Wright's method of staining, the leucocytes appeared in the microscopic field as gray blobs within which the ingested bacteria showed up as black dots. The index had to be determined at least daily for each patient, because Wright concluded that the rise and fall in the amount of opsonin was crucial in the proper use of vaccines.

He had observed that after each injection of vaccine the level of opsonin in the blood fell for one or more days, a negative phase, then rose gradually to a higher point than before, the positive phase. During the negative phase the patient's susceptibility to his bacteria was increased and if he was given another dose of vaccine at this time his condition grew worse. So it was vital that the physician keep constant track of the opsonic index to guide and control the treatment.

In the words of Shaw's Sir Colenso, "Inoculate when the patient is in the negative phase and you kill; inoculate when the patient is in the positive phase and you cure."

By applying this principle, much less simplistically formulated, Almroth Wright became "the father of vaccine therapy."

Previously the inoculation of vaccines had been considered a preventive measure only; it was the common sense of the day that there was no point, perhaps even harm, in injecting dead bacteria into a body already fighting swarms of the living germs — in adding poison, as it were, to already poisoned tissues. But Wright fixed on the fact that many infections were localized, did not involve the defenses of the entire body. Might not vaccination arouse and mobilize these general defenses? Soon he was maintaining and demonstrating that the use of vaccines in moderate doses at the proper times could be an effective treatment of infections already established.

Tuberculosis beckoned as a tough test of this idea. Thinking the general lack of success with Koch's tuberculin might have been due to haphazard inoculations that by mischance hit the negative opsonic phase, Wright decided to try Koch's vaccine again with proper spacing of the injections according to the index. By the time Gerald Webb came to his laboratory he was claiming substantial success in curing tuberculosis with tuberculin.

Not pulmonary tuberculosis. Medical politics at St. Mary's kept Wright from seeing much of this disease; his hospital practice was limited to the forsaken ones referred to his clinic from the wards as hopeless cases—unfortunates described by Gerald Webb as "the incurable refuse of the hospitals, patients who had passed uncured from the resplendent operating theatres to the Cimmerian obscurity of the out-patient departments." Among these castoffs Wright found tuberculous lesions and tuberculous joints aplenty on which to try his opsonic methods.

He had also found among them the many sufferers from boils with whom he had begun his vaccine therapy. In the search for vaccines the laboratory men had not neglected the common pus-producing bacteria, among them the clustering staphylococci that were considered the villains in such suppurating afflictions as abscesses, boils, carbuncles, acne, and pyorrhea.

Wright dismissed as useless the commercial vaccines available against these organisms; he thought the only effective agents were "autogenous vaccines" made from the patient's own pus. He taught his students how to make these vaccines and administer them according to the opsonic index. As the index rose the suppurative process would subside, he told them, and he convinced them by the results he achieved. The students, successive groups of them, broadcast their conviction throughout the medical world.

Wright's opsonic theories and methods did not escape criticism from his medical fellows but at this time the informed attacks on opsonism ran not so much to its validity as to its usefulness. Critics called the index too complex and calculating it too arduous to be practical; the ordinary physician would never have the time to use it even if he could understand it.

The difficulty of it did not faze Gerald Webb. In love with the laboratory since his undergraduate days in Denver, he embraced the new world of Wright's opsonins and vaccines with fervor. He called the cures he witnessed "no less than miracles" and Wright "a genius who has revolutionized the treatment of many diseases... and stands already on a level with such men as Pasteur and Jenner."

He enthusiastically accepted Wright's assurance that "we have, in the means for raising the anti-bacterial power of the blood, beyond all comparison the most valuable asset in medicine."

"It looks to me," wrote Webb, "as if the medical men of the future will wield the inoculating syringe, and look back upon the present physician, with his pill boxes and ointment pots, as we look back upon the practitioners of the Middle Ages." He said he was sure that *opsonic index* would soon be as familiar a term among doctors and nurses as *urinalysis*.

The monocled Wright was a demanding teacher; an intense worker himself, he had no patience with idlers. Gerald thought he personified Longfellow's lines about great men "toiling upward in the night."

Coming to the laboratory after a long morning in the clinic, Wright usually worked on at his bench until the early hours of the next day. He expected his assistants and students to do the same, said Gerald, "and some of them are occasionally found by the laboratory attendant the next morning, having fallen off their stools, asleep on the floor." But however worn out by the endless counting of black dots in gray blobs, the students deeply respected Wright and among themselves affectionately called him "the Proff."

After learning thoroughly how to calculate the index and make the vaccines — and, not least, how to blow molten glass into the form of a pipette, the slender glass tube with a hair-thin bore that Wright had devised to facilitate the handling of bacteria and leucocytes, impelling Webb to call him "the Wizard of the Pipette" — each student was assigned clinic patients to handle on his own in consultation with Wright.

One of several such assignments to Webb gave him reason to ponder the effects of exercise on tuberculosis. Some years earlier the patient had pierced his ankle with an old beef bone while walking through a butcher's refuse lot, and off and on ever since he had been incapacitated by a huge discharging sinus in the ankle. The opsonic index revealed the lesion to be tuberculous, but equally significant to Webb, calculations he made before and after the man took a long walk showed that the exercise had induced a negative phase from which it took the patient twenty-one hours to recover.

Gerald relished the shoptalk and banter that spiced the hard work in clinic and laboratory, where he was quickly credited with "an acute mind" and relied upon to keep the peace during disagreements. Since most of the students were young bachelors, he and Varina undertook to provide them with social diversions, inviting them to dinner in Maida Vale and guiding them on excursions to resort spots near London. Most of them became good friends who for years exchanged personal news and professional favors with Gerald Webb.

Another such friend was "Dr. A. May," one of Wright's assistants. A brawny, red-faced Irishman who had been a medical missionary in Rhodesia, Aylmer May, nicknamed Maisie, was the laugh-making life of the laboratory—until some crisis or mishap produced an outburst of profanity. Then he turned loudly censorious in pious outrage and it was up to Colorado, as he called Webb, to persuade him into good humor again.

Everybody in the laboratory from Wright down contributed blood to the pool from which was taken the normal blood needed for opsonic calculations. "We were all pricked like so many human pincushions." When presently discrepancies appeared in the index ratios, Wright decided it must be Webb's blood that was skewing the figures owing to his recent bout with bloodpoisoning.

Gerald was therefore faintly uneasy about himself when after three months with Wright he moved on for further study in Vienna. There some weeks later he read in the *Lancet* Sir Almroth Wright's account of a nearly fatal case of "tuberculous septicemia" that had yielded to opsonic treatment; the patient was Dr. A. May.

"It is a great satisfaction to know at last that it was not *my* blood that was abnormal," said Gerald.*

Subsequent letters from Dr. May told Webb that he was fully recovered and back in Victoria Falls as a medical missionary trying to unravel the mysteries of Blackwater fever.

Another lifetime friend from these London months was the newest addition to Wright's staff, a shy and silent young Scotsman named Alexander Fleming. They all called him "Little Flem" though he had more diplomas and gold medals in medicine than any of them. Two decades later, still in the St. Mary's laboratory as Wright's second in command, Fleming let a culture of staphylococci get moldy and so stumbled upon the incomparable boon of penicillin.

*This version of the May story comes from Webb's letters and papers. For a somewhat different telling of it, see André Maurois, *Life of Sir Alexander Fleming* (1959), p. 59.

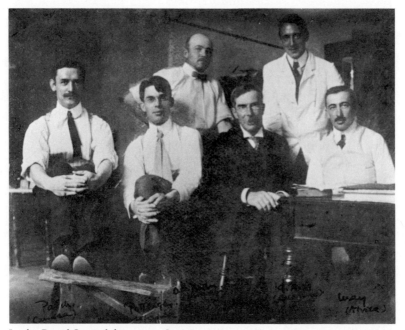

In the Praed Street laboratory, St. Mary's Hospital, London, 1906. Dr. Webb stands behind and between Almroth Wright and Aylmer May

Fortunately Fleming's long search for bactericidal substances had prepared him to recognize what the chance spore drifting in from Praed Street had done to his cocci. Almroth Wright refused to believe it; he remained stubbornly sure that only phagocytes could kill bacteria.

Why Gerald chose to continue his study in Vienna rather than in Paris or Berlin I do not know. The preeminence of "the Vienna School" in pathology and surgery had mostly faded away and its light was not luringly bright in the new medical science. In later years Gerald said of his Vienna period only that he "did clinical work, particularly in tuberculosis, with Lorenz, Covacs, Ghon and others at the Allgemeine Krankenhaus." But what he actually recalled on occasion back in Colorado Springs was a few principles and techniques of postoperative treatment he had learned in the surgical wards of Edmund von Neusser.

It was probably the attractions of Vienna itself that determined Gerald's choice. After all, he and Varina were supposed to be enjoying a holiday.

Historians say the grand old Austrian capital had gone decadent by now but this was not apparent to the Webbs. They delighted in Vienna's magnificent open spaces, woods, and parks, its historic buildings and broad avenues, its flourishing opera, its lighthearted people. One remembered night they saw the original cast in a performance of Franz Lehar's new hit, *The Merry Widow*; Gerald commented that the hero and heroine must have danced hundreds of miles that night.

Twice the Webbs' enjoyment was dimmed by saddening news. Margaret Hayes wrote to tell them of the death of Mrs. Jefferson Davis and a letter from Nell brought them word that Mater had died.

Gone was the staunch little mother on whom Gerald had relied so long for so much. Without the Varinae he would have felt bereft, forlorn. His sorrow was given an edge of pain by his sense that he had failed the proud Frances Susannah; he knew he had fallen far short of the high achievement in medicine she had expected of him.

He and Varina ended their relaxing stay in late September. Varina was some six months pregnant and they wanted to be back in Colorado Springs in good time for her confinement. Taking with them the Nurse Bianca who had been helping them look after Binks, they made their way slowly, with stopovers in St. Moritz and Paris, back to the French coast and boarded ship for home.

On 17 December 1906 Gerald's single regret was that he could not tell Mater he at last had a son—named Gerald Bertram Webb Jr. but to be called Gerry. He told everyone else, even professional correspondents of slight acquaintance, so overwhelming was his Englishman's pride in the birth of a man child.

VIII

A Foot on the Ladder

DR. WEBB returned from abroad to find Wright's opsonins and vaccines the medical topic of the day in the United States. The Proff himself was here, being lionized in eastern medical centers and giving lectures in Baltimore and Philadelphia which Gerald went to attend before completing the journey home. In Colorado the articles in medical journals and news relayed over the doctors' grapevine had teased curiosity to a tingling high.

Especially in Denver. Dr. Charles W. Powers wondered whether the opsonic index could help in surgery. Dr. Charles Denison, a stubborn defender of tuberculin therapy for tuberculosis, wanted to know just how the index made this more effective. Drs. William C. Mitchell and Benjamin H. Mathews, bacteriologists for the State Board of Health and St. Joseph's Hospital respectively, were trying to teach themselves how to use the new tool and admittedly making a botch of it. Dr. Joseph Steiner of the Agnes Phipps Memorial Sanatorium wanted to use Wright's vaccines but could not trust himself to make them properly. Dr. Henry Sewall as usual itched with questions about the new theories.

All these men wrote to Dr. Webb for answers since he alone in the area could explain and demonstrate Wright's difficult methods. He became the local man of the hour.

By urgent invitation he went, when baby Gerry was only four days old, to address the august Denver Academy of Medicine on "Wright and His Work on Blood and Opsonins, with Demonstrations of Some of the Techniques." And he so impressed his dignified hearers that they unbent enough, after duly ponderous deliberation, to make him, uniquely, a nonresident Fellow of the Academy.

In subsequent months he was called back to Denver to talk to the Medical Alumni Association of his alma mater, the Denver County Medical Society, the Colorado Nurses Association, the

Colorado Dental Society. He spoke at a banquet meeting of the El Paso County Medical Society, to the faculty and students of Colorado College, to a large public gathering at the First Presbyterian Church in Colorado Springs, at a dinner meeting of the city's elitist men's group called the Winter Night Club.

He proved to be an extremely effective public speaker. Those boyhood performances coached by Pater, reinforced by the lectures undertaken for Henry Sewall at the University of Denver, now came to his aid, giving him an easy presence at the podium along with the ability to achieve genuine rapport with his listeners. His baritone voice was warm and resonant and in American ears his English speech added overtones of uncommon cultivation to his words.

He was extraordinarily skillful in adapting his material to his audience, in translating scientific technicalities into plain English, in ranging far for mind-catching illustrations and analogies. Here for example is a part of his remarks to the public mass meeting at the church:

"[Much of our difficulty in finding a cure for tuberculosis comes from] the tuberculosis germ's unusual method of self-preservation. Thirty percent of the body weight of the tubercle bacillus is composed of wax which is laid chiefly around the outside of the germ like an overcoat. [When enough of this wax is extracted from a colony of the germs] it looks like beeswax, and just as our stomachs would find it hard to digest beeswax, so the white corpuscles of the blood, which can devour the germs of diseases like typhoid and pneumonia, have trouble digesting the wax of the tubercle bacillus.

"These white corpuscles are like individual microscopic animals. If we get a black eye it is the white corpuscles that come and eat up the debris and clotted blood. When a tadpole becomes a frog it is the white corpuscles that eat away the tail. When the elk or deer throw off their horns it is the white corpuscles that eat away the roots, allowing the antlers to be shed.

"These corpuscles contain in their little bodies ferments [enzymes] like pepsin, and one type of white corpuscles called lymphocytes contain in addition a ferment known as lipase, which can digest fats and wax. The white corpuscles of the cockroach are entirely of this type and it is impossible to cause tuberculosis in this insect even by injecting live tubercle bacilli. The bee-moth, which lays its eggs in the wax of the honeycomb and whose larvae when hatched feed on this wax, is also immune to the tubercle infection. One of the things we doctors must learn if we are to cure tuberculosis is how to increase the number of lymphocytes in the patient's blood."

Webb's talk to the Colorado dentists on the opsonic treatment of pyorrhea was more technical and more cautious. He summarized a late report from England that cast doubt both on staphylococcus as the sole cause of pyorrhea and on the effectiveness of vaccine therapy for it. "Much more evidence and experience are necessary before any definite opinion can be given," he concluded.

But what he reported of his own experience did not reinforce that warning. He had used Wright's methods on only one patient, he said, a young woman of twenty. From the pus welling up between her teeth he had grown a culture of staphylococcus albus, made a vaccine from it, and cured the trouble with two inoculations two weeks apart.*

Published in a professional journal for dentists, this paper was quickly picked up by an enterprising reporter in Brooklyn who made it the basis of a widely distributed Sunday supplement feature on "The Microbe of Toothlessness."

Dentistry had as yet made little headway against pyorrhea; loosening and loss of teeth was still a common and dreaded affliction even among the young. So the Brooklyn reporter played to the fears of many as he declaimed the horrors of the toothless state and the miraculous discovery of the microbe that caused it and of a vaccine to prevent it. Dr. Webb of Colorado Springs, he advised his readers, could now stop the falling out of teeth with only two injections of the vaccine.

Inevitably, urgent pleas for the vaccine, arriving from all over the country, were soon heightening the stack of Dr. Webb's daily mail.

Enough survives of that mail to reveal the swift growth and change in Dr. Webb's practice. When he resumed it in late 1906, despite his predominant interest in tuberculosis, that disease accounted for no more than a scant third of his patients. He was a general practitioner, treating all the ailments of the community. But in less

---

*This may not have been so primitive a state of the art as it seemed in later decades. In November 1980 the National Institutes of Health announced the development of a vaccine to prevent tooth decay that promised "to revolutionize dentistry by the end of the decade." The bacteria involved were identified as streptococcus mutans.

than three years he was busy primarily with infectious diseases. He had become a "specialist" in the new vaccine therapy and was in effect providing an extensive consulting and laboratory service in that therapy throughout Colorado and adjoining states.

This development came about naturally through increasing referrals of questions, problems, and patients from other doctors. During these years most rank-and-file physicians became at least vaguely aware that a new treatment was available for bacterial infections but few bothered to learn the tricky ins and outs of it. When a troublesome case came along...well, who's that chap—over in Colorado Springs, isn't he?—who knows all about this newfangled vaccine business? Oh yes, Webb. And off would go a query to Dr. Webb, to be followed usually, if not by the patient himself, by samples of blood and pus or sputum that would bring back a few days later a vial of vaccine with careful instructions for inoculation.

Imagine, for instance, the effects of a tale like the following, which Dr. A. C. Magruder of Colorado Springs spread around with gusto, then reported to a regional convention of ear, nose, and throat specialists, and finally published in the national journal *Laryngoscope.*

Mr. P. Merchant, a Springs businessman, went to see Dr. Magruder in late November 1906 complaining of a severe pain in his right ear. Diagnosing the trouble as acute inflammation, the doctor struggled for six weeks to find some treatment that would clear up the infection—while Mr. Merchant's pain in the ear became a violent headache, he lost much of his hearing, and the discharge of pus from the ear increased to a flow that soaked six wads of absorbent cotton daily.

By mid-January 1907 Merchant was frantic lest he not be able to keep an important business appointment in New York in early February, and Dr. Magruder: "In my despair, having heard Dr. Webb's lecture on the marked beneficial results obtained by Wright in these cases, I removed a specimen of pus from the ear and took the patient to Dr. Webb for treatment."

Webb identified the offending organism, checked the opsonic index, and made the appropriate vaccine, then injected the first small dose of it on 24 January. For two days the headache and discharge were worse, then they began to subside. On 28 January Dr. Webb gave the second inoculation. On 30 January the headache was gone, the ear was dry, the hearing was back to normal. On 1 February Mr. Merchant happily departed for New York, and ten months later he reported himself still free of pain and pus.

Dr. Magruder pointed the moral in summing up: "I am told by Dr. Webb that this is the first case of Suppurative Otitis Media treated opsonically in Colorado, and it is his opinion that it is the first case so treated in the United States. If I do not improve my method of treatment in this class of patients, Dr. Webb will get them all away from me."

As that story suggests, patients were referred to Dr. Webb not just for major infections like pneumonia, typhoid fever, influenza (which until World War I was thought to be caused by "the Pfeiffer bacillus") but in greater numbers for persisting ear, eye, and throat infections, boils, abscesses, old unhealing sores—and acne, acne, acne. (Staphylococcus soon gave place to "the Gilchrist bacillus" as the supposed cause of the ubiquitous pimples on the face.)

A huge lot of nasty stuff in capsules and bottles passed through the Colorado Springs post office on its way to and from the Webb office at 1222 North Cascade Avenue, where the tiresome calculations of the opsonic index mounted into the thousands.

This development is easy to explain in the local and regional area, where Dr. Webb was the first with the most in the expanding use of vaccines. Not so clear is why in early 1907 he was already receiving similar referrals from a few doctors in New York and Philadelphia. Those few became many, and the referrals focused on tuberculosis, as Dr. Webb of Colorado Springs won national recognition.

Gerald made his debut on the national stage when Henry Sewall secured a place for him on the program of the third annual meeting of the National Association for the Study and Prevention of Tuberculosis held in Washington DC in early May 1907.

This voluntary association, years later to be called the National Tuberculosis Association (the NTA as I shall designate it throughout hereafter), had come quietly into being in 1904 as an attempt by leaders of the eastern medical establishment to quiet the free-for-all that was developing among regional leagues as they all scrabbled jealously to become the national agency in the emerging crusade against tuberculosis.

By 1907 the NTA had absorbed its rivals and achieved a membership of twelve hundred, roughly three fourths medical men and one fourth laymen. Its purposes were broad—in summary to combat "the white plague" by all possible scientific, educational, and social means. Leadership remained in the hands of the eastern founders but to achieve the desired national scope they had elected to the board of directors selected physicians from throughout the country, including Dr. Sewall of Denver.

Announcements of the upcoming annual meeting told Dr. Sewall that the program would concentrate on phagocytosis and opsonism. Why should his protégé not be a participant? He told Gerald to join the NTA and register for the meeting, then sent off a letter to his old friend William Henry Welch, the Johns Hopkins pathologist who had a powerful hand in running most things medical in the East, including the NTA.

Sewall's letter was so late that the established sections of the program — clinical, pathological, and sociological — were filled but space remained in the newly added surgical section. The last week of April Gerald received a cordial note from the section chairman, William Stewart Halsted of Johns Hopkins, probably the greatest of America's surgeons:

"I am very much pleased to hear that you are to be in Washington for the meeting.... Dr. Rufus I. Cole of Baltimore is to read a paper before the Surgical Section on the result of his work with the opsonic treatment of tuberculous joints. We have heard so much of your contributions to this subject that I trust you will discuss his paper."

Gerald's acceptance of the invitation reached Baltimore barely in time for his name to appear on the printed program: "Discussion opened by Dr. G. B. Webb of Colorado Springs."

This was a heady first. At last Gerald Webb was associating with great men in American medicine. "It is exhilarating to be with all these giants," he wrote Varina Mea, "even if it does make one feel like a tiny grain of sand."

Some of the "giants" Gerald met on this occasion were:

Edward L. Trudeau, owner and director of the Trudeau Sanatorium and Trudeau Laboratory at Saranac Lake, the revered dean and first president of the NTA. Though often sickly and sour, Trudeau was already America's legend and symbol in tuberculosis research and sanatorium treatment.

Livingston Farrand, the remarkable executive secretary of the NTA, a physician who had been professor of psychology and anthropology at Columbia University. He was to become a neighbor of the Webbs as president of the University of Colorado, then head of the American Red Cross, and finally president of Cornell University.

The earnest, sober Lawrason Brown, consulting physician at the Trudeau Sanatorium. He was the initiator and editor of the *Journal of the Outdoor Life*, the NTA's magazine for laymen; the founder of the American Sanatorium Association as an affiliate of the NTA; and a meticulous laboratory worker who like his mentor Trudeau was doing much to prevent acceptance of the slipshod in tuberculosis research.

The genial and excitable Mazÿck P. Ravenel, a director of the NTA who was then on the staff of the Henry Phipps Research Institute in Philadelphia but was shortly to move to the University of Wisconsin as director of the State Hygienic Laboratory. He became a noted leader in the public health movement.

Also the prickly and combative S. Adolphus Knopf, an eminent clinician in New York City and a prodigious writer of articles and maker of speeches in English, French, and German. His pamphlet, *Tuberculosis as a Disease of the Masses and How to Combat It*, published in 1901, was translated into twenty-seven languages and attained a circulation second only to that of the Bible.

And, the most pregnant encounter of all for Gerald Webb, Arnold C. Klebs of Chicago, a member of the executive committee of the directors of the NTA.

Arnold was the son of the distinguished German pathologist Edwin Klebs, who as professor of pathology successively at Prague, Berne, and Zurich had first recognized the diphtheria bacillus, the typhoid bacillus, and the species of the tubercle bacillus. Unfortunately for his place in medical history he left it to others to prove that the bacteria he described actually caused the diseases he named. He migrated from Europe in 1895 to spend some years as professor of pathology at Rush Medical College in Chicago.

His son Arnold, of equally good mind and training but averse to spending his days hunched over a microscope, entered private practice as a specialist in the treatment of tuberculosis. Tall and handsome, sophisticated, sociable, this younger Klebs was universally popular in medical circles, where he was known as a fluent and provocative conversationalist in several languages on almost any subject and as a connoisseur of food and wine, books and music.

Arnold Klebs and Gerald Webb took an instant liking for each other when they met in Washington's New Willard Hotel in 1907, and on their train homeward they began a lasting friendship as they read together a recent article on serum therapy by the Nobel laureate Emil von Behring.

They also shared a fierce indignation about newspaper distortion of medical matters. Together they had heard and approved Adolphus Knopf's recommendation to the clinical section of the NTA meeting that morphine be used to deaden the pain of patients in the terminal stages of tuberculosis, so they were shocked by the outrageous report of his remarks in the *Philadelphia North American* under the headline "Kill Off Your Dying Consumptives, Says Famous Physician." Klebs was angrily sure that such a scare piece would be reprinted all over the country and would terrify thousands of tuberculous patients and their families.

As it was and did. A subsequent story in the *St. Louis Republic*, for instance, bore the heading "Consumptives, Fearing Execution, Bar Their Nurses." (The nationwide furore so exasperated Dr. Knopf that, spurred on by William Osler who had suffered similar newspaper calumny over a jocular comment on euthanasia, he brought suit against the Philadelphia paper and eventually won the case.)

Klebs had read a paper at the NTA meeting on "Mixed Infections"; he now learned that Webb knew more about this problem than he did. It was thought to be a striking discovery that the sputum and throat swabbings of tuberculous patients often contained more than one kind of bacteria and doctors were much exercised about how to treat such "parallel" infections.

Webb had learned in Wright's laboratory, he said, that "Germs are prone to hunt in couples. Influenza is usually complicated by the simultaneous effects of the pneumococcus. The growing of the influenza germ in an incubator is greatly aided if one adds a pus germ to it." He had pursued the problem in Colorado Springs and thought he had succeeded in reducing the amount of tuberculous sputum and nausea by vaccinating the patient against streptococcus infection and influenza as well as tuberculosis.

Klebs promptly invited his new friend to write a chapter on "Mixed and Concomitant Infections" for the book about tuberculosis he was preparing for publication the following year.

Gerald would appear in illustrious company. William Osler was writing the introduction, Edward Trudeau a chapter on treatment, Mazÿck Ravenel an essay on the tubercle bacillus. Adolphus

Knopf and Hermann Biggs, the influential New York pioneer in public health, were working up the section on prevention, Klebs himself the blueprint for building and managing a sanatorium.

This writing task and correspondence with Klebs helped to sustain Gerald as the euphoria engendered by the NTA meeting faded into discouraging awareness of the handicaps imposed by his professional isolation. None of the Colorado Springs doctors and only a few of the Denver men shared his compelling interest in laboratory medicine or his yearning to be more than "a tiny grain of sand" in their profession. Most of them, having lost all ambition when ill health disrupted their lives and sent them to Colorado, were content to be just practitioners—as were probably 99 percent of American physicians. Gerald, out of his own need for "the mutual reverberation of ideas," was often impatient with the apathy of his local colleagues.

He had heard much talk at the New Willard about the International Congress on Tuberculosis which was to be held in Washington the next year with the NTA as host and he wanted desperately to produce something that would earn him a place on the program. But how could he? He had no time, space, or equipment for laboratory work beyond the endless opsonic calculations and making of vaccines demanded by his practice. He had to rely on the part-time assistance of high school boys and students at Colorado College and found most of them too unreliable to be of much help.

True, Dr. William C. Mitchell of the State Board of Health, the university "professor" who had introduced Gerald to bacteriology, appeared from Denver for a couple of days a week, but he came only to learn the opsonic techniques—and he made such a slow business of understanding them that Dr. Webb, in exasperation one suspects, finally persuaded him to go study with Almroth Wright himself and made arrangements with the Proff to accept Mitchell as a postgraduate student for six weeks.

Another frustration for Gerald was the lack of adequate medical libraries in the state. English and American books and journals were no longer enough for his purposes; the best laboratory work was often reported only, or at least first, in French and German publications and even the current numbers of these, let alone back issues, were rarely to be found in Colorado.

Each time Gerald went to the capital he searched the libraries for items he wanted, but almost always in vain. At presumably the best of the collections, that of the Denver Academy of Medicine, he was so "repelled by the dirt and disarray" reflecting years of neglect that he gave up and fell back on the good-humored offices of Arnold Klebs, who tirelessly hunted up references for him and sent him reprints, books, and journals from Arnold's own library.

A letter from Klebs often brightened Gerald's day. Arnold wrote so spontaneously and gaily, was so full of news and gossip. He practiced well what he taught, that "there ought never to be one paragraph without a smile somewhere tucked into it."

He always had some matter to argue about too, if no more than the correct use of words. Why, for example, did Webb and the other Wrightists always say *vaccination* [from the Latin *vacca* meaning cow] when their work had nothing to do with cows. That word had been proper enough for Jenner when he was using cowpox but now surely one ought to say *inoculation*. Here Arnold's cause was lost before he espoused it; with the blessing of Pasteur long before, *vaccination* and *vaccine* had come to stay.

The correspondence often led to an exchange of gifts. Once Gerald sent Klebs a recording of the Quartet from *Rigoletto* and Arnold thanked him with a copy of *The Doctor's Dilemma*, telling how he had "giggled and chuckled" over Shaw's "buttered bacilli."

By autumn Gerald had his manuscript ready for review and went to Chicago for a face-to-face conference on "our book." He lodged with Arnold, who was a widower with only his nine-year-old daughter Sarah to share his home. Arnold listened sympathetically to his friend's problems and solved one of them by putting Gerald in touch with Richter of Milwaukee, a firm that handled orders for foreign books and journals, including back issues and items out of print. The service was expensive but greatly useful and time-saving.

The book remained a worry. Arnold had to struggle with his dilatory and cantankerous authors for many extra months and Gerald had to keep revising his chapter to incorporate new ideas and data. *Tuberculosis, a Treatise by American Authors*, a giant 939-page volume, finally appeared in the spring of 1909 and Arnold and his friends turned a luncheon session of the subsequent NTA meeting into a noisy and hilarious publication party.

Gerald Webb was there. And two days later he was in Bedford,

New York, serving as best man at Arnold's wedding.

The new Mrs. Klebs was soon Harriet to all Arnold's friends—except to Gerald Webb. Invariably in his subsequent letters Gerald referred to her deferentially as "the Madam." Not that she was so formidable; it was the term by which Gerald referred to all the wives of his professional friends. It was not in him to be easily casual and informal.

There was good reason for the warm relationship between the two men: A year earlier Arnold Klebs had shepherded Gerald Webb through a crucial public encounter with the great Robert Koch. The road to it was circuitous.

Three events in late 1907 dovetailed to put Gerald onto a promising track in research. The first, in mid-November, was an hour's notice to accompany a dying patient on his last journey home. The man's family promptly paid the doctor's bill for twenty-five hundred dollars and Gerald decided to use this "lucky fee" to build an adequate laboratory as an addition on the north side of the Cascade Avenue house. Varina amiably agreeing, he put the carpenters immediately to work.

At this same time, Dr. William Whitridge Williams arrived in Colorado Springs, bringing his tuberculous wife to Dr. Webb on referral by Dr. Charles Minor of Asheville, North Carolina.

Red-haired, tennis-loving "Billie" Williams, son of the professor of obstetrics who was shortly to become dean of the medical school at Johns Hopkins, was an able pathologist trained at Harvard by the extraordinary Theobald Smith, who has been called comparable in American medical science to Pasteur in France and Koch in Germany. Williams had been teaching pharmacology at Western Reserve University when his wife's poor health forced him to resign and take her first to Asheville and now to Dr. Webb.

Eager to be at work again, Williams gladly accepted Webb's invitation to become director of the new "Webb Tuberculosis Research Laboratory" when it was ready, his salary to be paid partly in treatment of his wife and partly from Webb's pocket.

On the night of 11 December the two men were hard at work in the office testing various stains for the tubercle bacillus when a second emergency summons sent Dr. Webb racing through the darkness to Kansas City.

Thomas F. Walsh, the multimillionaire owner of the famous

Camp Bird Gold Mine in Ouray, had been a carpenter in Colorado Springs before he struck it rich and rose high enough in the social scale to be presented with his wife at the court of Edward VII. Mrs. Walsh was a Springs girl whose mother, Mrs. A. J. Reed, had long been a patient of Dr. Webb's. Mrs. Reed had died this week in December and Mrs. Walsh and her little daughter Evalyn were in town for the funeral.*

Supposed also to be present were Mrs. Reed's widowed son-in-law, Samuel N. Lee, a prosperous building contractor in Kansas City, and his fifteen-year-old son Monroe, but Mr. Lee wired that he could not come because Monroe was gravely ill—dying, the doctors said, from typhoid fever.

Mrs. Walsh flew into action. She telephoned Dr. Webb, telephoned Superintendent Martin of the Rock Island Railway in Denver, telephoned the station master in Colorado Springs, telephoned Dr. Webb again. Within fifty-five minutes, at 11:00 P.M., she had the doctor setting off alone in a single Pullman car hooked onto the Rock Island's most powerful engine. Superintendent Martin had arranged for all other trains to be shunted onto sidings so that "Dr. Webb's Special" could run on cleared tracks and he had given the engineer carte blanche at the throttle.

Traveling in some stretches of the line at "the terrific speed" of eighty miles an hour, the Special pulled into the Kansas City station at 2:10 the following afternoon, having clipped more than four hours from the normal time for the run. And Dr. Webb was in time to be credited with saving Monroe Lee's life by the use of Almroth Wright's vaccine.

Mrs. Walsh and Evalyn came on from Colorado and Thomas Walsh from California to thank the doctor.

Neither Mr. Lee nor Mr. Walsh liked the bill he presented, however. They refused to pay it, even when half a year later he offered to reduce it by a thousand dollars if they would settle up by the end of the month. Gerald consulted Denver doctors, Addison Hayes, and Henry Hall about the fairness of the fee he asked and was urged by all of them to insist on the full amount. What that amount was

*The daughter grew up to become the glamorous Evalyn Walsh McLean, a much publicized Washington hostess and the owner of the fabled Hope diamond. Her husband was Ned McLean, publisher of the *Washington Post* and owner of the notorious hideaway "house on H Street" at which President Warren G. Harding and his cronies met to play poker and arrange their deals. Ned later became a patient of Dr. Webb's and Evalyn a frequent visitor to Colorado Springs.

and whether or not he was ever paid I do not know.

But he gained more than money from the trip. A great deal of publicity for one thing. Such special trains and cleared tracks for emergency runs were novel at the time and "the race with death," the record speed, the desire of the Rock Island to preen itself on the excellence of its roadbeds, the prominence of the Walshes and Mr. Lee, all combined to make the event a page-one story for midwestern and western newspapers. And every story carried Dr. Webb's name and picture and effusive testimony to his medical expertise.

More important, while in Kansas City Gerald met Professor M. A. Barber of the University of Kansas and spent a day in Barber's laboratory, from which he returned to Colorado Springs with a buzzing bee of an idea in his head.

Barber, an agricultural biologist, had devised a technique for isolating a single cell of yeast which he demonstrated to Webb, telling him the same method could readily be used to prick out a single bacterium. Gerald's imagination jumped to the possibility of substituting reduction of numbers for attenuation of virulence in vaccination.

Most vaccines then were prepared from killed bacteria, but a number of authorities, Koch and Trudeau among them, had become convinced that effective immunity would be achieved only by injecting living organisms whose power to reproduce and do damage had been weakened, attenuated, usually by growing them in successive cultures under adverse conditions. This conviction had not been tested in treatment because the use of live bacteria was considered too risky. The degree of virulence might not remain stable; an attenuated strain might reacquire strength in the human body so that injections meant to cure might kill instead.

But suppose that one could begin by injecting a single live bacillus and slowly, slowly increase the number—two, four, six, ten, and on into the hundreds. Might not the body develop immunity to the bacilli as it did to gradually increasing doses of snake venom and some vegetable poisons?

This echo of Henry Sewall's great discovery was the possibility that excited Gerald, and Bill Williams enthusiastically agreed that the idea was worth trying out—on animals first of course.

Impatiently Gerald prodded his builders into more speed and after weeks of maddening chaos—capsuled specimens of pus and sputum were lost, cultures misplaced, vials of precious vaccine broken, and inoculated rabbits got loose and scuttled away—the Webb Tuberculosis Research Laboratory was ready for occupancy in March 1908. With Bill Williams' assistance Dr. Webb set to work on his numbers game.

He had decided to begin, to practice as it were, with the anthrax bacillus because it was larger and easier to stain and therefore to count than its tubercle fellow. If he could immunize mice against the deadly anthrax he would move on to inject the tubercle bacillus into its highly susceptible host the guinea pig.

But he was stopped short at the start. Neither he nor Williams could duplicate Barber's technique. They could prepare the delicate "hanging drop" of anthrax emulsion but could only occasionally manage to draw off from it into their pipette the single thread they wanted, and they could not figure out at all how to keep the organism alive in the tube or how to flush it out into a mouse or onto a slide. Barber had done it all so deftly—by some sleight of hand it now seemed.

Refusing to be balked, Gerald telephoned to Kansas City: Would the professor please come to Colorado Springs and teach them how to isolate and inoculate a single organism? Barber gladly assented and spent a week in the new laboratory making sure the Coloradans were skilled enough to proceed on their own. In the process he became so interested in their project that upon returning home he initiated a parallel series of experiments in his own laboratory and made his findings available to supplement Webb's own.

Gerald was aiming for results he could report to the International Congress beginning in late September, but he had learned that he ought to lay public claim to his idea quickly lest someone else publish it first. Also he must let it be known that he would have something worth presenting to the Congress.

The NTA was holding its fourth annual meeting in Chicago in June. With Arnold Klebs's help Gerald secured time enough on the program to read "a brief preliminary report relating some experiments in immunizing mice against anthrax" and promising "that similar experiments relating to the production of immunity against tuberculosis in guinea pigs would be reported later."

Webb and Williams had as yet nothing even faintly conclusive to announce but the mere notion of beginning inoculations "with one living organism" was enough to create a stir—and to win for Dr.

Webb more than he had hoped for: an invitation from the high priest William Henry Welch, who was presiding over Section I of the upcoming Congress, to present his full report on the program of that section.

The Webb Laboratory was a-buzz with activity that summer. Gerald, now become that hard-driving captain of the polo team, produced an idea per day of what further must be done to make the report solid. They must nail down the practicability of Barber's method by applying it to a variety of organisms: the typhoid bacillus, streptococci and staphylococci, the bacillus of influenza. They must calculate the opsonic index before and after every injection in every animal. And they must begin the experiments with the tubercle bacillus and guinea pigs immediately, alongside the series on anthrax in mice.

But they could not secure a sufficient number of guinea pigs. All right, while waiting for the pigs (to come eventually from Henry Sewall's laboratory at the Jewish Home for Consumptives in Denver) they would start a series on rabbits; this would add variety to their findings.

All this required a tremendous amount of painstaking laboratory work and record-keeping, given the deadline against which the men were working. So Gerald commandeered the part-time assistance of Dr. G. W. Morse, a consumptive patient who was not yet able to resume practice but wanted a little work and income, and of Clarence W. Lieb, a trustworthy graduate of Colorado College who needed to increase his nest egg for further education.

Dr. Webb himself was assembling in odd moments the facts and references for a long introduction to the report tracing the history of the quest for immunity against tuberculosis, especially the experience with killed cultures versus living bacilli in vaccines. And he was keeping close track of five consumptive men upon whom he had boldly tried his minute doses, reasoning that since their bodies already contained millions of tubercle bacilli a few more could hardly hurt them and just might start up the development of resistance.

With two of the men, relatively mild cases, he stopped at five bacilli and no improvement occurred. The other three men he judged to be terminal cases and so increased their dosage gradually to five hundred bacilli. To his delight two of these men grew so much better that they were able to get up and around and even do light work. The third, a doctor, felt he had improved greatly though Gerald could demonstrate no change. "At least no harm has been done," he said.

Like virtually all laboratory workers of that day, Webb and Williams were better at spawning theories and contriving experiments than at arranging and interpreting their findings. The science of data analysis had yet to be born. Their tables, and Professor Barber's likewise, simply listed animal by animal and date by date the doses injected, tests made, and results observed: this guinea pig had lived free of tubercles, that one had died teeming with bacilli (or been stolen from its cage or lost to an epidemic of gastroenteritis).

By September their conclusions could be only negative or tentative: Mice were just too susceptible to anthrax to be immunized against it, whereas rabbits had too much natural immunity to the human tubercle bacillus to provide any suggestive results; the experimenters hoped for more valuable evidence from a new rabbit series using the bovine bacillus.

The guinea pigs yielded better findings: a mere twenty bacilli injected in a single dose would infect a guinea pig but in graduated doses beginning with one bacillus at least fifteen hundred bacilli could be inoculated without producing infection.

Adding these data to Dr. Webb's results with the tuberculous men, Webb and Williams were willing to say: "We feel that some immunity can be safely produced by beginning with the subcutaneous injection of one tubercle bacillus, and we regard such a method as harmless and more than probably beneficial to an already tuberculous man."

The report, by Webb and Williams "in conjunction with Prof. M. A. Barber," was still only a bunch of scattered notes and rough tables when it came time for Gerald to leave for the Congress; he would, as he said, "have to patch the scraps together" on the train and in Washington. But he set off confidently, carrying with him his official accreditation as an American delegate from the governor of Colorado.

This was the sixth of these international congresses on tuberculosis, the latest previous one having been held in Paris in 1905. Since the NTA had accumulated nothing like the funds needed to play host to such an international gathering, the Congress was being financed largely by the Russell Sage Foundation.

friend. He had problems of his own to worry about. The huge laboratories and full-time research men he had just seen made his own situation look hopeless, with only odd hours to work and Bill Williams to help—and as usual a hampering lack of money. Varina was pregnant again, expecting the new baby next April. With three children to support and a balance still to be repaid on the loan from Papa Hayes, Gerald knew he could not go on financing the work of the laboratory from his own income.

He had received some trifling donations from grateful patients but most of them had no understanding of what his "playing about" with mice and guinea pigs could have to do with getting them well.

The idea of contributing funds to endow medical research had entered the lexicon of philanthropy for only a rare few as yet. Even Edward Trudeau, consummate beggar that he had become, going twice annually to New York with hat and lists of possible donors in hand, made up his laboratory budgets more from personal gifts and charity to the poor than from support for his research.

Gerald sought aid from President Slocum of Colorado College whom he knew to be interested in his experiments, but moral support was all Slocum could spare him. He also addressed a deferential request to the grand old patron of the Springs, General William Palmer: "I know you have many claims upon your generosity but know also that you realize the benefit to Colorado Springs of a tuberculosis research laboratory."

He was too late. The valiant patriarch, almost completely paralyzed since breaking his neck in a fall from a stumbling cow pony two years before, died just a day or two after Gerald's letter was delivered to Glen Eyrie.

Reluctantly Gerald turned eastward and wrote to William Henry Welch, detailing his plight and asking for help from the Rockefeller Institute, of which Welch was a director and the preëminent adviser as to whose research should be subsidized.

"Opportunities for research in tuberculosis are unusual here," Webb told Welch, "and we have many doctors in the city with chronic tuberculosis who could work a few hours a day in the laboratory if only we could pay them a little. But we are so far from good libraries that our work necessitates a heavy subscription to medical journals which alone impoverishes me."

Again his plea was too late. The directors of the Institute had discontinued their individual grants-in-aid in order to concentrate their funds on expanding the Institute's own research programs.

Gerald applied finally to the American Medical Association, where he found an admiring friend at court. Dr. Alfred Stengel of Philadelphia, one of the easterners who had begun referring patients to Dr. Webb as an expert in opsonism, was both editor of the AMA's journal and chairman of its Committee on Research. It pleased him to make sure his able Colorado colleague was given assistance.

The grant was small, only a thousand dollars, but renewed annually for several years it kept the Webb Tuberculosis Research Laboratory in business until such time as personal contributions, principally a yearly check for one thousand dollars from Benjamin C. and Maria McKean Allen, financed its investigations.

IX

In Quest of Immunity

"It is to laboratory research that we must look for the solution of unsolved problems in tuberculosis, and for advances in our methods of prevention and treatment." So said Edward Trudeau near the turn of the century.

He spoke mostly in hope, for medical research was then barely beginning to take root in America. In the years 1900 to 1915 university medical faculties, spurred by the pioneering of a few—at Johns Hopkins, Pennsylvania, Harvard, Michigan—began to add research to teaching as their mission, and showers of philanthropy produced lavish endowments for research institutes on the French and German models.

At first, said Hans Zinsser, a participant in the development, space and equipment outran the brains available: "In many places half-trained people in the magnificent laboratories were sitting on sterile ideas like hens on boiled eggs." It took another decade or two for the manpower to catch up.

Here and there individuals like Henry Sewall, gaining access to the clinical laboratory of some hospital, conducted sporadic investigations on problems that teased them. But a private venture like the Webb Laboratory for Tuberculosis Research was rare and superbly daring.

The inspiration for it came from the Trudeau Laboratory at Saranac Lake, until then unique. Gerald Webb, alert to the parallel between the Adirondacks resort and Colorado Springs, did not fail to see what cachet the research laboratory added to Trudeau's sanatorium. It was his dream that his Webb Laboratory would in time make Colorado Springs an equivalent center of tuberculosis research in the West. Repeatedly, in public and in private, he invited the doctors of El Paso County to use the facilities of the laboratory

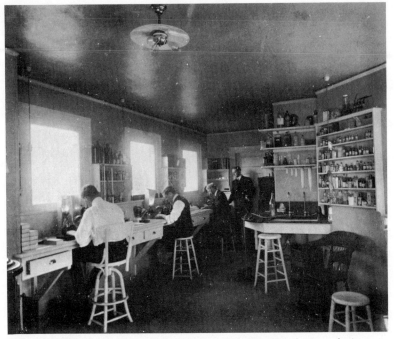

The Webb Tuberculosis Research Laboratory at 1222 North Cascade Avenue. *Left* to *right*, Dr. William W. Williams, Clarence Lieb, Professor M. A. Barber, and Dr. Webb

free of charge for any research project they wished to undertake.

But no one came. No one. Not even to sit on a boiled egg.

The only proposal was made by young Clarence Lieb. Webb and Williams had promised the International Congress they would repeat their live-germ series on rabbits using the bovine bacillus; Lieb asked permission to do this work independently as a thesis for a master's degree at Colorado College. Dr. Webb gladly assented.

In a year of painstaking experiments Lieb showed that by beginning with one bacillus at the time of the rabbit's birth and increasing the dosage slowly week by week he could keep an entire litter immune to a virulent bovine strain until well into adulthood. Highly pleased, Dr. Webb secured publication of Lieb's thesis in the *Journal of Medical Research* — and expansively promised to find supplemental funds to see the boy through his medical education at Harvard.

Gerald had cause to regret that impulse. Clarence took him at his word and for two years wrote periodically to ask for the promised help. For a while Helen Morley supplied the money, but when she became too engrossed in her several ailments to be bothered, the checks for twenty-five or fifty dollars at a time had to be squeezed, often most inconveniently, from Gerald's own bank account.

Still, when young Lieb proposed to borrow money in Cambridge for his second year's needs, Gerald advised him strongly against it. "When you begin practice you would find the burden of debt intolerable," wrote Dr. Webb, projecting his own painful experience. "Earn all the money you can for yourself and I will continue to send you what more you need."

Lieb proved worth it. For his last two years at Harvard he won laboratory assistantships to two of the university's noted physiologists, William T. Councilman and Walter B. Cannon, and by the time he received his medical degree *cum laude* in 1914 he had earned more than five thousand dollars and had a thousand dollars in the bank to carry him through his internship at the newly opened Peter Bent Brigham Hospital.

His close encounter with eastern provincialism mystified the young westerner. He asked Dr. Webb why the Harvard men were not at all interested in immunity or vaccination and why they considered nobody's research any good except their own and that of the Hopkins men.

Lieb had the grace to be forever grateful to Gerald Webb, repaying him with devoted friendship throughout his life. When Lieb had become an eminent clinician and philanthropist in New York City he wrote Dr. Webb, "For me you have always personified the ideal physician and I am glad to have had you as a model." And in the preface to one of his books he gave thanks to "a great physician, Gerald Bertram Webb of Colorado Springs, who directed my life into medical paths."

Webb's own attention in the fall of 1908 was diverted temporarily from the counting of tubercle bacilli by coincident epidemics of whooping cough and catarrhal bronchitis in Colorado Springs. Differentiating the two illnesses was sometimes difficult and Dr. Webb, reading in the *Archives of Internal Medicine* that whooping cough seemed always to be accompanied by an increase of lymphocytes in the patient's blood, thought he and Bill Williams ought to investigate this as a possible aid to diagnosis.

To his surprise they found the number of lymphocytes abnormally high in all the sick youngsters. What about children who were not sick? Yes, their counts were high too. And what of healthy adults? Theirs likewise. Even the rabbits and guinea pigs in Colorado Springs had elevated lymphocyte counts. Why? What phenomenon was this?

As Dr. Webb pondered the question several thoughts coalesced to give him a theory.

He knew that lymphocytes had been largely ignored in medical research because no one could imagine what purpose these white cells served. Under the microscope they appeared pale, passive things, lacking the dark granules that filled their phagocytic sisters and seeming just to drift aimlessly hither and yon, in and out of the bloodstream and the lymph nodes. "The wandering cells" they were called.

They were known to abound in the pus of abscesses and infected wounds, and Robert Koch had noticed they were present in force at the inflamed sites of tuberculin injections and in the tubercle walls around bacilli in the lungs. Following up on this observation, a few men, most recently Eugene L. Opie of the Rockefeller Institute, had suggested that the mysterious lymphocytes might play a part in the body's defense against the tubercle bacillus, perhaps because they were able to destroy its wax capsule.

Dr. Webb suddenly remembered the study he had started years ago with Louis Livingood of Johns Hopkins, the project aborted by Livingood's death at sea, a study of the comparative germ-killing power of the blood at sea level and at a high altitude.

This reminded him of the conviction he shared with his Rocky Mountain colleagues, that high altitude was beneficial in the treatment of tuberculosis. They still could offer no scientific evidence to support their belief. Might he have stumbled onto the physiological mechanism that produced the benefit they so often witnessed?

Excited by this hunch, Gerald Webb set out on what was to be a seven years' affair with lymphocytes.

He and Bill Williams began by testing for themselves the alleged power of lymphocytes to destroy the waxy overcoat of the tubercle bacillus. They transferred pus from an abscess, presumably full of active lymphocytes, onto the surface of a cake of beeswax and watched it unmistakably eat away the fatty substance. They asked their friend M. A. Barber, now become director of the laboratory of clinical pathology in the University of Kansas medical school, to send them a supply of cockroaches and grasshoppers, insects whose white cells were all lymphocytes. Patiently they squirted tubercle bacilli into one hind leg of each insect and after a day or so extracted from the other hind leg "juice" filled with lymphocytes they judged to contain tubercle bacilli in various stages of dissolution.

As for the bee moth whose larvae feed on the wax of the honeycomb, the Coloradans decided they could not possibly better the proof provided by the striking photographs just published by two Frenchmen, Marie and Fiessinger, showing conclusively that this moth's lymphocytes make short work of dissolving the protective wax coating of the tubercle bacillus.

Simultaneously the investigators were collecting comparative lymphocyte counts in every way they could think of. Dr. Webb combed the literature for records of such counts at sea level and found the highest of them, reported by the Frenchman Jolly, to be some 30 percent lower than those he had assembled from Colorado Springs. He asked Dr. Carl Hedblom of Harvard to send him blood smears from eighteen healthy Harvard students and Dr. Williams matched their lymphocyte counts with those of eighteen students at Colorado College. Again the Colorado counts ran about one third higher.

The two men startled many a patient and visitor arriving from homes at sea level with an urgent request for an immediate drop of blood, then carefully charted changes in the person's lymphocyte counts over a month or two. Without exception the count rose dramatically for two weeks, then dropped back to a constant level roughly a third higher than upon arrival.

The process worked also in reverse. In some thirty cases of Colorado Springs residents going to live at sea level for a while, again without exception the lymphocyte count dropped within a month by about 30 percent.

In one instance Dr. Webb was able to get his data going and coming. A Springs youth of frail body insisted, against his parents' wishes and the doctor's advice, upon entering college at Yale. Gerald took a blood sample before the boy left and asked him to send back a smear each week for a month. The usual drop in lymphocytes occurred. When four months later the lad was sent home from Yale with a diagnosis of incipient tuberculosis, Dr. Webb with double satisfaction watched his lymphocyte count climb again and his symptoms disappear.

All the while Dr. Webb was diligently searching the literature for even a suggestion that lymphocytes proliferate as altitude rises. All he could find was an account of a balloon ascension in France in 1901 from which the medical records included a significant rise in the proportion of lymphocytes in the crewmen's blood. But no attention had been paid to this observation. Gerald was certain he had made an original discovery.

He and Williams published a preliminary report of it in *Colorado Medicine* in April 1909 and Webb presented their findings in full at the fifth annual meeting of the NTA a month later.

In spite of all his tables and charts many in his audience were skeptical, among them one A. F. Basinger M.D. who detrained in Colorado Springs the following August with the admitted purpose of proving the tall blond Englishman a charlatan who was concocting false figures in order to draw tuberculous patients to his mountain city.

Dr. Webb courteously suggested that the doubter measure and chart the changes in his own blood.

When Dr. Basinger had watched his lymphocyte count per cubic millimeter of blood climb from 2400 on his arrival to 4200 in two weeks, then drop back to 3600 and remain there, he was willing to proclaim that this Coloradan was playing no tricks with his data. Basinger stayed on to work with Webb and Williams in the laboratory for more than a year and became co-author as well as prime exhibit in their next report to the NTA and the AMA.

If lymphocytosis (increase or proliferation of lymphocytes) might be of benefit to a tuberculous patient, how could it be artificially induced? Gerald recalled what he had learned from Edward von Neusser in Vienna about the work of the German surgeon August Bier, who had successfully treated chronic infections of bones and joints by applying tourniquets to produce hyperemia (an abnormal supply of blood) in the affected area. Might this procedure also induce an increase in lymphocytes?

Webb and Williams experimented first on themselves, then on fourteen volunteer patients, by applying tourniquets high on the thighs. On the average, in half an hour the number of lymphocytes had jumped by 18 percent, at the end of an hour by 75 percent.

They could not believe it. Could such marked proliferation really occur in so short a time? Dr. Webb wrote to ask W. E. Carnegie Dickson of the University of Edinburgh who had just published a book about bone marrow. Yes, replied Dickson reassuringly, cell division takes place rapidly in the marrow; their results were entirely plausible.

Too many of the volunteers had reacted badly to the tourniquet pressure, suffering faintness, dizziness, nausea, blurred vision; the procedure could be dangerous if not monitored closely. Might less constriction for a longer period do as well?

Ever resourceful, Gerald raided Varina's sewing basket for a length of inch-wide elastic and fashioned it into a pair of garters for the upper arms. These, he found, if worn day and night for two weeks would produce as much lymphocytosis as the tourniquets while causing the patient no discomfort.

He also, much to Edward Trudeau's amusement when Gerald told him of it, tried the homely old remedy of hot mustard foot baths daily, and they too were effective.

The ultimate question, of course, was whether the lymphocytosis induced by all this hyperemia actually improved resistance to tubercle bacilli. For an answer the experimenters turned again to rabbits. They inoculated thirty-one of these animals with big doses of a virulent strain of bovine bacilli provided by Webb's friend Ravenel in Wisconsin, then began inducing hyperemia with tourniquets.

It was an exasperating struggle; the critters would not cooperate. They were devilishly ingenious in ridding themselves of the rubber-tubing constrictors no matter how intricately these were harnessed to their bodies. Some were too weak to survive the daily treatment. And the fecundity of the breed interfered; some half a dozen of the females removed themselves from the experiment by producing litters of stillborn young.

In the dozen or so animals that provided usable data the results were ambiguous, so that Webb, Williams, and Basinger were probably stretching their evidence to conclude even that "Artifical marrow hyperemia...appears to hold in check a rapid bovine tuberculous process in rabbits."

Of their thirty-odd human subjects, all victims of advanced tuberculosis, they could say only that wearing of the arm garters produced in every case a marked increase in lymphocyte count. That this lymphocytosis had any appreciable effect on the subjects' precarious state of health they could not claim.

The next development added more éclat than substance to

Dr. Webb's work with lymphocytes. It derived from the Anglo-American Physiological Expedition to Pikes Peak in the summer of 1911.

This expedition to study "mountain sickness" was planned under the auspices of the Royal Society of London by John Scott Haldane and C. Gordon Douglas of Oxford and Yandell Henderson of Yale, all three "bully physiologists" according to Henry Sewall. Henderson had invited Sewall to join the team as the local expert on conditions at Pikes Peak. Not feeling well enough to accept, Sewall passed the invitation on to Gerald Webb with the comment, "It would be a great thing to have these men work among us and it would pay the nabobs of Colorado Springs to make a special effort to get them."

When Sewall's letter arrived in November 1910 Dr. Webb was in the midst of upheaval. As I shall explain presently, he was moving his laboratory into new quarters and was taking on a major new responsibility for Cragmor Sanatorium. And equally upsetting, Bill Williams was leaving him, to go into practice on his own as a clinical pathologist in Denver.

Luckily an able replacement was at hand in the person of Dr. George Burton Gilbert, another Johns Hopkins medical graduate who had been driven westward into Dr. Webb's care by tuberculosis. Trained in laboratory methods by Dr. John Jacob Abel, the noted pharmacologist and physiological chemist, Dr. Gilbert was to prove a valuable assistant and partner, highly intelligent, precise, painstaking. But at the moment he was new, he was still far from well, and he really preferred the bedside to the laboratory.

It was no time, then, for Dr. Webb to undertake an added project, especially one only tangentially related to his own research. So he nominated in his stead young Edward S. Schneider, a Yale Ph.D. who was professor of biology and hygiene at Colorado College.

The Expedition leaders amiably agreed to add Webb's study of lymphocyte changes to their own investigations, and Schneider secured for Gerald blood smears from each member of the group before, during, and after the team's six-week stay on the summit of the Peak.

Throughout this period Haldane's blood, owing to a chronic infection, was too abnormally full of leucocytes and, Gerald confided to Clarence Lieb, Douglas consumed too much hard liquor for either of them to provide a reliable blood picture. Nonetheless

Dr. Webb was able to say that in all the men the number of large lymphocytes showed "a very marked increase" (of from 50 to 60 percent, he told Lieb) at the 14,000-foot elevation of the Peak.

Webb's report, including a summary and bibliography of his previous studies of lymphocytosis, was presented to the Royal Society in 1912 and published in its *Transactions* the following year as an Appendix to the official report of the Expedition.

Gerald Webb blessed the timing of this publication when late in 1913 he received a letter from a friendly acquaintance, Dr. Karl Turban of Davos in Switzerland, the man whose classification of the stages in tuberculosis was then in widespread diagnostic use. Turban enclosed a reprint of an article by his two assistants, Baer and Engelsmann, which had just been published in the *Deutschen Archiv für Klinische Medizin*. The article reviewed Webb's work on lymphocytosis but gave credit for the original discovery that lymphocytes multiply at high elevations to a German Swiss physiologist by the name of Stäubli, whose findings the Davos men "thoroughly corroborated" with statistics of their own.

Gerald was dismayed. Was he to be involved in one of those disputes about prior discovery that dot the history of science?

He had read Stäubli's article when it appeared in a German journal in 1910 but had dismissed it as merely confirmation, on the basis of a small number of scattered observations, of his own discovery announced a year earlier. Now he replied promptly to Turban, pointing out the error, enclosing reprints of his 1909 reports to document it, and asking the doctor to make sure that Baer and Engelsmann corrected it. They never did.

On his own behalf Gerald began broadcasting the tale at conventions and in correspondence and asked friends who were editors of American medical journals to do all they could to make the true facts known. And whenever possible in speeches and papers he made occasion to cite his own relevant articles with dates, including always the one he had published abroad, the summary in the *Transactions* of the Royal Society.

All in vain. Nationalism was especially rampant in medical science at the time, keeping the French and the Germans, the disciples of Pasteur and those of Koch, jabbing jealously at each other and for the most part sniffing contempt at the laggard Americans. The Germans were not about to credit any other national with a discovery when they could plausibly assign it to one of their own.

The only European who ever cited the American Webb as the discoverer of the lymphocyte-altitude correlation was, not surprisingly, Albert Calmette of the Pasteur Institute in Paris.

After a while Gerald gave up pursuit of the credit he knew was his. Henry Sewall told him he might as well forget about it and get on with his work, as Sewall had done in the affair of his snake-venom antitoxin. A few years back Sewall had got a letter from somebody telling him of a German scientist who was publishing a book praising the American's work, but Sewall had lost the letter and could not remember the men's names. What did it matter? They both had better things to do than worry about what the Germans thought.

Meanwhile Edward Trudeau and his staff in the Adirondacks were urging the Webb team to expand their work with lymphocytosis in high places. Dr. E. R. Baldwin, Trudeau's second in command, made public the excitement felt at Saranac when he called the attention of the NTA to the promise and importance of Webb's findings. "I hope he and his associates will undertake a large-scale study and give us more facts."

Dr. Webb was willing to oblige, but not with much of his own time. Accumulating experience was making it clear that differentiating among white cells and especially among lymphocytes was trickier than it had seemed. Just before moving to Denver, Dr. Williams, in reporting the results of five hundred studies of white cells he had made in the Webb Laboratory, lamented the "chaotic state of affairs" and "contradictory conclusions" he had found in medical writings about classifying white cells.

A valid response to Baldwin's hope, then, seemed to call for Dr. Gilbert's special gift for taking pains, so Webb asked Gilbert to plan and supervise the new study, assigned him a team of two recuperating physician-patients plus one of Edward Schneider's graduate students, secured the cooperation of Dr. T. W. Hastings of Cornell University medical school, and sent Gilbert to New York to work out with Hastings' assistant Dr. Carolyn Rosenberg the identical methods to be used at both ends of the project.

The comparative findings from 100 Cornell students and 100 Colorado College students, all males, were reported by Doctors Staines, James, and Rosenberg in the *Archives of Internal Medicine* in 1914. Theirs was the most precise work and concise report to come as yet from Webb's laboratory, but the end results differed little from Webb's and Williams's earlier data: the Gilbert-Hastings team found the large lymphocytes in the circulating blood of early morning to number from 20 to 30 percent more in Colorado Springs than in New York.

Dr. Webb's curiosity had turned meanwhile to blood platelets. These are tiny pear-shaped floating bodies whose origin and function were still a mystery. It seemed to Gerald that they became more numerous in the presence of tuberculosis. Might they play some part in the immunity process?

Off and on for three years the laboratory team again counted endlessly: platelets at sea level, platelets in Colorado Springs, platelets in guinea pigs, in healthy humans, in tuberculous patients. Again they inoculated dozens of rabbits and guinea pigs, with virulent tubercle bacilli, with blood platelets, with the two mixed.

Dr. Webb summarized it all by telling his brethren in the NTA that the number of blood platelets did increase in tuberculous blood, and platelets like lymphocytes proliferated at high altitudes. He thought injecting platelets along with bacilli retarded the onset of infection. And he suggested that blood platelets contained opsonin which they released as they disintegrated.

That suggestion was an acknowledged echo of the man who more than any other determined the bias of Webb's research in these years: the man of flashing hunches, Elie Metchnikoff.

The flamboyant Russian, forced to flee his homeland by an egregious misadventure in his Odessa laboratory, was continuing his studies and disputes as subdirector of the Pasteur Institute in Paris. In 1908 he, along with Paul Ehrlich, was awarded the Nobel Prize for his work on immunity. This honor invested his thoughts and theories, set forth in his historic book *Immunity and Infectious Diseases*, with uncommon authority among groping immunologists.

Forced by the work of Almroth Wright to accept the existence and importance of antibodies, Metchnikoff ingeniously found a way to subordinate them to his cherished phagocytes. He announced "as a law" that antibodies are produced by the leucocytes, that they are elaborated within these cells and are set free into the blood serum only when the white cells themselves disintegrate.

Webb and Gilbert were not venturing implausibly far afield, then, when they suggested that platelets too might release antibodies when they die. Frequent references and quotations in

Webb's papers and letters show that he and his colleagues accepted as gospel the "laws" of immunity laid down by Metchnikoff.

All this while Gerald was continuing his efforts to induce immunity by graduated doses of live tubercle bacilli. He resumed those experiments in 1909, feeling ever more certain that no use of killed organisms would do better than Koch had done with tuberculin.

He explained his convictions to a New York physician: "I work with the live germs because no satisfactory immunity has ever been produced by the dead ones. The way I look at it, if a man wishes to win a prize fight he does not rely upon the development and dexterity he obtains by hitting a punching bag. He practises with a prize fighter. The punching bag is tuberculin and the prize fighter is the living bacillus."

But luck was not with him. Setting up an elaborate experiment with one hundred guinea pigs newly bought at a dollar apiece, he quickly lost almost the entire lot to successive sweeps of enteritis. It was little comfort that none of the dead animals showed any signs of tuberculosis at autopsy.

Of the two guinea pigs that survived the epidemic one was killed by a stray dog which Varina was befriending, leaving a single subject to receive in continued inoculations over a period of nine months a cumulative dose of some 42,000 bacilli. Remaining healthy and frisky, this guinea pig became a pet of the laboratory. "We named him Mithridates," Gerald told Arnold Klebs, "after the celebrated King of Pontus who made himself invulnerable to poison by taking repeated small doses."

Gerald was jubilant when for Christmas in 1910 an anonymous grateful patient gave him money to buy rhesus monkeys from a New York dealer—two successive lots of them, twenty-four in all. Monkeys were notoriously susceptible to tuberculosis; they ought to provide a real test of his live-germ theory. He did not have enough of them to expend any in establishing the minimum infective dose of bacilli, so—to the consternation of both Klebs and Trudeau— he guessed at it: if it took just twenty of his bacilli to infect a guinea pig it would probably take only a hundred or so to make a monkey sick.

The inoculations were proceeding smoothly when in the summer of 1911 disaster struck. Someone carelessly set the thermostat of the incubator too high and overnight all Webb's cultures, diligently kept going on an egg medium for years, literally cooked to death.

Webb and Gilbert immediately set about replacing them, by isolating new strains from tuberculous patients and by securing established strains from Saranac and elsewhere, but they could never find one of the same mild virulence. The nearest they came was a strain of which only ten would infect a guinea pig, too virulent to permit immunization by even the 1-2-3 sequence of doses. And most of the strains proved infuriatingly unstable, gaining or losing strength unpredictably, sometimes in the middle of an experiment.

Gerald was painfully embarrassed when he had to confess this "tragedy," as he called it—for example, to Hans Zinsser who, wanting to stock his new laboratory at Stanford University, wrote to ask for a culture of Webb's well-known strain. And to Edward Trudeau, who had once warned Webb that he must make allowance for varying virulence.

"I have learned my lesson about putting all my eggs in one basket," Gerald wrote Trudeau. Maybe, he came to think, the fluctuating virulence of tubercle bacilli was more important than their waxy overcoats in their resistance to vaccines. And later still he began to wonder whether maybe a guinea pig is not always a guinea pig; maybe they too vary significantly in their resistance.*

His monkeys did eventually give him the laugh on Trudeau. He continued inoculating them with the now more virulent strains until the number of bacilli injected in a dose rose into the high hundreds, in two animals to a cumulative total of half a million. Periodically he killed two or three monkeys and subjected their bodies and organs to all the accepted tests for tuberculosis. When the inoculated animals continued to show no evidence of infection, he felt he could safely call them immunized.

Edward Trudeau, following all this with skeptical interest, finally suggested that Webb put his surviving monkeys to an infallible test: inject each of them with a whopping dose of 100,000 bacilli all at once. If they still remained free of tuberculosis, one could be sure they had been truly immunized.

Gerald thought he knew of an equally effective test, one that could be doubly useful. He had learned that Dr. Herbert Fox, curator of the Philadelphia Zoo, was desperate for monkeys because he was losing them to tuberculosis as fast as the Zoo could buy

---

*Medical scientists today know there are several kinds of tubercle bacilli. They no longer speak of the tubercle bacillus as a single organism.

them. Early in 1913 Gerald shipped off his last two inoculated monkeys to do public service at the Zoo. Two years later Curator Fox wrote him that they were still alive and healthy.

Trudeau was loath to believe it. "I had half a dozen monkeys in the laboratory here once," he wrote Webb, "and they all developed tuberculosis fast and died of it before we could do any inoculating at all."

A thoughtful observer of Dr. Webb's work with the monkeys was one of his tuberculous patients, John Romanes, the son of George John Romanes, the English biologist who as an intimate friend of Charles Darwin had ranked second only to Thomas Huxley in popularizing Darwin's theories and who had endowed the distinguished Romanes Lecture at Oxford University.

The younger Romanes, a man of about Gerald's age, was himself a considerable scholar, "well posted in medical science." He was dying of tuberculosis and knew it. His Scottish wife also had the disease. They were worried about their two small sons, one aged three, the other nine months, neither infected as yet but both surely in grave danger. After watching the experiments in the Webb laboratory, Romanes one day asked Dr. Webb to inoculate these toddlers as he was inoculating the monkeys.

Gerald hesitated. He had been administering his graduated doses to severely tuberculous adults, forty of them, all volunteers, with marked benefit in some cases he thought, but dare he risk the experiment on uninfected children?

Well, what harm could it do? He would be introducing fewer bacilli into their bodies than they were probably inhaling daily from their environment. So he agreed to Romanes's request and began weekly inoculations of both children, using bacilli of relatively mild virulence and a cautiously slow gradation: 1-3-5-8 and on up to 150. He stopped at the thirteenth week and a cumulative total of 607 bacilli.

"I wouldn't think of doing that," commented Trudeau; "it's too risky, the benefit much too uncertain."

"Yes, it gave me many anxious days and nights," replied Webb. But he could add that the two little boys were free of infection six months later when, after their father's death, their mother took them back to Scotland. (Several years later Dr. Webb on a trip to Edinburgh went out of his way to visit the Romanes boys and was reassured to find them still untouched by tuberculosis.)

Gerald was emboldened to repeat his Romanes experiment on half a dozen other children who were living at a similar high risk of infection. All went well with the first five and he happily included them in the reports he was writing. Then matters went awry with the sixth; tubercular lesions appeared at the site of injection and in the axillary gland of the armpit.

Much alarmed, Gerald immediately removed the lesions and kept the child under close observation for more than a year. Telling the story in a letter to Arnold Klebs, he concluded, "I am happy to say this child is probably the best vaccinated person in the world today."

But the experience was sobering, daunting. Gerald felt he could never again inoculate either child or adult with living bacilli unless he could find a way to make such inoculation safe.

As a chance stab toward this end, he and Gilbert tried injecting guinea pigs with a mixture of blood platelets and tubercle bacilli. When this seemed to delay a little the onset of infection, Gerald thought hopefully again of his lymphocytes; maybe this was the way to make effective use of those defensive cells.

In repeated experiments he and Gilbert combined lymphocytes with tubercle bacilli, incubated the mixture briefly, then injected it into fifteen guinea pigs, at the same time inoculating eight control pigs with bacilli alone. It did not work. The lymphocytes did not diminish one whit the virulence of the bacilli; "the extent of infection was practically the same in both sets of pigs."

With this failure, reported in 1915, Gerald Webb ruefully abandoned his personal efforts to achieve immunity, either with lymphocytes or with graduated doses of live bacilli.

In later life, when reviewing his research for the author of an article in the *Journal of the Outdoor Life*, he said he had given up the inoculation of living virulent germs "as too dangerous for humans." But he said goodbye to lymphocytes with a profession of continued faith in them: "Each year we have been more and more impressed with the important part played by the lymphocytes in nature's defense against tuberculosis."

With that statement by Dr. Webb, according to Dr. David W. Talmage in his presidential address to the American Association of Immunologists in 1979, the word *lymphocyte* disappeared from the vocabulary of immunologists for more than thirty years. It did not appear in the *Journal of Immunology*, established in 1916, until

1948, when a young virologist, in unknowing echo of Dr. Webb's observations on whooping cough, reported that lymphocytosis occurs in the presence of viruses.

During the three succeeding decades an explosion of renewed attention, new theories, new techniques, and new discoveries made lymphocytes a predominant interest of immunologists, who by the mid-1970s had learned that these supposedly aimless "wandering" white cells are in fact the disciplined parents, patrolmen, messengers, warriors, and overall bosses—"the mastermind"—of the body's astonishing immune system, without which no one of us, nor our species, could survive in the sea of microbes that surrounds us. Unfortunately, Dr. Webb did not live to witness this vindication of his belief in the defensive role of lymphocytes.

Gerald Webb was no stranger to the disappointment he felt on giving up his personal quest for immunity to tuberculosis. For all his enthusiasm and the optimism of his public utterances he had frequently felt discouraged about his research, disheartened by its uncertain results. He knew in low moments that he was making no real headway, was amassing no sure proof of his theories. Once he confessed to Arnold Klebs, "We keep on running our heads against stone walls and reporting our bruises." And another time to Dr. Lewis Hamman, one of his friends at Johns Hopkins, "We are floundering about over our heads in several directions."

He was well aware too that he was moving against the contemporary thrust of the anti-tuberculosis movement. The NTA in these years had time for no more than a tolerant nod at research; it was wholly preoccupied with its elaborate programs of public education toward improving personal and public hygiene.

Dr. Webb did not object to these, he did his bit for them by giving lectures and writing articles for laymen, but to his professional colleagues he kept insisting that hygiene was not enough, that like smallpox, tuberculosis would never be conquered without an effective vaccine against it. He clung to Pasteur's assurance, and Almroth Wright's, that vaccines could free man from infectious diseases.

Few were so firm in this faith. It was attacked with vigor about 1913 under the banner of Dr. Victor C. Vaughan, bacteriologist turned biochemist and longtime dean of the University of Michigan medical school. After studying with Robert Koch in Berlin, Vaughan had established at Michigan one of the earliest university laboratories for the teaching of bacteriology. His subsequent research led him into preoccupation with "ferments" (i.e. enzymes), whose action he came to consider more important than antibodies in producing immunity.

He enunciated a "biological law" that when a cell is invaded by a foreign protein (e.g. a bacterium) the cell produces a ferment by which the alien protein is destroyed. From this law he derived the principle that since all vaccines contain a harmful bacterial protein such vaccines ought not to be used in prevention or therapy.

Vaughan's voice carried authority in American medicine and when in 1913 he published his theories of the chemistry of immunity in a book, *Protein Split Products in Relation to Immunity and Disease*, his disciples grew in number and in fervor. Gerald Webb was shaken by the storm.

Dr. Albert P. Francine of Philadelphia, in preparing to review Vaughan's book at a meeting of the faculty of the University of Pennsylvania medical school, wrote to ask Dr. Webb what counterarguments he as a well-known advocate of vaccines could offer.

"Are we still to consider opsonins an important factor in immunity?" Francine asked. "In view of Vaughan's studies, isn't the action of antibodies overshadowed by the much more powerful action of ferments? Don't you agree that we ought to give up the harmful use of tuberculins?"

Gerald replied with an admission of confusion: "I confess that your questions are beyond my depth. I have been reading Vaughan's book too, and cannot say that I know where I am now." He went on to restate the doctrine of phagocytosis stimulated by antibodies but for this transient moment could call it only "seeming" facts.

He was no more confused than immunologists generally were at the time. Their research was moving more or less blindly in all directions. The cellular immunology of Metchnikoff was going into decline, wrestled off center stage by the humoral school, the serologists, whose gradual elucidation of many mysteries in immunochemistry would dominate the field for decades.

Such matters were not only beyond Gerald Webb's scientific depth, they were remote from his predilections and convictions. His research had always been clinical rather than basic, directly aimed at finding a way to prevent tuberculosis or at least to improve the treatment of it. Now his interest was caught by new modes of therapy and his investigations centered on ways of immobilizing the diseased lungs.

What kept him going at research, when it was such a drain on his time and resources, caused him such frustration and fatigue?

He enjoyed it, for one thing. He liked the search for solutions to problems and puzzles. He liked the attitudes and concerns, the ambience, of the laboratory. Free to choose he would have spent his life in that milieu. Forced instead to engage in what an eighteenth-century predecessor called "the eternal chase after the damned guinea," he found diversion, escape from "the clamor of patients," in what Pasteur described as "the serene peace of laboratories and libraries."

He also believed in research, without reservation. Henry Sewall, Almroth Wright, and much reading had seen to that. He subscribed with the whole of heart and mind to the statement by Edward Trudeau with which this chapter began: only research could clear away the vast unknowns about disease and healing.

And he thought research offered the surest route to the high standing among his peers that he craved. Barely out of medical school in Denver he had told Mater that making some original discovery was the quickest way to fame, and over succeeding years he said again and again, "The greatest prize in medicine today is finding a way to immunize mankind against tuberculosis."

He wanted that prize with every cell of his being. He did not win it—but neither did anyone else. Calmette and Guérin came close with their BCG, as we shall see, and now, in 1983, it seems likely to be won by a research scientist working in the laboratory that memorializes Dr. Webb.

Since Webb could spare only limited time from his practice and since both Williams and Gilbert had better technical training than he, one is bound to wonder how much of the research reported under their joint names was actually Webb's.

Clearly, most of it. Dr. Webb was, beyond dispute, the creative and directing member of the team; he was also involved in every aspect of its work, down to surprisingly small and routine details. He was compulsively scrupulous about giving due public credit not only to Williams and Gilbert but to every transient assistant who worked on a project. He did not add his name to Clarence Lieb's report in 1909 although he made all the arrangements for its publication, nor to Williams's account of white cell studies in 1910 or the Gilbert-Hastings report on lymphocytosis in 1914.

Necessarily, most of the technical chores in the laboratory were done or supervised by Williams or Gilbert, but that the ideas were Webb's is certain from scattered evidence as to where and when and how he got them. His was the imaginative and resourceful mind that conceived the projects and solved the problems that arose about the equipment and methods.

Neither Williams nor Gilbert produced anything original on his own. The few single-author papers they published—Williams mostly, after his move to Denver—are merely technical reports of experiments done to try out some new diagnostic test or some therapeutic method or agent.

It was Webb who went to the many annual conventions of medical societies and listened to the endless papers and discussions, Webb who carried on a medical dialogue in extensive correspondence and exchange of reprints, Webb who did the diligent reading of medical journals and remembered what he had read when it could be useful. In 1912 he was subscribing personally to nineteen medical journals, seven of them American, six German, three French, and three British. He thought them essential because, as he told Trudeau, "Working alone here, it is so easy to get one's mind too much in a groove."

There can be no doubt either about who wrote the succession of joint reports. Webb's personal, discursive style, studded with literary quotations and allusions, is unmistakable, as are, in their individual papers, Gilbert's no-nonsense, almost cryptic concision and Williams's labored addiction to statistics.

And in his letters Webb was forever apologizing to a distant friend for some social sin of omission on a recent trip because he had been busy "patching together my scraps" for his paper. This piecing together was as likely to take place after as before the public presentation; Gerald habitually spoke *ad lib* from scattered notes or a brief outline, a few of which survive among his papers.

He was a trial to journal editors. More than one of them, confused or annoyed by the jumbled lists of emendations arriving from Colorado Springs, tried to explain that Dr. Webb could wait to submit a manuscript until his experiments were finished, his findings complete, instead of sending in a preliminary draft followed by a stream of updated additions and revisions. Gerald would apologize contritely for the extra trouble he caused, but he rarely managed to achieve a tidy *Finis*.

He added to editorial problems by being a pioneer in visual aids.

He liked to show lantern slides of charts and graphs to illustrate his reports, and arranging reproduction of these for publication was as yet an unfamiliar task for journal staffs.

After one such paper, on lymphocytosis, Dr. Myer Solis-Cohen of Philadelphia wrote to say he had been much impressed by Webb's presentation and to ask how his slides were prepared.

"I made those lantern slides myself," Dr. Webb replied, "using a Very pen dipped in India ink. I felt rather ashamed of them but am glad they pleased you. Any art store can cut the glass for you and doing the ruling and lettering is easy."

It may have been the journal editors who as the years went by tightened up Webb's style, made it, to the regret of a biographer, less personal and narrative, more coldly "scientific." On the other hand, Gerald himself, like his generation as a whole, became increasingly aware of what was scientifically acceptable. He soon dropped from his bibliography his early papers on syphilis, ingrown toenails, and the like, suggesting why he did so when he told a midwestern physician who requested a reprint of his article on Graves' disease, "I'm afraid it isn't very scientific."

He retained his characteristic use of analogy and metaphor, of anecdote and quotation, in the lectures and essays he wrote for the wider lay audience. Many of these were published in the NTA's *Journal of the Outdoor Life*, where they still make good reading. For instance, one he wrote on "Tuberculosis Carriers," the Typhoid Marys of consumption. He took the subject back to Pasteur's healthy guinea pigs that were spreading chicken cholera through his flocks, then found an analogy immediately at hand:

"Near me as I write is a coniferous forest. On many of the trees grows a parasite, the pine-tree mistletoe.

"Many trees are dead, others withering away as a result of the parasitic growth. Others, which may be designated 'mistletoe carriers,' are magnificent specimens, not in the least handicapped by the mistletoe they support, yet acting as hosts from which the parasite can send forth its seeds to other trees.

"The aim of all parasites is to perpetuate their species. They must not only have access to their victims but also egress from them. The ideal situation they can create for themselves, therefore, is the 'carrier,' a host which cannot destroy them but from which they can escape to other victims. Should all victims of tuberculosis die with the parasite inside them, there would be no more tuberculosis. . . .

"It cannot be denied that one result of the modern crusade against consumption has been to create an increasing number of tuberculosis carriers, and so from the microbes' viewpoint the campaign has been pro-tuberculosis. What chance have our children, who can be infected by only a few hundred bacilli, if they are exposed to an unrecognized tuberculosis carrier who can expectorate millions of bacilli a day?"

He found grist everywhere. One day on a trip to New York he dropped into the NTA headquarters for a chat with Livingston Farrand, executive secretary of the association and temporarily the editor of *Outdoor Life*. Farrand was in a fret; the printer's deadline for the next issue of the journal was upon him and he lacked copy enough to fill its pages. Gerald offered to write a piece on the spot, sat down at a vacated desk, and in an hour or so produced the needed copy.

He used familiar material—familiar to him but not to lay readers —about the waxy defense of the tubercle bacillus but added a new comparison with certain prairie shrubs that coat their stems with sticky wax to ward off predators.

Arnold Klebs, commenting on the interest and "erudition" of the piece, asked with a hint of skepticism, "Where did you learn about those remarkable prairie shrubs? Have you seen them?"

"No," answered Gerald. "I read about them in a government report on Agriculture."

Dr. Ronald J. Glasser, in his engrossing account of the immune system in *The Body Is the Hero*, published in 1975, pays tribute to the influential "immunologic insights of Bordet, Fleming, Zinsser, and Webb." Gerald Webb would have been justly gratified to find himself in such a company.

Jules Bordet was a brilliant Belgian scientist who, although he had studied with Koch and worked under Metchnikoff at the Pasteur Institute in Paris, chose for himself the pathway of Ehrlich into the mysteries of blood chemistry. The original discovery for which he was awarded the Nobel Prize in 1919 was the explanation of how the serum proteins he called alexin and we today call complement work with antibodies to destroy bacteria. Bordet knew there were at least three units of complement, we know there are nine; when in a fraction of a second they are all activated in sequence by an antibody, they literally blow a bacterium full of holes.

Alexander Fleming is known to the public for his discovery of the penicillin mold but for more than a decade before that lucky accident he had been urging, against the stubborn resistance of Almroth Wright, that there had to be more to the processes of immunity than the internal activities of phagocytes and serum factors, that the body had to have some defense *in all its parts* or else the microbes would have knocked out mankind long ago. He finally in the early 1920s found such a killer of bacteria in things like nasal mucous, saliva, and teardrops. He called it lysozyme; we have named it Immunoglobulin A, IgA for short. It stands guard along all the moist open channels into the body which blood cells and serum cannot protect.

Hans Zinsser became widely known as a teacher of immunology (finally at Harvard), as the author of important textbooks as well as the popular *Rats, Lice, and History*, and as an investigator of typhus in the field and of blood components in the laboratory. But more important, in 1925 he had the wit to see and courage to say that all the bits and pieces being discovered about the mechanisms of immunity were not antagonistic findings, not either-ors to be squabbled about, but instead were all parts of a single multilayered immune system. Some of those parts and almost everything about how they all work, separately and together, were unknown, even unimagined, at that time but Zinsser's insight offered a direction and pattern for subsequent thinking in immunology.

And Gerald Webb? What entitles him to a place in Dr. Glasser's quartet?

First, through his extensive practice and correspondence, his articles and addresses, he did more than any other single person to spread the gospel of vaccination among American physicians. And if we just imagine the horrors and terrors and devastated lives that have attended and still attend epidemic infections, we must recognize vaccination as one of medicine's greatest benefactions.

The recent eradication of smallpox from the earth is demonstration enough that Dr. Webb did well to preach so aggressively his faith that "With microbial vaccines we can rid mankind of infectious diseases." We can, if we will.

More specifically, Webb's idea of vaccinating with small doses of living virulent germs was considered a viable option for decades. It became a topic for discussion at meetings of medical societies all over the country. It was taken up enthusiastically not only by Doctors E. R. Baldwin, Lawrason Brown, and Allen Krause at the Trudeau Laboratory but by the great Theobald Smith, who carried approving word of it to Germany, impelling several German investigators to write Dr. Webb asking for reprints of his papers about it.

From that train of diffusion came the advocacy of Dr. H. Selter, a German immunologist who made a career of developing a live-germ vaccine à la Webb and who in the mid-1920s called Webb's work to witness in his spirited attack upon the competitive vaccine produced by the Frenchmen Calmette and Guérin. Calmette himself used Webb's small graduated doses in his experiments but his Bacillus Calmette-Guérin (the now widely used BCG) was an attenuated strain. (Of this more later.)

Hans Zinsser in his textbook *Infection and Resistance* published in 1914 described Webb's live-germ vaccination at length as an alternative to the use of dead bacteria or attentuated strains and retained it as such through half a dozen revisions, though in the edition of 1939, having come to the conclusion Webb had reached twenty-five years before, he recommended the method for use only in animal experimentation and never, never in treating human beings.

Second, Webb's long and intense preoccupation with those awesome lymphocytes can, from the viewpoint of the 1980s, be accounted a true immunologic insight. Dr. David Talmage has testified that "Webb's early research on the white blood cell is recognized by scientists throughout the world as the basis for many subsequent discoveries."

Not that his theories and findings about lymphocytes had enduring validity. The importance of any relationship between lymphocytosis and high altitude vanished as tuberculosis therapy turned from climate and open-air living to bedrest and various surgical procedures, then to effective new drugs. All his efforts to induce lymphocytosis by hyperemia were based on a false premise endorsed by the Scottish expert Dickson; lymphocytes do not multiply by division in the bone marrow (except when stimulated by antibody), nor do they die like other white cells; it seems we may be born with a lifetime's supply of them neatly stockpiled in the lymph nodes to await our need of them. And now that immunologists know how and why "rejection" takes place, it is clear why Webb's attempts to immunize with inoculations of alien lymphocytes were certain to fail.

Research must creep before it runs, stagger before it marches. Pioneers in a new field cannot be fairly judged on the basis of knowledge acquired after their time.

Dr. Webb's deepest insight was his prophetic perception of the vast potential of immunology itself. In the early years of the century when enormously more was unknown than known about it he kept saying, "The doctor of the future will be an immunologist."

Rarely has a prophecy come so true. Dr. Glasser described the state of medicine six decades later thus: "Medically speaking, we are living today in the age of immunology. The great majority of articles in the leading medical journals, the most discussed topic at great research symposiums, the main section of specialty boards in both medicine and pediatrics, the overwhelming thrust of all contemporary research and concern, indeed of all modern medical thought, are immunological."

X

The Blue Ribbon

"IT'S ONLY a nuisance now," Gerald said when late in 1909 he was nominated for the presidency of the El Paso County Medical Society the following year. A decade before, when he was elected secretary of the society, he had wanted the higher office badly as a rung up on his career. Now it would only interfere with his research.

He was elected unanimously—because if he were not, he told the nominating committee, he would not accept the post. He was riding his high horse again.

Earlier in the year Arnold Klebs had referred a westering patient to Webb but when the man arrived in Colorado Springs the friends with whom he was to live persuaded him to try their doctor instead, Dr. Charles Fox Gardiner. A few weeks later Klebs wrote that Dr. Gardiner had told the man Webb was a charlatan and a liar, that he had never studied medicine at Guy's Hospital as he claimed.

"Of course, I don't believe a word of this," said Klebs, "but I thought you ought to know what is being said."

Gerald was annoyed. He thought he had stilled those "poisonous slanders" from Gardiner. He wrote again for refutation from the registrar and Mr. Dunn at Guy's and told Klebs he would send him copies of their replies. "A lie will run miles while truth is putting on its boots. Fox is a good name for that man."

Hence Gerald's demand for a unanimous vote from the county's doctors. He was thin-skinned about Gardiner's charge because it came too close to truth; he knew his study of *medicine* at Guy's had been brief.

If there was jealousy on the part of Springs doctors other than Gardiner, Gerald and Varina (she was surely involved) did nothing to allay it by the lavish banquet they gave the society members to inaugurate Gerald's year as president. They really splurged.

The local *Gazette* said it was the most elaborate social function in the history of the city, that its cost had come close to a thousand dollars. The manager of the Antlers Hotel, gleeful at having such an opportunity, imported from New York the motif of the season there and in Paris: *jardin des fleurs.*

The sixty-nine guests dined sumptuously on oysters, pheasant, and venison as if in the showy garden of a large estate. Rows of vine-clad pillars suggested the verandahs of a southern mansion. Garlands of fresh red roses and carnations festooned the walls and gates of make-believe pathways and wreathed the miniature fountains that burbled on the tables to serve as coolers for the bottles of wine and champagne. Outsiders were allowed into the room before and after the banquet to view the splendors the Webbs had provided.

It was incidental that Dr. Webb addressed the meeting on "Pasteur and Lister."

Webb had already begun the yearly travels by which he hoped to counteract his isolation. The national medical societies scheduled their annual gatherings in leisurely sequence during May and June to permit members to attend a succession of conventions in a pleasant social round. In between meetings the doctors lunched and dined with friends, watched other doctors at work in their hospitals or sanatoriums, gave lectures to local medical societies, went sightseeing. Mingling in hotels and on trains, they got to know one another, formed friendships, and were welded ever more firmly into a professional fraternity.

Gerald Webb appreciated the value of all this and began early to participate. Every year he was on the road for several weeks in the spring, zigzagging from place to place in the appointed section of the country to report his latest research and renew and extend his web of acquaintance and friendship. Eventually he took a similar jaunt in the fall as well, arranging it usually around some speaking engagement as focus.

In 1911 the NTA held its seventh annual meeting in Denver, with a concluding day's session in Colorado Springs, which Gerald had arranged the year before as president of the local society. From the Springs most of the men went on together to the AMA meeting in Los Angeles.

This was an exhilarating time for Webb. The papers he read at the two meetings were well received. The presiding dignitary in Denver was the twinkling, amiable William Henry Welch; the president chosen to succeed him was Gerald's good friend Mazÿck Ravenel; the new vice-president was a Colorado colleague, G. Walter Holden, director of the Agnes Phipps Memorial Sanatorium in Denver. And Gerald himself was elected to a five-year term as a director of the NTA. He was in! And not yet forty.

The visitors clearly enjoyed themselves in Colorado Springs and, to judge from the letters they wrote Gerald afterward, gave equal place as highlights of the day to Webb's inoculated monkeys and the Garden of the Gods.

On the train to Los Angeles Gerald met for the first time Dr. William J. Mayo, the older of the two famous Minnesota brothers, and Dr. George Crile of Cleveland, one of the Mayos' chief rivals in goiter surgery, both of whom sent him patients from time to time thereafter. And he got acquainted with Dr. John B. Murphy, the brainy, blunt-spoken Chicago surgeon, a controversial innovator and gadfly who had invented the Murphy button, a revolutionary device for snapping tight shut the severed ends of the gut in intestinal surgery.

Murphy, who became president of the AMA in Los Angeles, was mightily taken with Webb. He had already sent him a few patients on the basis of his reputation in vaccine therapy; after meeting him he dispatched a stream of cases to Colorado Springs. Gerald reciprocated with referrals for surgery, many a jolly visit to Murphy's operating room, and gifts such as a pair of the arm garters he contrived for inducing lymphocytosis. He was often amused, sometimes moved to helpless laughter, by Murphy's tirades.

On this trip too Gerald began his close and lifelong friendship with Dr. James Alexander Miller of New York City, who had been reelected a director of the NTA.

Three years younger than Webb and a Princeton graduate who had taken his medical degree at Columbia, Miller had been a patient, then assistant and protégé of Edward Trudeau. He was now professor of medicine at the College of Physicians and Surgeons, a consulting physician in charge of the tuberculosis wards at Bellevue and Presbyterian hospitals, and an active trustee for a score of charitable organizations, including the Trudeau Sanatorium. Handsome and suave, a man of substantial means and social standing, Miller was nonetheless a serious and superior clinician. The mutual respect between him and Webb grew deep and lasting.

Gerald added trips to New Mexico and Minnesota that fall.

New Mexico, still a territory a year away from statehood, shared in the custom of health-seekers and had several respectable sanatoriums catering to the tuberculous. Dr. Webb served on the advisory boards of the two in the Gila Mountains near Silver City, the Sunnyside Sanatorium of Dr. LeRoy S. Peters and the New Mexico Cottage Sanatorium of Dr. Earl S. Bullock. It was "Bully" who asked him to address the convention of the New Mexico Medical Society in September. Knowing the ingrown nature of his audience, Webb gave them an elementary lesson on immunity—and they promptly elected him an honorary member of their society.

These New Mexican colleagues became troublesome after a while. They were all true believers in climate therapy for tuberculosis and when acceptance of this credo began to decline nationwide, they sought to bolster it by organizing southwestern doctors into a society committed to promoting it. They wanted Dr. Webb to join the society and lead it. "We need you," wrote Dr. Peters; "we must have you with us if we are to succeed."

Dr. Webb refused their petition, pleading as excuse that his research kept him too busy but suggesting his real reason when he warned several members of the group that their advocacy of climate must not be merely emotional and anecdotal, that it must be based on scientific findings if it was to be effective.

The trip to Minnesota was of a different order. Mrs. Leila Shields, a family friend as well as patient, was badly in need of gynecologic surgery. Making arrangements for Dr. John B. Murphy to do the operation in Chicago, Gerald was embarrassed when he had to cancel the appointment because Mrs. Shields balked. She was terrified at having "to submit to the knife" and equally at the thought of a strange man's using it. So Gerald took her instead to the Mayo Clinic where gynecology was the province of a gifted woman, Dr. Leda Stacy.

All went well and while Mrs. Shields recuperated Dr. Webb was free to join the scores of visiting physicians for whom the Mayo operating rooms were a recognized school in the new surgery. His most gratifying experience, though, was a long talk with Dr. Henry Plummer, the genius among the Mayo partners, "a queer fellow," not a surgeon but sure and flashing quick in clinical diagnosis.

The Seventh International Congress on Tuberculosis, supposed to convene in Rome in 1911, was postponed to the spring of the following year and Gerald had about decided he could not afford time or money to attend it when in February came a letter from NTA President Ravenel appointing him the U.S. Clinical Representative to the Congress. All right, thank you, he would go, but what would be his duties? Just to be a gracious guest and give a public lecture on American tuberculosis research.

"But what am I to say in *my* address?" added Ravenel. "I've got out of touch with immunity studies. Can you tell me what's been going on? Send me any suggestions you have as to what I should say."

Gerald's answer was merely to dispatch to Wisconsin a bundle of reprints of his own published papers—with the result that Ravenel's presidential address to the NTA that year was largely a laudatory review of Webb's research.

Gerald had already tentatively accepted invitations to speak that spring to the Chicago Medical Society, where he had become a favorite guest, and to the Laënnec Society in Baltimore. The latter was an organization of Johns Hopkins medical faculty and students who met once a month to hear and discuss papers by distinguished authorities on respiratory disease. Gerald's friend Dr. Lewis Hamman, head of the Johns Hopkins University Hospital, was in charge of the Laënnec programs for the year and offered Webb the honor of being one of the speakers.

No sooner had Gerald, after many letters back and forth, got his several dates set in convenient sequence than he thought he would have to cancel them all. He fell ill. Just a bothersome little cold, he thought at first, then acute bronchitis, then laryngitis. The physician could not seem to heal himself. Trying to do too much for too long had caught up with him. Not until a week before his first engagement did he feel able to tell his hosts yes, he would be on hand as scheduled.

On 20 March he spoke to the Chicago society, then spent a day in its library and another with Dr. Murphy; on 25 March he played the visiting lion for Dr. Hamman in Baltimore; on 28 March he sailed from New York for Europe with Livingston Farrand and his wife aboard the *Ivernia*.

He made things a bit easier for himself by using virtually the same speech throughout the trip, varying it only to fit the audience on each occasion. As published in the *Johns Hopkins Hospital Bulletin* it was long and impressive. "Studies in Tuberculosis" he called it, and he used it to state with force his mature ideas on tuberculosis research and to summarize in historical context the several series of experiments he had undertaken in Colorado Springs.

On the train up to New York Gerald found himself traveling with the philanthropist Henry Phipps, who was using the fortune he had made with Andrew Carnegie in steel to support munificently the Henry Phipps Research Institute in Philadelphia, dedicated from its beginning in 1903 to the extermination of tuberculosis. Phipps had made the journey to Baltimore solely to attend the Laënnec Society meeting, at which William Henry Welch introduced him to Gerald Webb.

What Phipps and Webb talked about on the train we may infer from the delivery next morning to Gerald's hotel room of a copy of Vallery-Radot's *Life of Pasteur*, the recently published translation from the French that William Osler said "reads like a fairy tale," plus a check for one thousand dollars in support of Webb's research, both gifts from Henry Phipps.

When the passengers on the *Ivernia* proved to be mostly wealthy old ladies, some embarrassingly flirtatious, others boringly voluble, Gerald escaped into the pages of his new book—and subsequently went about urging everyone to read Vallery-Radot on Pasteur. Nine months later he wrote Phipps that he had loaned his copy of the biography to a restless patient, who was so entranced by its story and so wholly converted by it to the worth of scientific research that he donated another thousand dollars to Webb's work.

Some unspecified delay made Webb and the Farrands two days late in reaching Rome, so that they missed the general audience which Pope Pius X granted to the delegates and were honored with a private audience all their own. Gerald confessed he found it "awe-inspiring."

At the grand reception in the Quirinal given for the delegates by King Humberto (Humbert II) and his Queen, Gerald was impressed only by the number of "flunkeys" in splendored livery who scurried about everywhere in the palace; he thought there must be two of them for every guest.

The dominant topics of discussion at this Congress were clinical: heliotherapy (treatment by sunlight) and artificial pneumothorax (collapse of the diseased lung by introducing gas into the chest cavity). Gerald had intended to go on to Vienna after the Congress but its discussions changed his mind. He stayed on in Rome a few days to watch Forlanini, the Italian surgeon who had invented pneumothorax, carry out the procedure, then set off on an extensive tour of Swiss sanatoriums. At Davos he made the acquaintance of Dr. Karl Turban—without learning about the unpleasant surprise Turban's assistants Baer and Englesmann were preparing for him. He stayed longest in Leysin to witness Rollier's use of sunlight to cure tuberculosis of bones and joints.

A quick journey to Paris gave him a day with Metchnikoff at the Pasteur Institute but this was a disappointment. The lively old lion, aged sixty-seven now, had done with twisting facts to support his theories of immunity; he had turned his impulsive illogic loose upon two new sciences, one of old age which he named gerontology, the other of death which he called thanatology. Neither was of much interest to Webb.

He next cut back to Frankfurt-am-Main for a longer stay, his first, with the merry, mercurial German Paul Ehrlich at the Institute for Experimental Therapy. He felt at home in Ehrlich's untidy office, where stacks of books and papers piled higgledy-piggledy on every surface left not even a chair to sit on and where the air was a reeking fog of smoke from the chemist's endless cigars.

Gerald counted it worth the entire trip when he won from Ehrlich the promise to send him for use in Colorado Springs a goodly supply of salvarsan, "606," the new "magic bullet" against syphilis which it was almost impossible to buy because Ehrlich was zealously guarding it from misuse by incompetent practitioners.

Crossing the Channel for a quick visit to his family in Cheltenham, Gerald spent a day in London with Sir Almroth Wright and Alexander Fleming and another day in Oxford delivering to John Scott Haldane the manuscript of his Appendix to the Royal Society report of the Anglo-American Expedition to Pikes Peak. He did not get back to Colorado Springs until early June.

One thing he had not made time for on his trip was a visit to Arnold and Harriet Klebs. Two years earlier Arnold had abandoned what he called "the hustle and bustle" of America, moved to Switzerland, and shifted from medical practice to collecting books and writing medical history. His home—first Montolivet in Ouchy, then Las Terrasses in Nyon—had become a favorite European way station for his many medical friends. He and Gerald had maintained their intensive correspondence and he kept urging Gerald to come see them. At last he was coming.

When he did not appear and they received his excuses from Colorado Springs, Arnold was hurt and angry. "I am still sore at you for passing us by," he wrote Gerald that fall from Washington where he was attending a conference on demography. "We shan't have any more time to visit you now than you could spare for us when you were in Switzerland."

Why *did* Gerald skip the Klebses on this trip? No more than Arnold can we accept his excuse that he was too hurried, too tightly booked; he found ample time for what he wanted to do.

There had been a few minor disagreements between the two men, mostly over the index to Arnold's big book which Arnold had compiled and Gerald thought inadequate. And a mutual friend had told Gerald that Arnold said a doctor in active practice could not expect to achieve anything worthwhile in research and ought not to try it. This would have irritated Gerald, but was hardly enough to weigh against all that Klebs had done for him.

Varina may have influenced Gerald's attitude. Although as far as we know she never met Arnold she is said to have developed a strong dislike of him, to have decided he was too conceited, too glib and flippant, to be trustworthy.

In later years Gerald tended to blame Klebs's unguarded tongue for his prior discovery problem. He had written Arnold in great excitement about his hunch that lymphocytosis occurs when altitude rises, had even asked Arnold's help in finding any earlier suggestion of the idea in the literature, and he came to feel certain that Klebs in his characteristic garrulity had spread word of it in Switzerland, thus putting Stäubli, Baer, and Engelsmann on the track of it. Whether or not this suspicion was justified, it could not have influenced Gerald's behavior in 1912, more than a year before he was aware of the problem.

The breach was real. It was papered over in a year or two and the men saw and wrote each other sporadically throughout their lives, but their friendship never regained its former strength and warmth.

Questions may have been asked about how Gerald Webb could act as United States representative to the Rome Congress when he was still a British citizen, or his own conscience may have been troubled by the anomaly. Whatever the prod, a few months after his return home he reactivated his long-dormant application for American citizenship and was awarded his naturalization papers on 16 December 1912. He was thereafter a more concerned patriot, more actively interested in American traditions and monuments, than many a native-born son of the nation.

The long European trip was travel enough for that year. Besides, Gerald owed Dr. Gilbert, who had been looking after his patients all this while, a rest and in September sent him off for a month's vacation at Thomasville, not far from Gerald's and Varina's favorite resort at Woods Lake.

The next spring Gerald felt obliged to forgo the NTA meeting in May because Varina was due to be delivered of another child that month, but he spent most of April in Chicago and New York — investigating the value of "the Friedmann cure," one of the medical nine-day-wonders of the time — and in June he went north to Minneapolis for the AMA convention.

There on 19 June 1913 Dr. Webb participated in the birth and christening of a new medical society, the American Association of Immunologists, and was elected its first president.

The idea of such a society had come to Dr. Martin J. Synnott of Montclair, New Jersey, the year before. Synnott like Webb was a former student in the Praed Street laboratories and a devoted disciple of Sir Almroth Wright. He decided that organizing the American and Canadian doctors who had studied with Wright into a "Society of Vaccine Therapists" would be of benefit to them all. Among those whose opinion and support he sought was of course Gerald Webb.

Webb was uneasy about Synnott's proposal; he saw serious flaws in it. It was too narrowly focused, too restrictive; surely it ought to include research men as well as therapists. And it left no room for shifting directions as knowledge expanded — no room for the future.

Gerald knew that Wright's theories and methods were already under scientific attack in Europe, so widely that London wags had dubbed the great man Sir "Almost" Wright, and in America it looked as though vaccine therapy might be retreating into shadow behind the glitter of Victor Vaughan's and the serologists' chemistry. Who knew what tomorrow's dominant practice and theory would be? If Synnott's society was to survive and be useful beyond the immediate present it must have a wider compass, more flexibility; there must be more stretch in it.

So Webb suggested to Synnott that eligibility for membership in the society be broadened to include men who had studied with the likes of Koch, Metchnikoff, and Ehrlich as well as Wright's students, and that the organization be called the American Association of Immunologists. Synnott agreed.

From "vaccine therapists" to "immunologists"! Quite a transfiguration!

Where had Webb got his word *immunologists*?

For convenience I have been using *immunology* and *immunologist* anachronistically. As far as the makers of the Oxford English Dictionary can determine, *immunology* did not come into existence until 1910 when it was coined to translate the word *Immunitätslehre* in the title of a German book. Its first discovered use in medical discourse was in the *Journal of the AMA* in 1911 as the title of an article in defense of animal experimentation written by Dr. Frederick Gay of the University of California, a former pupil and colleague of Jules Bordet at the Pasteur Institute. Dr. Webb, who knew Gay, read the article and recognized the usefulness of the noun. From *immunology* to *immunologist* was no step at all.

Dr. David Talmage, president of the AAI in 1979, thinks it likely that Webb's choice of the word for the society's name, which led to its use three years later in the title of the society's official organ the *Journal of Immunology*, was responsible for its coming into common usage to designate the vital new branch of medical science. Hans Zinsser did not use *immunology* in his textbook on the subject in 1914; "science of immunity" was his term throughout. But Victor Vaughan was using it in his *Journal of Laboratory and Clinical Medicine* in 1916.

At the first meeting of the AAI Doctors Webb and Synnott both quoted Sir Almroth Wright as saying, "The doctor of the future will be an immunologist." But they were wrong.

What Wright said, on the title pages of his books, was "The doctor of the future will be an *immunisator*." A clumsy word, from such a master of languages. Nor did he mean by it "an immunologist." So expansive a concept was beyond Wright's thinking, as Alexander Fleming learned again and again to his frustration. Wright meant "an immunizer," "an inoculator," i.e. a vaccine therapist — no more than that. Gerald Webb was using the word *immunisator* in this sense in his papers in 1911. It was he who during the succeeding two years discerned the farther horizons implied by *immunologist*.

The "Objects" of the AAI as stated on its first letterhead in 1913 were more of a compromise than its name with Synnott's original idea: "To unite the physicians of the United States and Canada who are engaged in the scientific study of immunity and bacterial therapy. To study the problems of immunology, and to promote by concerted efforts scientific research in this department. To spread a correct knowledge of vaccine therapy and immunology among general practitioners."

The AAI had collected sixty charter members by the time of its first annual meeting in Atlantic City on 22 June 1914. Dr. Webb presided and Dr. Synnott as secretary-treasurer jubilantly summarized the inception of the society, predicting that it would become "one of the most important medical organizations on this continent." As indeed it has.

Aside from Victor C. Vaughan none of the speakers at this first meeting was notably science-minded. Webb's effort to recruit charter members may be surmised from the presence of Dr. T. W. Hastings of Cornell, Dr. Lewis Hamman of Johns Hopkins, Dr. William Whitridge Williams of Denver (who characteristically read a paper on the technique and reliability of the Abderhalden test for pregnancy), and Dr. George Burton Gilbert of Colorado Springs.

Perhaps because of Vaughan's presence the papers and discussions were about evenly divided between vaccine therapy and his protein ferments—and among cancer, arthritis, and tuberculosis. When tuberculin came under attack Webb was firm: no one, he said, could work with Wright in his St. Mary's clinic and not be convinced that tuberculin could be effective. And he stubbornly held the ground for antibodies.

He must have won Vaughan's respect despite their disagreement, for two years later Vaughan named him an associate editor of the *Journal of Laboratory and Clinical Medicine* of which Vaughan was editor-in-chief. Webb became the only member of the nine-man editorial board who was not a professor of medicine in a university. Among his editorial colleagues were Hans Zinsser and Frederick Gay.

Dr. Webb's presidential address on the "History of Immunity" was an exercise in diplomacy, distributing good words for everybody—except the drug houses, which he castigated for advertising to physicians their dangerous "phylacogens" for use in vaccinations. He paid tribute to immunologists from Jenner and Pasteur down to "the brilliant work of Victor Vaughan," with the puzzling exception of Metchnikoff. Had the great Russian gone so quickly into eclipse?

Dr. Webb was reelected for a second term and was in the chair again at the second annual meeting of the AAI in Washington on 10 May 1915. Going once more to history for his second presidential address, he spoke on "Pasteur," pleading in justification that "immunologists cannot hear too much or too often of this, their greatest master." What he chose to point out about the master reveals much of Webb himself.

Pasteur was fortunate, he said, in having "a reserved father of slow and careful mind," a mother "full of enthusiasm and imagination," a wife "who was willing that the laboratory should be put before everything else." The great man "rarely visited a theater or went out socially, feeling like the philosopher who said 'I am never bored except when I am being entertained.' He read only good books, especially selected biographies. He advised students to 'Worship great men.'"

In a timely reference, Europe being then nine months into the Great War, Webb quoted Pasteur's lament during the Franco-Prussian War: "I cannot concentrate on my work. This war has sent my brains to grass. Might and right struggle for the world; right which constitutes and preserves society; might which overcomes nations and bleeds them to death."

The tilt at this second meeting was all the way toward vaccine therapy. Webb and Gilbert described their efforts to immunize with mixtures of lymphocytes and tubercle bacilli, but the two dominant topics were narrowly clinical: the difficulties of administering the Wassermann test for syphilis, and the use of vaccines to alleviate hay fever.

Dr. Webb participated with some asperity in the discussion of the latter subject. Vaccination could not be expected to succeed in hay fever, he said, if doctors always assumed the offending pollen came from grasses; other plants could cause it. In his experience the allergy often derived from cottonwood trees. And one must always watch out for a dangerous anaphylactic response. One of his laboratory workers had caused him great alarm by going into a near fatal reaction to inoculation with cottonwood pollen.

He added that he thought it a reproach to the medical profession that doctors could do so little for the common cold. He suggested that vaccines helped so rarely in this affliction because the colds were not caused by the bacteria thought to be at fault; he had heard recently that these colds, and perhaps grippe and influenza too, might be caused by filter passers (i.e. viruses), in which case vaccines were not the remedy.

On the whole Dr. Webb might have thought at this meeting of the AAI that he had wandered instead into a session of some state medical society. He could hardly have emerged feeling sanguine about the association's prospects.

He secured publication of the proceedings of his two meetings in the *Medical Record*, of which his perennial correspondent Dr. George Mannheimer of New York City was editor, and joined Dr. Synnott and others in establishing the *Journal of Immunology* the following year, but he was glad to turn over the presidential reins to Dr. J. W. Jobling of the Vanderbilt School of Medicine in Nashville. Although he remained a member of the AAI for many years, he had nothing to do with its affairs thereafter.

Dr. Webb was truly an itinerant that year of 1915. Before the AAI meeting he had gone to address state medical societies in Wisconsin, Kansas, and Louisiana and made the rounds for ten days in New York City. After the meeting he gave himself a vacation jaunt to Cuba and Panama. In June he set off westward to read papers at the NTA meeting in Seattle and the AMA meeting in San Francisco. And in December he made a two-week tour of sanatoriums in southern California, Arizona, and New Mexico.

On his mind all the while was a nagging concern about his pending nomination for what he considered "the blue ribbon in American medicine."

On the way home from the AAI meeting in Atlantic City in 1914 he had ridden part of the way with Dr. Joseph L. Miller of Chicago, editor of the *Archives of Internal Medicine*, who had been one of the first easterners to refer patients to Webb for vaccine therapy. Three of Dr. Miller's tuberculous patients were now under Dr. Webb's care in Colorado Springs, and as the train rolled toward Chicago the two men discussed the possibility that one of the three had also a fungus infection. Dr. Miller said not one word of what he had done at the convention of the Association of American Physicians from which he was returning. Extraordinary, exemplary restraint.

For the next day Gerald received a note from Henry Sewall,

newly elected president of the Association, telling him that Dr. Miller had nominated him for membership at the recent meeting.

In response to Gerald's note of humble thanks Dr. Miller said he had been "only partly responsible" for the nomination, and Gerald told Varina he was sure he owed the honor principally to the influence of Dr. Sewall.

An honor it undoubtedly was. The Association of American Physicians was an elite body, its membership limited to 150 carefully selected physicians and medical scientists. According to William Henry Welch, one of its founders in 1886 and its president in 1901, it grew out of the mediocrity that prevailed in medical practice, education, and organization in the 1880s. Its founders hoped "to create a society without medical politics, where no one cared who the officers were and where one would find fellow workers in medicine and pathology capable of intelligently understanding and discussing the papers presented and from whom one could learn."

Membership in the Association was still, said Welch in 1927, "the high ambition of aspiring young clinicians and pathologists" in spite of all the specialized medical societies that had come into being. It was certainly "the high ambition" of Gerald Webb in the 1910s.

Perhaps he valued it too highly, so that he felt himself unworthy of this "blue ribbon," for he did an astonishingly bad job of selling himself when Dr. Miller asked him to write out his qualifications for submission to the secretary of the Association. He responded with only a haphazard and meager list of his published articles — without a single accompanying word about his laboratory or his research or anything else he had done. Dr. Miller had to write a second time to extract even minimal information about his education and study abroad.

It may have been in medical education that Gerald feared he would be found wanting. He wrote, significantly, "I became a medical student at the age of 19. Cheltenham General Hospital 1890. Guy's Hospital, London, Oct. 1891 to Dec. 1894. University of Denver, 1895 to graduation in 1896. Winner of class prize in medicine."

He made no mention of his licentiate in dentistry at Guy's. For study abroad he listed his five months' "Special Courses" in Vienna first, his three months in Wright's laboratory second. He said nothing of his presidency of the American Association of Immunologists though he did report his directorship in the NTA. Perhaps he thought the great men in the Association of American Physicians would look askance at much emphasis on Wright and vaccine therapy.

They did take their time in scrutinizing his nomination; he was left without word about it for nearly two years. But on 10 May 1916 he jubilantly wrote his brother Frank from Atlantic City, "Today I was elected to membership in the Association of American Physicians, the most exclusive medical body in the United States."

He was actually elected to associate membership, a routine sort of probationary status. As he teasingly explained to Varina, "This means that if in five years I 'prove good' I become a full member, so you see I shall have to read medical journals at night!!"

It was anticlimax for Gerald when in October of that same year he was granted membership also in the American Climatological Association.* Years before, when he was consumed with jealousy of Dr. Edwin Solly who shone in "the Climatological," Webb coveted this membership; now his enthusiasm was muted. The society's members were too socially elitist, its meetings too frivolous, for his mature taste. The jokes passed around to raucous laughter at its gatherings he thought vulgar and unfunny; "they're not for your ears," he told Varina.

His first participation in a meeting of the Association of American Physicians came the following year, again in Atlantic City. A letter to Varina tells the story:

"Such a feast of medical wisdom should certainly last me a year. Your blown egg with the shell shattered is the way my brain felt after three days of medical papers from 9 a.m. to midnight. The meetings have been at Hotel Traymore, the most magnificent hotel here. It is a mile away from the Chelsea [where he was staying] so I have walked to it and back three times a day so as to give my brain a rest at meal times. I had no paper to give but took part in one discussion, showing lantern slides, and received many expressions of satisfaction from the wise men later. All the Rockefeller, Johns Hopkins, Harvard etc men are here and it is fine to come in contact

---

*This society kept changing its name to keep up with shifting emphases in medicine. In the 1920s it became the American Climatological and Clinical Association. In the 1930s it reversed the adjectives to become the American Clinical and Climatological Association. Its journal was never one of Dr. Webb's favorite outlets for his papers.

with these intellects even if it makes you feel like a grain of sand."

That grain of sand again! In time the "intellects" would elect the "grain of sand" their president.

The Association meetings were as usual concentrated interludes in rounds of social doings, some professional in purpose, others for Gerald's personal pleasure.

The biggest such personal event of his spring trip in 1916 was an invitation to dinner at Sagamore Hill, the famous home of Theodore Roosevelt near Oyster Bay on Long Island. Gerald scurried around New York City half a day hunting a large portrait photograph of the former president which he took along for Roosevelt to autograph for the Webb ménage.

He was awed by the site of the storied house, which sat in splendid isolation on the very top of the hill, overlooking on one side the waters of the bay and Long Island Sound and on the other verdant meadows and belts of woodland clothed in what Roosevelt called "the blossom-spray of spring." He told Varina of the few special moments when he stood in silence with his host on the piazza of Sagamore Hill and watched "the sun sink away beyond the imposing stretches of darkening waters."

He found "the Colonel" in vigorous form, "cussing at the Kaiser and the Germans," Gerald wrote his brother Frank, and at President Wilson for whose shilly-shallying about the war he felt fiery contempt. "I asked him if he had heard of the Wilson tango: one step forward, one step back; hesitation, side step. He told me that when the war was young the Kaiser sent one of his attachés from Washington to remind Roosevelt of the good times they had shared at Potsdam, etc. Roosevelt said 'Yes, he recalled them with great pleasure and he also recalled the good times he had had with Albert in Belgium!' He is in daily communication with your European crowned heads and gave me a letter to read that had come that day from one of your kings."

The two-year-old war was on everyone's mind and lips during this trip. Argument was fierce as to whether or not the United States should enter the conflict. Gerald had no doubt that it should and was impatient at its delay.

In Washington he spent three hours one day sitting in Congress listening to the House debate on preparedness: "it was painful." At the Surgeon General's Library he ran into Arnold Klebs and went home with him for lunch. Arnold and Harriet were living in Washington for the duration of the war, but Arnold was strongly pro-German and outspokenly bitter about the Allies, giving Gerald another painful time.

Invited to dinner, casually he thought, by the mother of one of his patients, he found himself instead at a large and formal party from which all the guests were going on afterward to a fund-raising gala for British Relief. He was "amazed" by their attitude: "They are all more pro-ally than the English themselves."

But at dinner the next night his hostess, Mrs. Richard Townsend, the cousin of another patient, was defiantly loyal to her friend Count von Bernstorff, the German ambassador. "None of the other ladies of Washington will be friends with her because they all ostracize Von Bernstorff. She has a magnificent home, like a palace. I have dined before with one footman behind each chair but she had two! There were so many flunkeys in the house it reminded me of my visit to the King and Queen of Italy at the Quirinal in Rome!!"

At dinner another night with the Braden Kyles to recall his and Dr. Kyle's days as fellow students in Wright's laboratory, he met Margaret Wilson, the President's daughter. "She is a most delightful girl and a real live one. At one-twenty in the morning she brought me home in one of the White House cars, so I felt I was 'very near' the President!!"

One morning he walked from his hotel, the Shoreham, with Dr. Farrand to see "the new Lincoln monument—impressive," then "went on a pilgrimage as a true American citizen to Mt. Vernon and came back by boat. Wonderful and delightful. This is such a very beautiful time of year to be in Washington and the city is going to be in 20 years the most beautiful in the world."

Returning to New York, before taking the train for home he spent a day at the Rockefeller Institute, where he was pleased to find "Smillie," who had worked with Clarence Lieb in the Webb Laboratory, doing well as an assistant to the chief Simon Flexner, and where he played chess again with Hideyo Noguchi, the eminent Japanese bacteriologist on the senior Institute staff. They had last played when Noguchi was Webb's guest in Colorado Springs.

That was in September 1914. Livingston Farrand had been installed as president of the University of Colorado in June of that year and, eager to establish a closer relationship between the state's doctors and the university, he sought to spark up the meeting of the state medical society in Boulder that fall. Wanting to secure a distinguished speaker for the banquet session, he thought of Noguchi, who was much in the medical news at the time for his exhaustive study of spirochetes and the improvement he had made in smallpox vaccine.

But Farrand was unwilling himself to approach Noguchi. The scientist—an Oriental who had learned he must make his way in Occidental society, as he usually closed his letters, "with bent neck" —was notoriously difficult, an unstable mixture of arrogance and obsequious humility. Personal communication with him was so awkward that even his colleagues at the Institute preferred to avoid dealing with him. Farrand, knowing that Gerald Webb was one of the few persons Noguchi got on with, asked Webb to persuade the man to come to Boulder.

Gerald was soon wondering why he had agreed to do so. Noguchi found a repetitive succession of questions to ask before he finally accepted the invitation to Boulder and to visit Webb in Colorado Springs on the way, and then it took letter upon letter to explain to his satisfaction the travel and fee arrangements. To the last minute Gerald, as he warned Farrand, was not sure Noguchi would appear where and when he was supposed to.

He did, and he told Farrand he had enjoyed his stay in Colorado Springs and thought highly of Webb's efforts to immunize with live bacilli. But Gerald knew that what pleased Noguchi most was the chess they played. Noguchi was addicted to the game but was such an impulsive and excitable player that he could rarely find a willing opponent outside his family.

Chess diverted Webb again on his spring trip in 1917. At the Manhattan Chess Club in New York he was one of ten or so men chosen to play an exhibition match with the French champion Janowski and another with the American champion Marshall. He played them both to a draw.

The United States had declared war against Germany on 6 April, just as Gerald was leaving Colorado Springs, and he witnessed the first flush of romantic patriotism on every hand. "You never saw so many and such huge flags as are flying everywhere here," he wrote Varina. "Everything in the East seems well-organized, just waiting for Congress to get through talking. At Dr. Miller's house for dinner the other night I met a munitions manufacturer who told us lots of interesting things about what's going on in Russia. I went to

TB Association headquarters to ask if there is anything I can do. The shortage of doctors on the other side worries me. I hope lots of young ones will go from this side."

He went one afternoon to check up on Laura Gilpin, the daughter of his Springs friend Frank Gilpin, who had shifted from managing the Broadmoor Casino to handcrafting fine furniture, pieces of which have become treasured heirlooms in old Springs families. Laura, in her mid-twenties, was now a student of photography in New York and her father was uneasy about her. Gerald was able to reassure him that Laura was healthy and happy. "She has a comfortable apartment and enjoys her life here. It is amazing how cheaply she and the other girls can live."

But they could afford few extras, so Gerald took Laura and a friend to see the first-night performance by the great English actor-manager Sir Herbert Beerbohm Tree in his final role as the principal in *Colonel Newcombe*. "Tree's performance was grand and the Colonel's toast to the British Navy brought down the house."

Across the aisle was a Springs family friend, Mrs. Frenaye, who provided the thrill of the evening for young Laura by introducing Gerald and his guests to her own guest, Ethel Barrymore. In time Laura Gilpin was the source of just such thrills for others. She had starch as well as great talent; though she long knew hardship and struggle she became one of America's truly distinguished photographers.

"I sometimes think New York is a suburb of Colorado Springs," Gerald told Varina. Having a quick lunch with Dr. Miller, he found at the next table Amelia Scudder, who insisted he have dinner with her, and waving greetings from across the restaurant was Mrs. George Stebbins, a Springs patient who was stopping over in Gotham on her way to Seal Harbor for the summer. She invited him to dinner to meet an English kinsman, Dr. Henry Drysdale Dakin, well-known at the time for his antiseptic Dakin's solution which Dr. Alexis Carrel, Rockefeller Institute surgeon and Nobel laureate in 1912, was using to blessed effect in the treatment of wounds on the European battlefields.

Gerald turned gossip in writing Varina about Dr. Dakin. He was becoming an American citizen, said Gerald, because he had married the rich widow of Dr. Christian A. Herter, a biochemist who, having inherited a fortune from his interior decorator father, had main-

tained an elaborately fitted laboratory on the top floor of his palatial New York home. "Dakin inherits the laboratory with the widow," wrote Gerald.

He had promised Varina he would not linger long in New York
but would go quickly on to Atlantic City for "a long lazy loaf" before the meeting of the Association of American Physicians, so he
grew increasingly defensive as his stay stretched from a few days
into two weeks. From New York he went to Boston for a day's observation of Dr. Richard Cabot in his pathology laboratory at the
Massachusetts General Hospital. Dr. Cabot had begun publishing
his postmortem findings the year before; Gerald was a charter sub-
scriber and he and Varina read the grisly reports together.

Setting off finally for Atlantic City he stopped overnight at Princeton "to visit the renowned Dr. Theobald Smith in charge of the
Rockefeller Institute Animal Research Center near there. I learned
much wisdom from him. He is the biggest man in research probably in any country today, is of the Pasteur-Koch-Ehrlich type."

Also visiting Smith was Dr. T. W. Hastings of Cornell. To extend
this chance meeting over the weekend, Dr. Hastings and his wife
drove Gerald on to Atlantic City—through a drab New Jersey
countryside "of once painted wooden houses all now badly in need
of paint."

Settled at the Chelsea for ten days of loafing, Gerald grew restless.
The weather was "raw and cold," Atlantic City was "decidedly
shoddy in many spots," and the Chelsea was full of the same kind
of old ladies he had encountered on the *Ivernia*: "it's an old ladies
home from which I see no hope of rescue."

He escaped again into a book, this time "a thrilling and most
satisfying life of Florence Nightingale." He went for daily eight-mile
hikes along the boardwalk and took lessons in a sport new to him,
trapshooting. "I'm getting so lazy I don't think I'll be able to go
back to work again." After a week he was joined on his boardwalk
treks by another physician come for a rest, Dr. William S. Thayer,
physician-in-chief at the Johns Hopkins University Hospital.

After the brain-fagging Physicians' meeting Gerald went south
to North Carolina for a short visit to Dr. Charles Minor's sanatorium in Asheville, turned westward to Nashville for the NTA convention, then on to Memphis to address the doctors of Tennessee.

He whipped up a storm in Memphis. Looking in on the municipal tuberculosis hospital, he was so appalled by what he found there that he lashed out at the town's citizens and officials with unaccustomed lack of restraint.

How dare they consign human beings to such a "black hole of misery"? Did they expect anyone to get well in such "a place of desolation and neglect"? People could only go there to die. It would be better for them not to have a hospital at all. Nor could they put the blame onto the hospital's nurses; these women were doing their best "under the shameful conditions"; they showed "heroic courage" even to try to work in such "a dreadful place."

The city's newspapers gave columns of space to this arraignment "by a nationally known tuberculosis expert" and followed up, under such headlines as "Black Hole in Memphis Must Go," with columns more of their own castigation of the local government. "People are talking about nothing but the hospital since Dr. Webb's stinging indictment," said the *Commercial Advertiser*. "The politicians are uneasy."

Dr. Webb left them to it. Having vented his outrage he departed for home, after nearly two months of "butterfly existence" and "dormouse life" on the road.

Gerald always said he disliked all this traveling, that he was lonesome and homesick away from his family, that the long trips exhausted him and he was in need of recuperation when he got back home. All his "strenuous lunchings and dinings" were "necessary for the sake of the practice," he told Varina.

We may wonder how much salt to shake on these plaints. Gerald Webb was so much a traveler all his life that he must have found his journeys more satisfying than not. He certainly enjoyed seeing the sights, visiting museums, going to the theater, looking up old friends.

But there is no doubt that he always kept his eye firmly on the ball. He did not shirk attendance at convention sessions or visits to centers of medical progress. He did not let the medical leaders forget him or new developments escape his personal witnessing. Through his travels as well as his research and papers and correspondence he built and maintained a network of professional contacts that brought him recognition and reputation — and a growing practice in referred patients.

At the Chelsea in 1917 he seriously considered heading for home right after the Physicians' meeting. Would it really matter if he skipped the NTA convention this year and said no to the speech in Memphis? But in the end he kept both engagements. "If I go to Memphis I may as well go to Nashville on the way," he wrote Varina, "and I ought to go to Memphis for business and Cragmor reasons. We ought to get more patients from that section than we do."

XI

The Clamor of Patients

DR. EDWIN SOLLY could not savor the fruit of his ambition to build the grandest of sanatoriums in Colorado Springs; his plans had been too often and too far pared down from the elegant Sun Palace with which he and Thomas MacLaren had started. The community had responded to his pleas for funds with little more than talk.

When at last Cragmor Sanatorium was built the number of its rooms had been cut from 100 to 24; its massive central block had dwindled to what Gerald Webb called a cottage; its sweeping wings had been slimmed into plain two-storied "pavilions" housing just eight persons each; its clustered individual cabins were reduced to only a scattered eight, its cost scaled down from Solly's grandiose $350,000 to about $40,000. But each room retained its large open sleeping porch and the immediately surrounding acres were beautified with gardens and walkways.

Shortly after Cragmor opened its doors to patients on 20 June 1905, Dr. Solly collapsed into "neurasthenia," exhausted by his prolonged struggle with bankers and contractors and undoubtedly by his frustration and disappointment. He sought recovery eventually in Asheville, North Carolina, where he died at the age of sixty-one on 19 November 1906.

Colorado Springs eulogized and mourned its long-time mover and shaker, then quickly forgot him—and Cragmor too. With no one really to care or take effective charge, the sanatorium went literally to ruin. The patients moved elsewhere, the buildings became the prey of vandals and looters, the gardens and grounds grew back to weeds.

After a while the bankers woke up to the appalling deterioration of the property and prodded the trustees to do something about it. So they ordered the necessary repair and refurnishing of the buildings and persuaded a troika of local doctors to reopen and run the sanatorium: Will Howard Swan, Henry C. Hoagland, and Charles Fox Gardiner.

Gerald Webb did not approve. He told William Otis, who still owned land near Cragmor, that he had advised against this arrangement because he did not think the sanatorium could succeed without an experienced manager in residence, that as a mere adjunct to private city practices it was sure to fail.

He did not tell Otis that Dr. Swan was the only one of the medical threesome whose professional competence he respected. He had no love for Dr. Gardiner of course, was quite blind to the man's virtues. He thought Gardiner's insistence that tuberculosis victims live outdoors day and night at any temperature and in any kind of weather was fanatical and cruel.

Dr. Hoagland merely amused him: Henry must have been well trained at the University of Pennsylvania but he treated tuberculous patients like foie gras geese in France, grossly force-feeding them in the absurd notion that enormous weight gain alone would cure them. And Henry was so vain! In a sickroom, Gerald said to Clarence Lieb, he spent more time viewing himself from all angles in the mirror than in examining the patient.

But Dr. Swan was an able physician whom Gerald respected and sometimes called in consultation on puzzling cases. Swan paid little attention to medical squabbles and not much more to advancing medical science, but he gave his patients wise and devoted care. Always congenial and courteously pleasant company, Swan was nonetheless a loner, preferring to roam the mountainside in solitude rather than chatter and imbibe at social gatherings.

Gerald's prediction about Cragmor came true. The triumvirate soon found their sanatorium responsibilities a distraction and a financial burden. To keep Cragmor's beds occupied they had to transfer their private patients to "the san" and forgo their fees, since the weekly charge for a Cragmor room included the physician's care. By the early spring of 1910 the doctors, and the trustees too, were ready to quit their venture. Cragmor was offered for sale.

Addison Hayes now took charge of the situation. Cragmor must not be allowed to close again; it was potentially too big an asset for Colorado Springs. And he thought it would be a fine gift for his son-in-law.

But Gerald thought otherwise. He remained convinced that the physician-in-charge must live at Cragmor, which he had no desire to do. Nor did he want to give up his flourishing practice or exchange his research for sanatorium management. Besides, he knew his limitations; he was the least likely person to undertake the orderly running of any enterprise or the inevitable haggling over financial details. He couldn't even keep his own office tidy or be firm about the collection of his own bills.

But he did want Cragmor to grow and prosper and himself to be a part of it. The Trudeau model of sanatorium cum laboratory was again on his mind. If they could find the right person to take over the sanatorium it would be a great stride toward realizing his dream of Colorado Springs as the Saranac Lake of the West.

He thought he might know that right person: Dr. Alexius M. Forster, the young medal winner he had met at the International Congress in Washington in 1908.

Alexius Forster was another of the Johns Hopkins medical graduates whose careers had been interrupted by the onset of tuberculosis. He had betaken himself to Saranac Lake, where as his illness diminished he earned his keep as one of Trudeau's assistants and began to learn the basics of running a sanatorium. Upon his return to Baltimore he was given a junior teaching post at Johns Hopkins and named superintendent of Eudowood Sanatorium, one of the oldest in the United States, located at Towson near Baltimore.

At Eudowood Dr. Forster, becoming interested in the problems of convalescents, conceived and developed a "farm colony" in which patients worked in the fields and gardens when they were able as an aid to their rehabilitation as well as to the sanatorium's budget. The spectacular success of this program won Forster his honors at the International Congress and also a growing national reputation as clones of his colony sprang up across the country.

Forster, now twenty-nine years old, of medium height and slender build, mustachioed, endowed with dark good looks and an engaging manner, had just left Baltimore for a post as sanatorium superintendent in Louisville, Kentucky. Going to Colorado Springs for an anti-tuberculosis conference sponsored by the NTA in 1909, he had paid a visit to Dr. Webb, who took him on a tour of the city's sanatoriums including Cragmor. When the two met again at the NTA convention in May 1910 Gerald was abrim with enthusiasm about the prospects for Cragmor.

Forster should buy it, he urged; with his experience he could make it a great success. Forster ruefully replied that sanatorium men were not paid enough to let them buy anything beyond necessities. That need be no problem, said Webb; Mr. Hayes and his friends would buy the place and Forster could pay them back as the sanatorium prospered.

Dismissing the idea as just a friendly gesture on Webb's part, Forster forgot all about it as he plunged into his new work in Louisville. He was astonished when a month later he received a laconic telegram: "Cragmor is yours. G.B.W."

Well! What made Webb so sure he wanted it? He considered his opportunities to be good, his future assured, in Louisville. Why should he move to Colorado?

On second thought, Colorado Springs was a world-famous resort for the tuberculous and Dr. Webb was becoming a well-known authority on the disease. Cragmor might indeed have exceptional possibilities. What terms were they offering?

Dr. Forster took the next train to Colorado Springs, where he learned that on Dr. Webb's recommendation Cragmor had been bought in the expectation that he would come out and take charge of it.

Dr. Webb told what happened in a letter of 22 June 1910 to William Otis:

"Cragmor, on which forty-three thousand dollars actual cash was expended we were able to pick up for seven thousand. Joel Hayes, Leila Shields, Helen Morley, and Dr. Bill Williams made up the pool [suggesting that it was as much Gerald Webb as Addison Hayes who tapped his friends for funds]....I have learned from my travels to European and Eastern sanatoria that the success of such an institution depends on the man who is in charge. Dr. Forster is just such a man and Dr. Trudeau told me in Saranac Lake last November that he considers the career of Dr. Forster in sanatorium work the most remarkable he has seen. Dr. Forster came out here last Sunday week and looked over the situation and promised to pay 7% interest on an invested amount of not more than ten thousand before taking any salary himself. We need another two thousand to put the place in repair and to meet the first two or three months running expenses. Mr. Hayes said I should tell you that the nine thousand invested would be treated as preferred stock....I do hope you will be able to help us in the next two or three months."

Mr. Otis obliged.

Dr. Forster secured Cragmor, then, by promising to pay 7 percent interest on invested capital of $9,000. The newspapers said he bought it for $50,000. Somebody was making the story better by adding the initial $43,000 to the actual resale price. Dr. Forster was in no financial position to assume the larger indebtedness.

Feeling honor-bound to stay on at his Louisville job until a successor could be found, Forster did not enter upon his commitment to Cragmor until September. During the interim the sanatorium was the responsibility of Doctors Webb and Williams and it made them hustle. It may have been the hectic pace of those weeks, and perhaps the prospect of added bedside duties at Cragmor, that gave Bill Williams the final push into private laboratory practice in Denver.

Although Gerald wrote to several friends in the East seeking a replacement for Williams, he began to see that he had at hand the man he wanted. His convalescent patient Dr. George Burton Gilbert had found part-time work on the staff at Cragmor, and as Gerald watched him tend the patients he saw that Gilbert was very good indeed. Certainly his training at Johns Hopkins could not be bettered. Why look further?

Dr. Gilbert joined him in practice in November 1910 and became his full legal partner in October 1914. The two men worked harmoniously and affectionately together for more than thirty years.

In one of the Cragmor beds in 1910 Dr. Webb found a young man of twenty-seven years who especially stirred his compassion and soon won his respect and affection. Here truly was "an intellect in splints."

James Johnston Waring, born in Savannah, Georgia, had graduated from Yale, then moved to Johns Hopkins for training in medicine. During his third year there he contracted tuberculosis. A year at the Trudeau Sanatorium did him no good; he remembered it as a time of great anxiety, misery, and self-pity—"I was one of the damndest psychoneurotics ever." When he arrived in Colorado Springs he was so dreadfully ill he had to be carried from the train on a stretcher. He was taken to Cragmor where Will Swan became his doctor. Now he was safely on the road to recovery.

Dr. Lewis Hamman later told Webb that Jim Waring was the most promising student he had seen in all his years at the Hopkins.

Waring was a warm and friendly person, intelligent, witty, a constant and ranging reader, and when he was well a "compleat angler." From William Osler and Harvey Cushing at Johns Hopkins he had caught an absorbing interest in medical history and a lifelong devotion to Leewenhoek, "the father of microbiology." Webb and Waring, kindred spirits from their first encounter, fell into the habit of long companionable talks and fed each other's intellectual interests.

When Waring was able to leave Cragmor two years later he decided to remain in Colorado and resumed his medical studies at the University of Colorado medical school in Denver, where he received his medical degree in 1913. Dr. Webb then found work for him with Dr. Walter Holden at the Agnes Phipps Memorial Sanatorium and recommended him for a post as assistant to Dr. Sherman Bonney.

Taken to lunch "on shad roe, asparagus, and strawberry shortcake" by Bonney, Jim learned that the doctor was seeking a man merely to do his laboratory work. "A lab man I am not and do not want to be," Waring wrote Gerald. "I want to work with him in all aspects of his practice as Gilbert does with you."

When Dr. Bonney would not change his mind Jim daringly established his own private practice and supplemented it with a teaching post on the medical faculty of the University of Colorado. (It was said by now that, considering all the recovering consumptives on that faculty, it must be "the best example ever of the survival of the *un*fit.") Dr. Waring married Ruth Porter of Denver, who bore him two daughters and made herself his devoted partner, in fishing as well as all other aspects of his life.

Dr. Forster must at first have wondered whether his decision to leave Louisville had been wise. Doctors Webb and Gilbert remained with him as consulting physicians and for the first time Cragmor's facilities were opened to use by all the local doctors, but the beds filled slowly that first fall and winter.

Even when full occupancy and a waiting list were achieved the following summer, the sanatorium's capacity proved too small to carry a reasonable overhead at its charge of thirty-five dollars per week per room. Forster himself had to keep the books, plan the menus, help with the nursing, even tend the furnaces and carry out the rubbish. By these labors he managed to avoid financial loss the next two years but neither he nor the investors made any money. Cragmor *must* be enlarged.

At the first hint from Addison Hayes that this might actually be done Dr. Forster seems to have lost touch with reality. He outdid Edwin Solly in the compass and grandeur of his dreams, the magnificence of the plans he ordered drawn up, the extravagant rhetoric of his public announcements. The monies he thought to spend soared to half a million dollars and beyond.

The daring of his scheme and his airy self-assurance about it mesmerized his sponsors, including Mr. Hayes and Dr. Webb, into approval for a time. Fortunately the aberration vanished in a few months, prudence returned, and they all agreed to settle for the possible.

The Cragmor Sanatorium Company was incorporated in January 1913 by Addison Hayes, William Otis, Henry C. Hall, A. E. Carlton, Alexius Forster, Gerald Webb, and William Williams. With the $100,000 subscribed in stock a new "Main Building" (Solly's central block) was constructed in 1914 to increase the capacity of Cragmor to sixty patients and provide kitchen and diningroom facilities for one hundred and fifty — the optimal number, Forster thought, for an ideal sanatorium. Patients' quarters to accommodate that number were to be added later as income permitted.

The company now became the owner of Cragmor and Dr. Forster went on salary as resident director. With all its beds continuously occupied and patients always waiting for admission, he was able to make a modest annual profit which he applied to improvements and expansion. The stockholders never did receive any return on their investment.

Throughout this new beginning for Cragmor Gerald Webb behaved like an eager father toward it, doing his utmost to advance its fortunes. He talked and wrote about it constantly, enclosed its announcements and rate cards in his letters, touted its advantages to all referring doctors and prospective patients. On his many travels he kept it in mind, seeking patients for it and studying sanatoriums for ideas to improve it. He placed those of his own patients who could afford the luxuries of Cragmor in its beds — at substantial financial sacrifice, since the sanatorium's fees continued to include the physicians' services.

Equally important, Dr. Webb shed upon Cragmor Sanatorium some of the personal renown he was acquiring. He adopted it as the place of his professional affiliation, listing it wherever another might use the name of the university, hospital, or institute at which he worked. He involved Dr. Forster in some of his clinical studies and included him as co-author of the published reports. And above all, from 1911 to 1917 Webb indited his research papers, not as before "From the Webb Tuberculosis Research Laboratory," but instead "From the Laboratory of Cragmor Sanatorium."

Since in addition to all those who read the journals in which the papers were published, Dr. Webb personally distributed five hundred or more reprints of each paper, this inditement was in itself a repeated reminder worldwide of the existence and excellence of Cragmor.

Whether the shift of Webb's laboratory to the sanatorium was physical fact or a calculated fiction is uncertain.

We know that Dr. Webb removed his research from 1222 North Cascade Avenue at about the time Bill Williams left him, in late 1910, a few months after he acquired his first lot of rhesus monkeys.

He had to do so. His family was growing, as was Varina's collection of pets. Little Margaret and Gerry, aged five and three, were active youngsters, into everything. He could lock them out of the laboratory with its hazardous vials and capsules and cultures but neither they nor Varina's dogs and cats could be kept safely away from the shed full of fascinating animals in the backyard—fascinating but inoculated, infectious, prone to get loose. Varina could not tolerate the danger. Margaret as an adult had only a faint memory of monkeys in the yard where she played, so they must have been gone by the time she was five or six.

But where did they go? To the Laboratory of Cragmor Sanatorium? It would seem likely, given the new provenance Dr. Webb began declaring for his research reports at this time, and there was certainly room to tuck their cages away somewhere on the unused acres of the place. But there seems to be no record or memory of their ever having been there, although animal experimentation on the premises could hardly have gone unremarked by Cragmor patients and staff.

Dr. Forster was not the kind of research man to consider infected animals an added amenity at his sanatorium. Nowhere in all his glowing newspaper descriptions of a prospering and expanding Cragmor is there any mention of a laboratory, or of an operating room, yet both of necessity existed, for clinical procedures if nothing more.

In 1915 Dr. Webb moved his offices from his home to the Burns Building downtown and some years later his research animals return to the light of record in the basement of that building, where his sons were assigned the task of feeding them. But by that time he had abandoned his efforts to develop a live-germ tuberculosis vaccine. Just where he and Dr. Gilbert did all their reported work with guinea pigs and rabbits and monkeys, just where John Romanes and Hideyo Noguchi, Doctors Mayo, Crile, Murphy, and all other medical visitors observed it so admiringly, remains a mystery.

Doctors Forster and Webb felt only relief when soon after Cragmor's new start another sanatorium opened its doors out where the mountains meet the prairies, this one about a mile east of town on Boulder Road. It was named Sunnyrest and was built, under public pressure, by the Colorado Springs Board of Associated Charities.

Both Dr. Solly and Dr. Forster had encountered opposition when descriptions of Cragmor's luxurious accommodations, service, and food, as well as the high fees it would charge—at first $25, then $35 a week in comparison, say, to $15 a week at Glockner and $5 at the Trudeau Sanatorium—made it clear that no poor man need apply at its doors. Many in Colorado Springs, seeing tuberculous derelicts wandering the streets with at best a rundown hovel to sleep in and only such food as they could scrounge, thought what the city needed was a charity sanatorium for the indigent, not one to pamper the rich.

Dr. Solly had answered tactfully with a utopian promise: when Cragmor was prospering it would support a refuge for the tuberculous poor out of its profits, at no cost to the city. Dr. Forster in his turn countered with defiance; the nation had numerous city and county sanatoriums for the poor, more every year, he said, but few places where the affluent could pay for proper care and comfort.

Neither response stilled the controversy. Colorado Springs had become a hotbed of the "Consumption Terror"—also called phthisiophobia—that was sweeping the nation as awareness of the infectious nature of tuberculosis seeped through the populace. The NTA was doing its chosen work too well.

As a major part of its program of public education the national office of the NTA was sending a traveling exhibit to scores of cities around the country and encouraging its local chapters and committees to stage similar exhibits of their own. The traveling exhibit was an informative collection of photographs and pamphlets promoting good sanitation and hygiene, giving instructions for the proper use of handkerchiefs and sputum cups, offering blueprints for sleeping porches and sanatoriums, but all this was much too sober and dull for many local sponsors; they submerged it in more titillating items of their own devising which, with the aid of quack nostrum barkers lured to the exhibit as bears to honey, made it into a rousing old-time medicine show.

Appropriately, since in some small communities the exhibit was set out in the back room of a neighborhood saloon, the sponsors borrowed the crude methods of the temperance movement designed to induce the utmost in fear. They displayed such items, the grislier the better, as plaster models of open mouths emitting the gushing blood of hemorrhage and specimens of cheesy lungs eaten into ragged holes by swarming bacilli made to look like maggots. They used huge jars filled with colored beads alongside rows of garishly painted skeletons to portray graphically the annual toll in death from tuberculosis, while flashing red lights signaled second by second the dispatch of another soul into eternity by the dread white plague.

The public, having become enamored of world and state fairs, went by the hundreds of thousands, perhaps millions, to see these exhibits. In Milwaukee alone attendance is said to have passed one hundred thousand.

The sequel in many communities was disaster for the tuberculous. They were made outcasts, barred from employment, hounded out of town or county, segregated in ill-tended pesthouses. State legislatures enacted severe laws against them—e.g. the Oklahoma law that revoked the license of any physician who attended a consumptive patient.

That law aroused Dr. Adolphus Knopf to militant defense against the ignorant injustice of all this phthisiophobia. He invited Dr. Webb to join him and Gerald responded with his written assurance that a doctor was not made tuberculous or a carrier of bacilli merely by treating consumptives.

Dr. Webb was also asked to support the crusades of the terror-stricken. An anxious mother in Kansas pled for his help in ridding her county's schools of tuberculous teachers, and a lawyer in Ohio sought his testimony to the danger of trolley cars, since riders in them ran so grave a risk of being shut in with a coughing consumptive. Many a letter from a prospective patient or one of his worried relatives, sometimes even his local doctor, asked Webb whether it would be safe to bring family members, especially children, to live among the many infected residents of Colorado Springs.

One George Murray of Kansas City, informed of his tuberculous brother's death in a Colorado Springs boardinghouse, wrote to thank Dr. and Mrs. Webb for their kindnesses and added, "Be sure to include in your bill the cost of fumigating the house where he stayed."

It was all sadly reminiscent of the rampant terror in southern Europe a century earlier when in Spain and Italy fear-crazed townspeople burned down the houses of consumptives and made bonfires of all their possessions — when the frail and cough-racked Paganini was turned summarily out into the street by his frightened landlord in Naples, when the tuberculous Chopin was not only driven from his hotel room and banished from the island of Majorca but was asked to pay the cost of the bed he had slept in because the hotelkeeper was required by law to burn it.

Colorado Springs was not immune to the new wave of fear. It was one of the first cities to sponsor the NTA exhibit when this was made available west of the Mississippi in 1909. A month-long "conference" of addresses, demonstrations, and discussions was held in conjunction with the exhibit in October; Dr. Webb's address to the public mass meeting in the church which I quoted earlier was a feature of this conference and it was the occasion for Dr. Forster's first visit to Colorado Springs.

Upwards of ten thousand came from all over the state and beyond to see and hear. The unforeseen effect was an explosive outbreak of pent-up hostility against the city's consumptives. Before the conference was over the city fathers instead of proudly promoting it were trying frantically to hush up sensational newpaper accounts of it.

Some of the speeches turned out to be emotional tirades against careless coughing and "promiscuous expectoration." The discussions degenerated into brawling arguments. Outside the halls loud shouting matches ended in street fights between those who urged "driving the dirty lungers out of town" or at least forcing them to wear bells around their necks and those more sensible who thought it would be protection enough to eliminate public drinking cups, disinfect public telephones, keep coughers off the streetcars, and prohibit open-air markets in which fruits and vegetables acquired "all the bugs in the dust."

The fever from fear raged on for many months after the conference had ended. Indigent consumptives who could not hide themselves were taunted and harassed with mounting cruelty. Angry placards appeared. "Segregate the Lungers" read one, but where they were already segregated in clusters of Gardiner tents set up in the park another sign labeled them "A Menace to the Community" and schoolchildren marched around them chanting "Unclean, unclean, better dead and never seen."

The city council sought to defuse the tensions by replacing communal drinking cups with sanitary fountains at the soda springs, requiring the registration of all consumptives, hiring inspectors to collect dust from public thoroughfares and analyze it for bacilli, and imposing fines on those caught spitting in public. Whereupon busybody vigilantes took to riding the trolley cars and patrolling streets and stores in search of violators. Abuse of the luckless lungers became a common and savage pastime.

In November 1909 the Board of Associated Charities, seeking to remove from sight the cause of all the uproar, appointed Irving Bonbright chairman of a subsidiary board urgently charged with finding a site, raising funds, and building a municipal sanatorium for the indigent.

By March 1910 the sum of $25,000 had been collected, $15,000 for the building and $10,000 for two years' operating expenses. Mr. Bonbright himself had contributed $3,000, his brothers another $1500, Chaloner B. Schley and Mrs. Benjamin C. Allen $1000 apiece. Young Jim Waring put in $10, Gerald B. Webb $50, Addison Hayes and Helen Morley $100 each. The sale of Christmas Seals added $1800. Gifts in kind to the Furnishing Committee poured in, ranging from jars of juices and jellies, potted meats and oysters, to brooms and towels, nightcaps and nightshirts, hot water bottles and knitted slippers, a piano and a music box.

Locating an acceptable site was not so easy. Mr. Bonbright found two in succession that he thought suitable but the neighborhoods of both rose up in wrathful determination not to be contaminated by the proximity of contagion. When their cause was emphatically endorsed by the Merchants' Association the city council passed an ordinance forbidding the construction of a sanatorium within the city limits. Mr. Bonbright then bought a plot of twenty acres "with a beautiful view of the vista of the Rocky Mountains" a mile outside of town.

As the twin wings of Sunnyrest Sanatorium, providing porch rooms for twenty patients plus five beds in an infirmary, rose toward opening on 1 April 1911 the eighteen-month excess of fear and frenzy drained away and Colorado Springs emerged from its bout of inhumanity to show again, a reporter said, its "sense of brotherhood."

The building of Sunnyrest can only have provided the excuse for this simmering down; its twenty-five beds hardly dented the problem of indigent patients.

The trustees persuaded the Kaiserwerth Deaconesses of Buffalo, New York, who already operated a boardinghouse in Colorado Springs, to undertake the management of Sunnyrest and the motherhouse sent four sisters under the direction of Sister Ida Pobschell to perform the housekeeping and nursing chores. For medical supervision the trustees named three consulting physicians: Doctors Gerald B. Webb, Henry C. Hoagland, and P. O. Hanford, an able young newcomer.

Gerald welcomed the chance to give his services to Sunnyrest patients. He had taken little part in the preceding commotion. Professionally he could only applaud the better sanitation it effected but personally he was moved to indignation and compassion by the undeserved plight of the hapless victims of tuberculosis who were being hounded like lepers. It made him feel uneasy about his commitment to Cragmor which so obviously flouted their needs. Taking care of some of them at Sunnyrest would assuage his guilt.

For many years faithful service gratis at the municipal sanatorium and a shorter span as unpaid medical consultant to the children's ward at Beth-El Hospital were the publicly visible part of Dr. Webb's charitable activity.

He did not wholly approve one measure taken by the city council. When he sent in the names of his tuberculous patients as required for the new registration he slyly added an innocent-sounding suggestion: "Since many of these people work in city stores and offices, ought not their places of occupation to be registered and published as well as their names and residences?" He knew the businessmen would howl in outrage at any such requirement.

He was feeling annoyed just then with these gentlemen and their agents in city government.

During the summer of 1910 Colorado Springs was struck by a sudden epidemic of scarlet fever—some seventy cases in just two weeks—and Webb set about tracking down the source of it. He traced the microorganism to the milk supply and thence, he was sure, to a couple of cows dying of puerperal fever on a dairy farm near town. He reported these facts to the city health officers and urged them to inspect the dairy and issue a bulletin advising residents to boil all milk before drinking it.

The health men refused to do any such thing; the city council forcefully advised silence about the epidemic; the newspapers cooperated fully in the hush-up. They all said the action Dr. Webb wanted would damage the tourist business which was being battered enough by the anti-consumptive furor.

All Gerald could do was fume in frustration and vent his anger to friends like Ravenel and Farrand and to neighboring doctors when the epidemic spread to their communities and they sought his advice.

This was only the first of Dr. Webb's confrontations with the powers-that-be in civic affairs. A few years later during a rabies epidemic he tried to get them to warn and instruct the people, tell citizens how to recognize the symptoms and how to handle a crazed dog, but the officials again preferred to soft-pedal the danger lest it drive tourists away.

For the same reason they ignored Webb's repeated pleas for quarantine measures and an isolation hospital to protect the community against virulent contagions. They did maintain a small building at the poor farm to house smallpox victims but they chose to look away from any other threat to health. Gerald learned to be cynical about the way elected officials defined the public interest.

The new sanatoriums could by no means accommodate all Dr. Webb's patients. Most of them were neither poor enough for Sunnyrest nor rich enough for Cragmor.

"Miss Lincoln's friends, all school teachers, are furnishing the money for her trip to see you, so I hope you will find her a cheap place to live," wrote Dr. Millikan of Springfield, Illinois.

"This poor woman is a widow, without a relative in the world. She has enough to live on but not much more, I think. Can you get her a modest room?" asked Dr. Dearborn of Milwaukee.

"Mr. Riley's uncle, a farmer of small means, is paying his way while he's sick, so he won't be able to pay much for lodgings," reported Dr. Simpson of Memphis.

And so on by the dozens.

Some doctors were steady suppliers, notably one Dr. Daniel Morton of St. Joseph, Missouri, who sometimes referred three or four patients in a single long and rambling letter. He was clearly a fatherly family doctor, more fussing than effective. His diagnoses were frequently far off the mark, calling tuberculosis what Dr. Webb found to be asthma or anemia or in one instance hookworm.

Typical from Dr. Morton was young Harold, "a deserving boy who has been a fine son to his sick father and mother. They were poor people and he gave up his schooling to earn their bread and butter. Since they died he has been too sick to do any heavy work. He will have to get some light work there and a room that won't cost more than $6 or 7 a week. I know you will help him."

And one Mr. Warner: "He has deep mental depression, feels terror and panic at the thought of tuberculosis. So don't tell him he has it. Just build up his general health. He's a poor man and can't pay you much. You'll have to put him in some inexpensive place."

Another doctor who sent Webb a stream of patients was Joseph L. Miller of Chicago, the man who nominated him for "the blue ribbon." Miller seems to have had remarkable faith in the healing powers of Dr. Webb and the Colorado climate. One time he wrote that he was sending out a favorite trained nurse "because she won't stay quiet here. I want to get her out of this climate and into your hands. Mrs. P. D. Armour is interested in her and will pay her expenses for as long as she needs to stay." And the very next day he announced the coming of "an employee of the Iten Biscuit Company which has agreed to pay his expenses for three months if they can be kept at a moderate figure."

Willy-nilly, Gerald had to run a sort of housing bureau for free. And sometimes an employment service as well.

The bedridden he placed on the sleeping porches of Glockner Sanatorium, often to the limit of its capacity. Able-bodied milder or convalescent cases he distributed among several ranches roundabout. For most of the others he had to use the town's boardinghouses though he loathed most of them—"draughty, dirty places, little better than pest houses, with rickety beds and too little or too heavy food." He had three or four favorites among the landladies, good-hearted motherly women who couldn't help taking excellent care of their lodgers; their rooms he kept constantly filled.

A few wealthy men who disdained living with the herd even at Cragmor he settled in suites at the Antlers Hotel. To parents or spouses who came along to take personal care of their sick ones he recommended renting at thirty dollars a month "one of the attractive small bungalows that abound here."

When business was more than normally brisk Gerald was a veritable juggler, shifting patients from room to room to keep them pacified until the place of their choice or his choice for them had a vacancy.

Neither Sunnyrest nor Cragmor quite measured up to Dr. Webb's idea of what a sanatorium should be. He was disturbed to find Sister Ida content to provide her patients with merely custodial care. When he gently suggested that it was bad for them to lie abed or sit around idle all day, she stubbornly refused to do more than feed them and keep them clean. He asked Dr. Forster to go with him to talk to her about their need for distraction from gloomy brooding about their illness, but Sister Ida only listened and stood mute. So Gerald asked the trustees to send her on a trip to eastern sanatoriums to observe what she ought to be doing, but the men said no, they had to hoard their meager reserve in order to be sure of maintaining Sunnyrest for its initial two years.

Fortunately Dr. Forster had more effect on Sister Ida than Dr. Webb thought. The pocket-sized garden cultivated by the sisters in Sunnyrest's first summer became flourishing fields of truck and grains in its second, with a "hennery" to provide eggs and a herd of cows to give milk besides, all tended by the patients—a mini-version of Forster's farm colony.

At Cragmor the trouble as Dr. Webb saw it was the reverse of inactivity. When he went to call on patients for whom he had pre-scribed rest and quiet, he was as likely as not to find them if adolescents racing noisily through the halls or around the grounds, if adults playing croquet on the lawn or card games in the lounge, all gaily whooping it up to the limit of their strength. He had to don his severest manner and exert all his authority to return them to bed and, he hoped, keep them there awhile.

An example appears in Douglas R. McKay's story of Cragmor titled *Asylum of the Gilded Pill* (1983). It comes from an interview with a man who had been a patient at Cragmor in his youth:

"Dr. Webb was very stern with us. One day he took hold of my arm as I was running down the hallway in my pajamas. 'Young man, do you want to recover your health?' he asked. I was surprised by the earnestness of the question. Dr. Webb looked straight into my eyes while he spoke.

"'Yes, sir. Yes, I certainly do,' I mumbled.

"'Then turn around and go back to your room. Go to bed and stay there for six months!'

"Saying that, he turned and walked away. I went back to my bed and I stayed there for six months. Lord, there was something about that man that commanded respect."

Dr. Forster was too naturally easygoing to be a successful disciplinarian. Besides, he wanted Cragmor to become known as a lively, gladsome place in which to chase the cure. He firmly believed that a cheerful and contented mind was indispensable to recovery from tuberculosis. Why, then, hold the patient to a boring regimen he did not enjoy? Why forbid him simple pleasures in the distracting company of his kind? Why not let *him* decide how much and what kind of activity he could tolerate?

Dr. Webb was too experienced a clinician to trust the wisdom of patients that far. Most of them, he thought, were heedlessly self-indulgent, incapable of self-discipline, ignorant if not stupid about what was necessary to get them well again. His highest praise, rarely bestowed, was "He is a patient who uses his head."

One tuberculous patient who at first did *not* use her head was fragile Constance Pulitzer, the younger daughter of the newspaper titan Joseph Pulitzer. By the time her father died, in 1911 when she was twenty-two, she had been in Colorado Springs as Gerald Webb's patient for two years, probably because she was kin to Varina Webb.

Constance's mother Kate was the daughter of the impeccable Judge William Worthington Davis of Georgetown, a distant cousin of Jefferson Davis. Joseph and Kate Pulitzer occasionally visited Varina and Jefferson Davis at Beauvoir and for long periods in New York and Paris acted as surrogate parents to their younger daughter Varina Anne, whom her doting family called Winnie and who, because she was born during the war with the North, was affectionately known throughout the South as "the Daughter of the Confederacy." When the widowed Varina Howell Davis moved to New York, Joseph Pulitzer quietly contributed to her support by

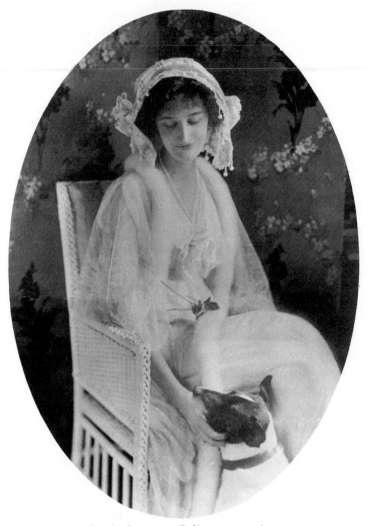

Cousin Constance Pulitzer as a patient

putting her on salary as a feature writer for his *Sunday World*, though his editors could rarely use what she wrote.

All this kept Kate Pulitzer intermittently in touch with Winnie's older sister Maggie, Margaret Davis Hayes, and because of this family connection the Pulitzers sent Constance to Gerald Webb when she became ill.

She bought the house at 1221 North Cascade Avenue across the street from the Webbs, but she seldom alighted there for long. Gerald put her in touch with Dr. James A. Miller as a good physician

to see when she was in New York and for several years the correspondence between the two doctors carried a refrain: Where is
Constance? How is she?

She would be off for a merry whirl in London or on the Riviera,
at Bar Harbor or Lake Tahoe, in some Mediterranean or Caribbean
resort, from which she would return home exhausted, in fever,
coughing blood.

No one should have expected otherwise. Constance had been
reared in a continual hullabaloo of comings and goings. Her whole
family, all eight of them, were feverish globetrotters. A group of
them might gather for a brief joint sojourn at one of their three
homes but soon would scatter to the four winds again. Her manic-
depressive father hurried off to Switzerland the day after she was
born and did not manage to see her again until she was two. When
he was at home for short spells during her adolescence no one knew
in the morning whether that day he would be lovingly lenient and
generous or a raging irrational tyrant. Her beautiful and spirited
mother was too preoccupied with fashion and the social spin to
provide much stability or good judgment.

So Constance on her own in Colorado Springs was just doing
what was normal to her.

She was a nagging worry to Gerald. Away on a trip he peppered
his letters to Varina with instructions: "Make sure you see Constance every day, to keep her quiet if you can." "Is Constance still
there? Try to make her behave." "Do take some more books over
to Constance. She might like Osler's *Alabama Student.* Or maybe
that life of Florence Nightingale. Something you think will keep
her resting."

Fortunately for all of them Constance was an eager reader, thanks
largely to her father. Being practically blind for most of his adult
life, Joseph Pulitzer maintained a corps of secretaries part of whose
job it was to read to him the hundred or so books he consumed each
year — and to send copies of those he liked to his children, especially to Constance who shared his interest in history and biography.

In time Constance learned what was required of her and became,
Gerald reported to Jim Miller, "a truly good patient, making every
effort for recovery." She fell in love with another of Webb's patients,
William Gray Elmslie, son of a British judge and a graduate of Oxford University who had been her brother Herbert's tutor and one
of her father's secretaries. She married him, bore him three chil-

dren, and moved them all into a larger house on Wood Avenue. She remained Gerald's patient and a cherished friend of the family, affectionately called Cousin Constance by the Webb children.

Doctors Webb and Miller briefly shared another young and headstrong patient, Allan Ryan, son of the notorious New York financier Thomas Fortune Ryan. When Dr. Miller announced the boy's coming to Webb he commented tersely: "Allan has been in the Adirondacks for two months without benefit. He has been spoiled by too much money and rebels against any restraint. He smokes and drinks too much. His father's secretary is bringing him out and he will have a good nurse with him. You will have to work upon his mind. He's a great bluff. He shuns medical supervision."

Gerald managed to keep the restless young man in Colorado Springs for three months before he threw a tantrum and dragged his nurse back to New York, presumably to revisit Dr. Miller. He did not show up and Miller and Webb again played the game of Where is he? until months later two letters reaching Webb in the same mail answered their question. An obscure doctor in New York wrote to boast that he was "curing" Allan Ryan with hydrotherapy and the distinguished Dr. Hermann Biggs, writing to refer a patient to Webb, incidentally thanked him for sending Allan Ryan to see him. Gerald had done no such thing. He and Miller agreed that young Ryan would come to a fool's end.

Gerald had somewhat better luck with a woman patient Dr. Trudeau sent him from Saranac Lake. After taking an up-and-down course for more than a year her disease quieted enough for her to get up and about with reasonable comfort and she decided to live permanently in Colorado Springs. Gerald had been keeping Trudeau informed of her progress and wrote to tell him of this decision, concluding, "I don't think she will ever be really well but as a creaking hinge she will probably outlive the two of us."

Trudeau replied, "You have done well with that lady. When she was here she had no patience but was in and out of the place every couple of months, always expecting to be cured overnight. Too many expect that."

So they did. One is struck by all the coming and going, the continual moving about from place to place. Rarely did a patient stay under treatment more than six months before departing to try someone and someplace else. Half the patients Dr. James A. Miller sent to Webb had spent a previous period in the Adirondacks, mostly at Saranac Lake, and the traffic from Asheville, North Carolina, was equally heavy. Many came to Colorado Springs for the winter and returned home for the summer or vice versa, depending on whether they lived up north or down south. Webb's letters to referring doctors were full of comments like this: "I have told his mother that the boy should stay here and take daily sun baths on his open porch until he gains more strength, but he wants to go home and she cannot control him."

A great many of the patients sent to Dr. Webb at this time were children and he often said the youngsters were easier to handle than their anxious, addled, weakly indulgent parents.

Dr. Webb's research and his methods of treatment ran hand in hand. Not only did he administer his graduated doses of live-germ vaccine in selected cases but he kept Varina busy making arm garters for his patients to wear and nurses on the run with his prescriptions of hot mustard foot baths three times a week. He had such faith in the garters that he scattered sample pairs of them all over the country as gifts to his professional colleagues.

But for the most part he stuck with the therapies in general use at the time. "We have no special modes of treatment beyond those used by good physicians everywhere," he wrote an inquiring physician. "We have found no specific to cure tuberculosis."

He told the assembled doctors of Louisiana in 1915, "Our first measure is rest in bed, as absolute as possible, in the open air. In breathing a normal person 'opens and shuts' the lungs nearly 30,000 times a day. By rest we aim to make the breathing as shallow as possible, imitating almost that of a bear in hibernation.... We maintain rest until the temperature has remained normal for two to three weeks. Then we permit the patient to sit up and gradually return to daily walks. It is rare, however, for a patient not to have a slight relapse. When this occurs the rest in bed is again enforced. No patient is allowed to get up with even as slight a temperature rise as 99°. This rest phase of the cure can take from a few weeks to two or more years."

That is what he said. He was describing his ideal regimen of the moment, which he did not often achieve in practice, and he had come only slowly to define it. Five years earlier his definition of rest was likely to be "a few hours' nap in the afternoon" or "take it easy for a while" or "you must be lazy this winter."

The practice of alternating brisk exercise with spells of rest which had prevailed since the mid-1800s when Dettweiler established it at his sanatorium in the German Alps was slow to fade away, especially for one like Dr. Webb who had thought the best rest cure for nervous patients was to keep them the busiest folk in town. As late as 1913 he was allowing a patient sent him by Dr. John H. Lowman of Cleveland to continue her daily hour of singing practice.

Reasonably typical of his use of rest in the earlier years was the case of Richard Robinson, a young man referred to him in 1911 by Dr. Adam Webster, president of the Illinois State Board of Health. He was obviously pleased to inform Dr. Webster, "Richard is himself again. After two months of ups and downs his temperature stayed normal for two weeks and I allowed him to get up for outdoor exercise. He enjoys it and is doing well."

Alas, a month later poor Richard was back in bed. "He went duck hunting," Webb told Dr. Webster. "His car stalled in the snow and he spent hours digging it out. His temperature rose again, so I have prescribed another period of bedrest."

Dr. Webb's primary emphasis lingered long on breathing deep in the open air. But he never succumbed to use of the Gardiner tepee tent which became almost ubiquitous in Colorado Springs and its environs, appearing even on the grounds of Cragmor for a while during the regime of the troika before Forster.

Dr. Gardiner in his early years of practice "above the timberline" on the western slopes of the Rockies had been struck by the extraordinary sweet freshness of the air in Indian tepees, which he thought was maintained by upward circulation that carried all impurities out through the hole at the top. When he moved to Colorado Springs and acquired many tuberculous patients he remembered that tepee air and designed a tent on the Indian model as the perfect home for consumptives. He arranged with a local company to manufacture the tents for him and sold them by the hundreds everywhere in Colorado.

By the time the reign of the tents faded away thousands of wretched patients consigned to them had shivered under their blankets, teeth clattering, through endless icy winter nights and sweltered through the hot ones of summer in their cramped quarters. Dr. Gardiner's daughter as an adult remembered resentfully the horrible discomfort of living in those tents. "It was worse than the disease," she said.

Dr. Webb refused to inflict such misery in the name of therapy.

Like Edwin Solly and the nabobs of the NTA he preferred the sleeping porch. Were those open porches really much less cold, much more comfortable than a Gardiner tent? Apparently so, for in time every hospital and sanatorium and virtually every private home in Colorado Springs, including Webb's own, was adorned with one or more of these protruding annexes, some of which are still to be seen on the older houses of the city.

After hearing Rollier in Rome in 1912 and visiting his sanatorium at Leysin, Dr. Webb added "the sunlight treatment" to his arsenal. Rollier made him for a time a true believer in the ancient cult of heliotherapy. He adopted the Swiss doctor's method of using mirrors to reflect sunlight into the throat to treat laryngeal and esophageal tuberculosis and began prescribing the sunbath for most patients. He thought it was of great benefit in pulmonary tuberculosis and capable of "miracles of cure" in tuberculosis of bones and joints.

A published photograph of that day shows one of Webb's patients, a teenage boy, lying naked, except for a hat to shade his head, on a narrow patch of grass between a house foundation on one side and a three-foot wall of snow on the other. The picture was captioned "Sunbath in a Snowdrift." Despite the snow "the temperature in the sun may be 90°," said Webb. "Summer or winter patients can remain from four to six hours bathing in the sun, and, to paraphrase Homer, 'become cured by the arrows of Apollo.'"

At Cragmor the niches and bays formed by a crenated wall on the flat roof of Main Building were favorite spots for the prescribed sunbaths, as were grassy crannies screened by shrubbery here and there around the grounds. Such secluded areas and the recommended minimum of clothing were an invitation to illicit lovemaking and scandalous affairs among the patients, much to Gerald Webb's puritanical distaste.

After several years Webb's enthusiasm for sunbathing waned. "While finding it to be of much benefit to our patients, we are not yet able to share the high degree of optimism for the method which is held by Rollier," he said.

Watching, reading, pondering, Dr. Webb came slowly to accept prolonged and absolute rest in bed as his "first measure" of treatment. He could not fail to wonder why he had to cope with so many relapses, by no means all "slight" ones. Many of the patients he and other doctors dismissed as "cured" when they had gained strength and weight and that magic goal, a normal temperature, turned up someplace not long thereafter as ill as before. Dr. James Miller's repeated plaint, "He is on the ragged edge of disease again," described a condition that was discouragingly commonplace. "It is the nature of the disease to relapse," said Webb.

The problem was all the more worrisome, he thought, because these patients in between their bouts of active illness were likely to be that menace to public health he talked and wrote about so much, tuberculosis carriers.

It was one of Webb's teenage patients who made him question the inevitability of all those relapses. The lad had lain uncomplaining in bed for six months and, his temperature at last being normal, Dr. Webb told him he could get up and begin to exercise. The boy thought about it awhile, then said he guessed he wouldn't. "If six months in bed has made me better, another six months might make me well." He made so extraordinary a recovery after his year of bedrest that Dr. Webb took the lesson to heart. "Out of the mouths of babes..." he said.

Forlanini's artificial pneumothorax hammered the lesson home. Gerald saw the operation in use everywhere he went in Europe after watching the Italian surgeon do it himself in Rome. By injecting nitrogen into the chest cavity to increase the pressure within the pleura the doctor forced the diseased lung to collapse and so to rest from its 30,000 labors a day as long as the pressure was maintained by repeated injections.

The procedure was introduced into the American East by Dr. Lewis Hamman and his associates at Johns Hopkins Hospital and Eudowood Sanatorium, and Gerald Webb is credited with bringing it to the West.* He certainly made haste to try it. He did not return to Colorado Springs until June 1912 but by mid-July he was applying it in five cases, using an apparatus he had rigged up himself by following the description and illustration published in the London *Lancet.*

Actually, as he was quickly informed, long before Forlanini won fame with artificial pneumothorax Dr. John B. Murphy invented the method and described and recommended it to the doctors of Colorado assembled in Denver in 1898. Dr. Webb promptly con-

*See Dr. L. Fred Ayvazian, "The Fifty-Five Trudeau Medalists" in *American Review of Respiratory Disease*, vol. 121, no. 4 (April 1980), p. 8.

gratulated his Chicago friend "on the reinstatement of your idea."

Webb also introduced a modification in Forlanini's method. During his visit to John Scott Haldane in Oxford on his way home from Rome he told the British physiologist about the exciting new surgical treatment and Haldane wondered why Forlanini was bothering to use nitrogen. Plain air filtered through cotton would do as well, he said, and it would cost far less.

Would it? Gerald wrote to ask Dr. Lewis Hamman. Were they using nitrogen at the Hopkins? Why? Why not air?

Hamman was nonplussed. Yes, they were using nitrogen, but no one knew why. To be honest, no one had given the matter a second thought. They had all just assumed that nitrogen would be absorbed more slowly and so would permit fewer injections.

Gerald decided to find out. Dr. Gilbert and his assistants were just finishing their study of lymphocytes and altitude, so he asked them to undertake the necessary series of comparative gas analyses. Their first discovery was startling: they could not buy pure nitrogen. In the best of the commercial products the cylinder contained only 85 percent nitrogen; the remainder was oxygen. All right, they would make their own. Webb himself hunted up a book that described how to do it and assembled the necessary materials and equipment.

Eureka! The nitrogen they collected at the end of his process proved to be 99.46 percent pure.

(They later had an identical experience with oxygen. When the commercial tanks tested only from 70 to 80 percent oxygen, they made their own and consistently achieved a product assaying above 99 percent.)

The team now began their comparative series, working first on big dogs, then on patients. Webb, Gilbert, and Forster withdrew samples from the chest before and after injecting either nitrogen or filtered air; their assistants analyzed the samples in Dr. Schneider's chemistry laboratory at Colorado College and kept meticulous records.

The results proved Haldane's conjecture to the hilt. Thirty-six hours after injection the mixture of gases in the pleural cavity was the same whether the material injected had been nitrogen, air, or in a few cases oxygen.

When Dr. Webb reported this experiment to the American Medical Association in 1914 he also summarized his experience with eighty-three patients—all in advanced stages of tuberculosis—in whom he had induced pneumothorax and maintained it with nine hundred injections of gas. He judged the benefit to have been "great" in a third of the cases with lesser degrees of improvement in another third. The remaining third had presented him with a variety of hampering adhesions, effusions, hemorrhages, and in one case nearly fatal air embolism.

He thought that with proper precautions the danger of the procedure itself was negligible. Its greatest drawbacks were the need to keep the lung compressed by repeated injections over a long period of time and the uncertainty as to what would happen when the artificial collapse was ended. He concluded: "For the present, every known method should be very thoroughly tried out before suggesting pneumothorax to our patients."

In the discussion that followed, with Dr. Lewis Hamman in the chair, the hottest argument was between those who agreed with Webb that pneumothorax should be a last resort and those who, echoing Dr. John B. Murphy, insisted that its failures and complications arose because it had not been applied early enough; it should not be reserved for advanced cases but should be used as soon as a diagnosis of tuberculosis was made.

Dr. Hamman stood firmly with Webb. He confessed that at Johns Hopkins and Eudowood they were still groping for an answer as to how long collapse of the lung should be maintained. They were certain it took at least a year of it just to relieve the worst symptoms. And they had learned that sometimes the collapsed lung would not re-expand and the patient suffered permanent loss of function in that lung.

Dr. Webb ended the discussion with a quiet warning against overenthusiasm: "We may be inflicting upon some of our patients a remedy worse than the disease, by reason of the treatment being so long drawn out and the possibilities of complications."

He continued to use artificial pneumothorax but he liked it less and less. And when more severe surgical procedures were introduced—thoracoplasty and phrenicectomy by name—after seeing them tried a few times he would have nothing to do with them; he thought they were too drastic and not noticeably more successful.

He finally found a simple substitute that he considered just as effective in many cases. Dr. John B. Murphy sent him a patient with the recommendation that he treat her with pneumothorax. His examination showed heavy cavitation in her right lung, no disease in her left. He put her to bed at Cragmor and went next morning to begin the injections of air. She was still asleep on her open porch and he paused in the doorway to observe her.

She was lying on her left side, the healthy lung pressed down by her weight against the bed and so partially at rest, while her diseased lung, uppermost and unrestrained, was doing its full 12,000 movements in ten hours of sleep. The very lung that needed rest the most, the one he was intending to collapse to give it rest, was doing most of the work.

He went quietly away to think this over and discuss it with Dr. Forster. They discovered that most of their patients had this habit of sleeping on the healthier side, claiming that lying on the sick side was less comfortable; it made them cough more and bring up more sputum.

Dr. Webb persuaded Murphy's patient to let him postpone pneumothorax while she tried sleeping and resting on her right side. She adjusted readily to the change and began slowly to improve. After two and a half years Dr. Webb pronounced her healthy again and sent her back to Chicago. When he looked her up there sixteen years later she was still alive and well.

Not all patients responded to this "postural rest," as Webb called it. Some, because of "resistance, impatient temperament, or intolerance of initial discomfort," could not be trained to lie on the diseased side and a few hemorrhaged when they attempted it, but enough improved to justify trying it before resorting to more drastic treatment.

Dr. Webb added the use of a small firm pillow under the arm on the resting side to increase restraint of motion, and for those with disease in both lungs he prescribed lying on the back with a one-pound load of shot bags arranged on the chest to achieve a measure of compression. This little burden, he discovered, also induced more thorough rest because patients hesitated to move lest they dislodge it.

Webb described his use of postural rest to the AMA in 1916 and returned to it in talks and papers again and again in succeeding years as immediate resort to surgery became the fashion in treating tuberculosis. He never felt obliged to apologize for the simpler, homelier measures he advised. They might be less spectacular than collapsing a lung or sawing out a section of ribs but they were also less damaging. If they succeeded they saved the patient pain and risk.

Yes, postural rest took long years to do its work, he admitted, but so did proper healing of the diseased lungs after surgery.

One reason Dr. Webb could never join the rush to the operating room was his inhibiting awareness of how often the diagnosis of tuberculosis was in error. Dr. Morton of Missouri was by no means the only physician who saw tuberculosis in every case of frail body, persistent cough, or pain somewhere near the chest. It seemed to Gerald he was forever finding the true source of supposed consumption in some systemic disorder like anemia or in the heart or the gallbladder, even a few times in the appendix—though more often in those days of the appendicitis fad errors about that disease were tilted the other way.

"In the last six years several hundred cases of pulmonary tuberculosis have passed through our hands at Cragmor Sanatorium," Doctors Webb, Gilbert, and Forster reported to the NTA in 1917. "Among them we have seen many previous errors in diagnosis, the most common being the mistaken diagnosis of appendicitis. Three cases had been diagnosed as hysteria. One case was thought to be gall stones, one a case of syphilitic crisis. Several had been mistaken for tuberculosis of the caecum and appendix."

Commonly overlooked, said the Cragmor men, was diaphragmatic pleurisy. Out of sixty-one cases of that disorder, "appendicitis was diagnosed nine times and two cases were operated on. Ulcer of the stomach was diagnosed twice and one of those was operated on. In addition diaphragmatic pleurisy had been mistakenly diagnosed as lumbago, neuritis, liver abscess, peritonitis, kidney stones, and so on."

Ways of making more accurate and earlier diagnoses became Webb's foremost clinical quest.

He gradually gave up reliance on tuberculin tests and analysis of sputum. Exposure to tuberculosis was so widespread that almost everyone reacted positively to tuberculin, and "it is not a mild bygone infection but active infection *now* we are looking for," he said. And finding bacilli in the sputum was no help; by the time they appeared there the disease was so advanced its presence was obvious.

He tended to rely more and more on what he could hear and feel within the chest, especially the râles (rough raspy sounds) he could hear through the stethoscope as the patient took deep breaths. He tapped and thumped poor Dr. Gilbert again and again to improve his technique in percussion and refine his interpretation of the body sounds it produced.

He was ahead of his time in assigning prime importance to exhaustive case histories. He wearied some patients, gratified others, by his endless probing questions about not only their own health records but those too of their families and forebears. And he listened to the answers, no matter how rambling and irrelevant they seemed; "a helpful clue may drop from a passing few words," he said.

In time he became a reluctant advocate of X-ray examinations of the chest, although he thought them of value only to confirm and define gross lesions in the lungs; "They fail entirely to reveal the manifestations of early or mild pulmonary tuberculosis."

But they certainly had their uses. A sixteen-year-old Texan named David Arnold was referred to Webb with a diagnosis of consumption by an Amarillo doctor. David's wheezing and coughing were severe but did not, Webb thought, add up to tuberculosis. He called in Dr. L. G. Brown, a local colleague who was specializing in X-ray work. Brown said the X-ray revealed a foreign object, a carpet tack perhaps, lodged crosswise in the left bronchus. Removing it might be tricky, so Dr. Webb sent David on up to Minnesota with a letter to Dr. Charles H. Mayo.

Yes, the carpet tack was there, wrote Dr. Mayo, but he wanted Dr. Plummer to go over the boy before he removed it and Dr. Plummer was away on a trip.

Four days later a telegram arrived: "Plummer back but your patient can't be found. Has he returned to you? Mayo."

Unable to locate the boy in Colorado Springs, Gerald telephoned his home in Amarillo. Yes, David was there, said his mother. He had got tired of waiting in Rochester and so "rode the rails" home. Their local surgeon had removed the tack and the boy was convalescing nicely in the Amarillo hospital.

The incident was not wholly profitless for Dr. Webb. In early November 1913 Luther J. Abbott came to his office. A tall emaciated man aged forty-five, Mr. Abbott had been wandering from one sanatorium to another in the Southwest for two years, seeking relief from a persistent cough that had forced him to resign his professorship of history at a state college in Oklahoma and had reduced his weight to little more than a hundred pounds. The cause of the cough had eluded the many doctors he had consulted but most of them said it must be tuberculosis. So he had come to Colorado Springs and Dr. Webb.

Gerald was uncertain too until he palpated the trachea. His manipulation brought on a paroxysm of coughing. He heard a familiar wheezy rasp in that cough and suddenly remembered the boy from Amarillo.

"Have you ever swallowed a foreign object—a tack, or anything like that?"

"No-o-o, I don't think so."

But Mrs. Abbott, sitting nearby, called out. "Luther! You never found that band from your tooth. Remember?"

Three years earlier their Oklahoma dentist had let the little gold band from a crowned tooth fall into Luther's throat and he swallowed it. When it gave him no immediate trouble he assumed it had passed on out through the alimentary canal and forgot about it.

"It may have gone into a bronchial tube instead of your stomach," said Dr. Webb. "That could be what's causing your cough."

He called in Dr. Brown to do an X-ray examination, which showed something, probably the gold band, blocking the bronchus near the right lung.

What could they do about it? Mr. Abbott's condition was critical.

Gerald had recently read a journal article about a new instrument called a bronchoscope which had been devised in Germany. It was a flexible tube about twelve inches long that could be pushed down the throat and maneuvered into the bronchial passages. Through it the surgeon could pass a smaller tube carrying a tiny mirror and light bulb and along this inner tube he could slide a slender forceps to grasp and withdraw any object in the air passages. The article said that so far only three surgeons in America had learned to use the bronchoscope and one of the three was Dr. E. Fletcher Ingals of Rush Medical College and Presbyterian Hospital in Chicago.

Dr. Webb told Mr. Abbott of this possible treatment but warned him that the new procedure carried out so near the lung could be fatal. Luther replied that his life had been worth nothing for a long time anyway. He left the next day for Chicago.

On 28 November Dr. Ingals tried for two and a half hours to get hold of that thin scrap of gold. In vain. The bronchial tissue and blood vessels had grown all round and through the circlet, almost closing off the breathing passage entirely. Mr. Abbott, conscious throughout the operation done under local anesthesia, was exhausted but begged Dr. Ingals to try again. The surgeon was willing but said bluntly he no longer expected to succeed.

On 3 December he went after the strip of gold again. And got it.

Mr. Abbott was ecstatic. His cough was soon gone and he began rapidly to regain the pounds he had lost. He returned to the house he had rented on Cheyenne Avenue in Colorado Springs and shared the tale of his "miracle" with everyone, including a special meeting of the El Paso County Medical Society. His gratitude to Dr. Webb was rapturous.

The dramatic story of the strange dental accident and the wondrous new bronchoscope was featured in newspapers throughout the Midwest, all the accounts giving admiring credit to Dr. Webb of Colorado Springs for diagnosing correctly what "had baffled dozens of doctors before him."

Although it seems clear that Dr. Webb had become a specialist in tuberculosis he refused to call himself that. He always insisted that his specialty was internal medicine. Certainly at this period his practice still included a goodly proportion of general medicine.

As knowledge and use of vaccine therapy spread among physicians the number of patients referred to Webb for this treatment declined, but as late as 1915 he was still sending out capsules and bottles of vaccine. No longer for pyorrhea and seldom for ear, nose, and eye infections—for those he now thought leucocytosis induced by hyperemia was equally effective—but wearisomely still for acne.

"The acne bacillus is extremely hard to grow," he wrote Dr. Tyndale of Salt Lake City, "but send me another capsule from the pustules and I'll try again to secure a vaccine for you." It would take about two weeks to grow the culture, he said, and the vaccine would cost twenty-five dollars.

He had given up entirely his use of the opsonic index. He had decided an experienced clinician could tell as well from observation as by the index when it was safe to inoculate and was not surprised to hear that Sir Almroth Wright himself had quit advocating the index because he had concluded that in most hands it was unreliable.

The bulk of Webb's general practice now consisted of injuries and illnesses among his tuberculous patients and their families and among his longtime patients and old friends. These folk brought him all their broken bones and lacerated limbs, their myriad aches and pains and discomforts. And their venereal diseases. He was still having to cope regularly with cases of syphilis. By late 1913 he had exhausted the supply of salvarsan Ehrlich had given him, still could not buy any in Colorado, and was writing friends east and south to ask if they had some they could share with him.

He often felt drained to the dregs of energy and spirit by the interminable succession of patients with all their varied complaints and demands. Sometimes he voiced his weariness to friends, once vividly to Dr. James Hart, his early mentor and ally, with whom he continued to exchange long letters and occasional visits. Dr. Hart had finally settled in Geneva, New York, where his tuberculous wife seemed most at peace though chronically ailing still. In 1913 he sent Webb a specimen of her sputum for analysis and Gerald reported back that her bacillus was now much attenuated:

"It is evident that although she cannot beat him out, she has made a cripple of him. Tell her I believe a bodily infirmity can be a good thing for a human being; it keeps them out of a lot of trouble—and also from overwork. I often wish I had something like her headaches to enable me to get away from the clamor of patients. I think I will have to cook up some chronic disease to act as a safety valve for me."

What troubled him most was a case of heart disease or of cancer. "As you know," he wrote his good friend Dr. Frederick Tice of Chicago, "heart conditions baffle me. I don't know much about the heart or anything about cancer or what to do about them." Nor could anyone else at the time tell him much that was useful about either of them.

When in 1915 he learned about the new electrocardiograph he wrote posthaste to ask Dr. Hamman whether it was a machine a physician could use in his office laboratory. "If you think so, please order one sent to me COD, and tell me about your experience with it."

Equally ignorant of it, Dr. Hamman passed Webb's letter on to "the heart man" at Johns Hopkins and relayed back his "expert" opinion: "He thinks the electrocardiograph is too difficult to use and too technical to interpret to be used outside a hospital. Also it has to be imported and costs $1500 to install. He suggests you use a polygraph at $100 instead."

Gerald certainly was at a loss about cancer when Margaret Davis Hayes suffered and died from it in 1909, but six years later he was abreast if not ahead of his time in treating it. Dr. Emile Dupuy, a

French surgeon who had become Gerald's friend during visits to his tuberculous daughter whom he had placed in Webb's care, sent him from Paris a young woman upon whom Dupuy had operated for breast cancer. She was a friend of his daughter and he thought their reunion in Colorado Springs would be good for both of them. Also, "I don't know anyone better to entrust her to." Gerald prescribed a series of X-ray treatments administered by Dr. Brown.

After fifteen of these he thought it advisable to get another opinion and sent her to Dr. Powers in Denver. Powers judiciously averred that X-ray therapy might have been a good idea but it should be discontinued now; she should of course be thoroughly examined every three months—"preferably by a surgeon like myself." Dr. Powers was not a modest man, nor a shy one.

Gerald no longer did any but the simplest minor surgery. He had grown wise far beyond the brash new medical graduate who cockily ventured to operate for brain tumor and aneurysm of the aorta. True, in 1909 he dared to do, or at least assist in doing, a blood transfusion, which was then a novel and risky procedure carried out by direct transfer of the blood from donor to recipient. He described the exploit to Dr. Powers: "We slipped the husband's radial artery directly into his wife's vein, thinking Carrel's technique better than Crile's, although I made exact hemolytic determinations [blood typing?] according to Crile's instructions."

(Dr. Alexis Carrel had only just perfected the method of suturing veins and arteries for which he received the Nobel Prize three years later. Karl Landsteiner did not complete his delineation of basic blood groups until 1902 and much essential information about them remained unknown into the 1920s. We may wonder whether by good luck Webb's husband and wife survived his daring.)

But not long thereafter Gerald was referring to others virtually all his surgery, including the appendectomies and tonsillectomies then so much in vogue. He distributed the cases according to kind among Dr. Murphy of Chicago, the Mayo brothers of Minnesota, Dr. Crile of Cleveland, and Dr. Powers of Denver. For lesser surgery and those patients who could not afford the great men's fees he turned to his able neighbor Dr. P. O. Hanford.

As often as not Dr. Powers made the trip down to Colorado Springs to perform his surgery on Webb's patients and as late as 1914 he was still, like the early horse-and-buggy surgeons, doing many of these operations in the patients' homes.

One such operation was on young McKean Allen, the son of Benjamin and Maria Allen, Gerald's generous benefactors. McKean had slipped from the top of a high hip roof on a rancher's barn and grabbed hold of a live wire to brake his fall. After three years of Dr. Webb's ministrations he had recovered from all his injuries except for one twisted foot. Dr. Powers, examining the foot in his Denver office, thought he could set it straight and arranged to do so in the Allens' kitchen, with Dr. Webb acting as his assistant and Dr. Hanford giving the anesthetic. Powers bossily sent Gerald minute instructions as to what sterile clothing, basins, sponges, instruments, and solutions he should have ready and how he should prepare the makeshift operating room.

Powers repeated this behavior when he performed an appendectomy on Constance Pulitzer, this time at Beth-El Hospital. All went well and he immediately informed Webb that his surgeon's fee was $850. As usual Gerald added the fees for himself and Dr. Hanford and submitted the total as a single bill to the patient. Constance promptly paid him and went off to California to recuperate, but Gerald, arranging for a similar operation on a Miss Schofield who lived a few doors down North Cascade Avenue from Constance, hinted that Miss Pulitzer's bill might have been excessive and that Miss Schofield should not be charged so much.

Dr. Powers' reply was prolix. He set his fees, he said, according to the standard in New York, where surgeons charged well-to-do patients from $500 to $1000 for an operation in the city, $1000 for an operation out of town if the trip took them only half a day and $1500 if they had to stay overnight. In Chicago and Baltimore the fees were much higher. Webb must remember that Miss Pulitzer was a woman of wealth who was well known in elite circles in New York and elsewhere. Of course he would charge Miss Schofield less because of her lesser means, but it certainly was awkward when patients lived in the same neighborhood and could compare fees.

Webb himself was not charging enough, Powers said, for all the responsibility he bore as attending physician in charge of postoperative care; he must remember he was an established physician and not an immature student such as most surgeons used to assist them. It was just scandalous that he had charged the wealthy Benjamin Allens only $125 for all he had done on McKean's foot.

Well! Gerald huffily wrote back that hereafter Dr. Powers must send his own bill directly to the patient and he and Dr. Hanford would do the same—implying that he was no longer willing to bear the onus for Powers' outsize fees.

Three weeks later he wrote Powers in real distress. The surgeon's bill to Miss Schofield was much too high. "She cannot afford to pay it, has already discharged her nurse, and is having a severe nervous upset. I have cancelled my bill to her and think you must reduce yours."

"The part of medicine I detest is the sending of bills," he added.

Whereas, we may suspect, Dr. Powers enjoyed that part of it.

He did reduce Miss Schofield's bill, "substantially" he said. But he was unrepentant. Without taking breath he began preparing Gerald for trouble over the appendectomy they were doing on "the Tiffany boy." Mrs. Tiffany's New York doctor had warned him "she is the rich-but-hard-up kind, always ready and able to buy an expensive string of pearls but never able to pay her medical bills. She hasn't paid him anything for more than a year. He advised me to charge $3000 up for my services. You and Hanford should ask full value too because there will be delay and possibly litigation."

There was. A year later the three doctors sued Mrs. Tiffany for payment and it was almost another year before they collected—Dr. Webb $1000, Dr. Hanford $1500, Dr. Powers an undisclosed amount.

Gerald needed a good many such substantial fees to compensate for all the bills he canceled or never sent. His private charity was extensive; he belonged to the "don't mark them down in the book; they're poor folk" school. Frequently he dipped into his pocket to give a needy patient a few helpful dollars or even on occasion a sizable loan. Some of these came back to him unexpectedly years or decades later with a reminiscently grateful letter; more of them probably were never repaid.

Webb must have collected something somehow for all the patients he tended at Cragmor but it was not by direct payment to him. The sanatorium's weekly cost included his and Dr. Gilbert's services as well as Dr. Forster's. For non-Cragmor patients the fees he quoted were $10 for his initial examination, $2 or $3 per subsequent visit, $3 for each inoculation; he estimated the total cost of his treatment of tuberculosis at about $12 a month. His roster of patients included an extraordinary number of fellow physicians and to them and their families it was his policy to make no charge at all. "I am always glad to do anything I can to help a member of the profession," he said.

Still, he earned enough to support his growing family with increasing ease, to pay Dr. Gilbert and maintain a well-equipped office and clinical laboratory, to defray the costs of all his buying of books and journals and all his traveling. His income must have been substantial, but it came, it seems, from the number of his patients, not from charging them greedy fees.

Added to the wearying "clamor of patients" was the enormous chore of Gerald's correspondence. He loathed it. Keeping each referring doctor informed of his patient's progress or lack of it; replying to all the parents and spouses, brothers and sisters, uncles, aunts, and cousins who inquired anxiously and often how their loved ones were doing; staying in touch with colleagues about research and publication, association affairs, convention schedules, and all the rest—it was just too much.

Early on he bought a typewriter and began hiring a succession of part-time secretaries from among his recuperating women patients. Most of these were patently unskilled and inefficient, quite unable to manage either spelling or grammar. Off and on they embarrassed Dr. Webb, as when one sent the frank comments on NTA affairs he wrote Dr. Miller of New York to Dr. Miller of Chicago instead, or when another kept Dr. McIntyre of Cripple Creek waiting impatiently for Webb's report of an insurance examination while it wended its way to and from Dr. McIntyre of Lake Charles, Louisiana.

Dr. Webb could hardly complain. He was no model of disciplined order himself. He could never get to the bottom of his stack of letters-to-be-answered in the few hours or half a day he allotted to dictation once or twice a week and fresh arrivals went on top of those unanswered, so that he was continually having to explain: "I have just unearthed your letter of [weeks, even months, ago] from the pile of papers on my desk" or "I will answer the questions you asked a while back when I can find your letter again. It has got lost in the papers on my desk."

He was unashamed about this failing. "Procrastination is my besetting sin," he told several friends who twitted him about it. More than once his delay cost him a patient, as when Dr. Edwin Locke of Boston wrote him after three tries, "I began to think my patient would be dead before you answered my inquiry about accommodations at Cragmor, so I have sent him to Dr. Bullock in New Mexico instead."

Gerald must have found communication through secretaries inhibiting, an affront to his privateness, for many of his dictated letters were uncharacteristically brief and stiff, even at times inadequate to the question or situation they dealt with. Often when the typed transcripts came to him for signing he penned in freer, less stilted additions. Unfortunately we have no copies of these more relaxed postscripts; only a few that were never mailed and the responses to those that were reveal their existence.

That Dr. Webb had an effective "bedside manner" cannot be doubted but it was not the compound of spurious cheer and false, formula charm the term suggests. He was no chin-chucker or arm-squeezer, seldom even a handshaker. Patients said they listened expectantly each day for the sound of his voice in the hall or his slightly halting footsteps approaching their door, but not because he brought them chatty gossip or the latest risqué story. The farthest off-color he could go was his habitual comment in season that "Winter is lingering in the lap of Spring this year." He was a proper son of Victorian, not Edwardian, England.

He tried always to bring a bedrest patient something new to think about: a book from his library or a newspaper clipping to read, a poet's couplet or quatrain to ponder and memorize, an unusual bit of lore about a flower he had picked or a bird or butterfly he had seen on his way that morning.

Besides his natural reserve Gerald knew the need for caution and restraint. The aggravated sexuality and flushed hunger for romance of many tuberculous patients were a medical commonplace at the time, the passive dependency of others equally so. Dr. Webb's female patients were just waiting to fall in love with their handsome courtly doctor, or at least to make of him what we nowadays call "a father figure." He sought to avoid both involvements and learned to walk the line between inviting personal intimacy and imparting faith and courage.

His own experience had given him genuine understanding in the sickroom. He once said that standing by during Jenny's long ordeal had made him "know and *feel* the moods" of his patients — their loneliness and fear, restless boredom, overwhelming despair — and the helpless anxiety of their families. This true compassion somehow came through the formality of his manner as an inspiriting, sustaining concern.

The virtual idolatry this evoked in some patients is perhaps expressed in a few lines of verse, undated and anonymous, on an otherwise blank sheet that lies among his correspondence for 1914:

> Dr. Webb,
> "You have power like strong, deep rivers running,
> Carrying fresh life and force into the sea—
> And calmness like the ease in mountains wide.
> You are so vital, you attract like light
> Lesser creatures, frailer ones, wan and weak,
> That only know in you they find their strength."
>
> Sincerely yours, A patient.

XII

A Full House

BY ALL available accounts and evidence, Gerald's wife and children adored him too. In the time he could spare for them he was an enlivening, nourishing presence in their midst. They in turn anchored his busy life in a loving, diverting home. Only fleetingly did he think of all they cost him. As when in telling Varina about the splendid laboratory Dr. Christian Herter had outfitted for himself on an upper floor of his New York City house, he added, "I'm sure there weren't five little Herters!"

"Quoth the Raven, 'Never More!'" was Gerald's vow when his second son and fifth child, named Joel Addison Hayes for Varina's father, was born 2 May 1913. And Varina underscored the pledge by posing the baby with a raven for his first photograph.

There could have been more—Gerald was approaching forty-two and Varina had just turned thirty-five when Joel arrived—but the parents agreed that five were enough. Gerald meant it as more than a clever figure of speech when he told his friends, "We now have a full house, three queens and two kings."

The two immediately preceding queens were Frances Robine, born 11 April 1909 and named for Mater and a favorite English niece, and Eleanor Leila Constance, born 1 November 1911 and given the names of Gerald's sister Nell and the two family friends who became her godmothers, Constance Pulitzer and Leila Shields. The girls were called Robine and Leila; only Joel was allowed to keep his baptismal first name in family use. Gerald Junior was still Gerry but Margaret had undergone another change.

When she was four she was taken one day to visit her nurse Bianca whom Varina had sent to help out at the Hayes house when Mrs. Hayes was ill. Someone called her Binks. Bianca flashed into anger. "You are not Binks! You are Margaret! When you get home you tell your mother *you are Margaret*!" The child tried to obey

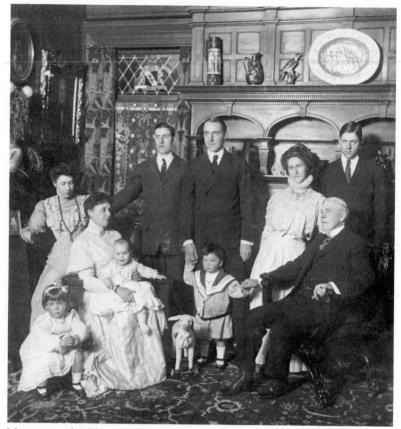

Margaret and Addison Hayes with their family, 1909. Baby Robine is on her grandmother's lap, Marka and Gerry at her knees. In the semicircle behind are, *left* to *right*, Varina, Jefferson Hayes-Davis, Gerald, Lucy, and William

but the nearest her little tongue could come to "Margaret" was "Mar-ka" and Marka she became and remained, creating a favored name for girls in succeeding generations of the family.

Margaret Hayes's illness cast a shadow over the Webbs throughout the first half of 1909. When Gerald discovered cancer in her breast he sent her to Dr. Francis Kinnicut, a New York surgeon of repute, who pronounced the growth inoperable, metastasis already begun, and death likely within the year.

That was in January. Addison Hayes was away, in Coronado Beach, California, the resort to which he usually took his asthma during Colorado's winter. He began preparations to return home immediately but Gerald advised him to wait:

"Dear Daddie: I think it would be most unwise of you to return at present. You are only just now getting better of your annoying cough. The worst feature with Mamie [Mommy] just now is her mental condition, but I am glad to say she has taken my advice and is out driving this morning. Her unfortunate condition is spreading but it will be a long time yet before it becomes desperate. The weather is as treacherous as ever and the grippe epidemic is becoming worse. It will be better for you to stay away some weeks longer. We all feel you cannot accumulate too much reserve strength, especially nervous strength, as you will have very trying times before you this summer. With all good wishes, Gerald."

The trying times came sooner than Gerald expected. A harrowing crisis in trust developed. Mrs. Hayes expected Gerald to pull her through this sickness as he always had done before and when nothing he tried made her better, she grew querulous and reproachful. He felt pressed to desperate measures, even to hopes about quack nostrums, especially one called Radium-Thor which was lavishly promoted by a Dr. Stillman Bailey of Chicago. Gerald wrote to ask Arnold Klebs about it: "A member of my wife's family has developed this disease and I am especially anxious to know if there is any value in this remedy."

Arnold's reply was sarcastic: "Nobody knows this 'Skillman' Bailey. His radium-thor does as much good in cancer as antiphlogistine in tuberculosis. But perhaps you feel hopeful about antiphlogistine. Do you know of a cure for baldness? I hear many reports from all sorts of people about such cures. Knowing now of your interest in these matters perhaps you can advise me. I am reminded that the great von Behring once tried Fleckwasser for dissolving tubercle bacilli!"

This letter may well have contributed to the dislike Varina felt for Arnold. He was happily preparing to marry Harriet and move to Switzerland at the time but that hardly excused such insensitivity to his friend's distress.

The family could only stand by helplessly. "Fortunately," said Gerald, "there is much work to do." He was busy with his new research into lymphocytes and his exploding practice in vaccine therapy and Varina was soon preoccupied with the new baby Robine. At times Margaret Hayes, in pain and frightened by the nearing shadow, thought them uncaring. Her death came on 18 July 1909. She was fifty-four.

The sadness was doubled for Gerald. Less than a week later, on 24 July, his sister Sophie died in London, of tuberculosis, ironically. She was fifty-three.

Margaret Hayes's will, unchanged since she had made it twenty-nine years before, left her Mississippi real estate and her personal property, the latter valued at $20,000 for probate, to her husband, with the provision that at his death it all be divided equally among her children. Mr. Hayes chose to anticipate this division to some extent, so that Varina received an immediate legacy of $2,000. She and Gerald knew exactly what they wanted to do with it.

Since their marriage they had managed to get away each summer to spend a week or two in the camp at Woods Lake to which they had gone for their honeymoon, up in the high mountains some two hundred miles west of Colorado Springs. The country thereabouts was wild, the accommodations "rough and primitive," but they enjoyed the solitude and recommended the place to friends as "wholly delightful."

Now, though, the children were becoming too many to be either taken along or left behind. So they used Varina's legacy to buy from William Otis a plot of unspoiled wilderness ten miles north of town (the site is now part of the grounds of the United States Air Force Academy) and to build in a sunlit clearing among its virgin pines a cabin-camp as a summer home. They named it "Ausflug," signifying a place to flee to, escape to, but the harsh German word did not long survive the outbreak of World War I; both being fervidly anti-Hun they replaced it with the more poetic and American "Tall Timbers."

As soon as the weather warmed enough, or in later years when school was out, Gerald moved Varina and "the bairns" to this retreat, where, he said, "the children can run wild and get brown as Indians." He drove out to join them some nights, on weekends, and for a vacation month in August.

Such divided living would have been difficult without the motor car. Gerald, sparked by the obsessive enthusiasm of his brothers Wilfred and Roland for the new horseless carriage, was among the first residents of Colorado Springs to own one. He took to it avidly, loved to tinker with its innards, did not mind the inconvenience of cranking it up or of stopping about every second trip to patch a puncture or a blowout. By 1909 he was driving a "Hup-mobile."

Dr. Webb and his big open car filled with a growing bevy of lively children became a familiar sight in town.

But the auto gave Varina no pleasure. For quite a while she refused even to ride in the noisy, dusty, jouncing thing, preferring to stick to her spirited horse and stylish carriage; these might be slower but she was sure they were safer too. In time she succumbed to the convenience of the automobile but she never did learn to drive one.

Varina was not gadget-minded. She accepted electric lighting and indoor plumbing but for a long time she resisted such innovations as the electric refrigerator and vacuum cleaner, even the kerosene kitchen stove. The old icebox, woodburning kitchen range, broom and carpet beater were good enough for her. Besides, she enjoyed such homely routines as the thrice-weekly coming of the iceman with his big sparkling bluish blocks to be swung with huge tongs or a canvas sling into the kitchen sink and there chipped into pieces of proper size and shape to fill the melted-empty spaces of the cooling chamber. New was seldom better for Varina.

She rejoiced in the casual freedoms of life at Tall Timbers. For Gerald the place was a diverting new toy. He plunged into additions and improvements, writing here and there to sportsmen and university deans of agriculture for advice on how to build a proper privy and dig an "earth hopper" for garbage disposal, how to make the cabin secure against animal intrusion, where to find good seeds for exotic wildflowers and native grasses.

He and Varina took the children for long walks in the woods, by their own enjoyment teaching the youngsters the fun of getting to know the various trees and plants and flowers, the birds and their songs and calls, the ways of the shy animals that were their neighbors in the forest. Always, of course, watching out for the ubiquitous rattlesnakes!

Leila never forgot how her father gently restrained her when in childish excitement at coming upon a stand of bluebells she greedily reached out to snatch up all the pretty flowers. Just pick one, he told her; that would be enough to take home and look at closely. If she left the others to go to seed they would make more flowers for her to enjoy next year.

The August vacations were half busman's holidays for Gerald. He used them to catch up on his correspondence ("Being on vacation I have time now to tell you how your patient is doing"), write his essays ("Near me as I write is a coniferous forest" — in which he found those mistletoe carriers), plan his research, schedule his trips for the coming fall. But at least during these few weeks he was physically present as husband and father for more hours of the day than in Colorado Springs.

Varina would certainly have liked to see more of him, to share more of his time, have more of his help in rearing the children, but she took cheerfully and understandingly what she could have. Gerald was appreciative of this; he paid tribute to her when in itemizing Pasteur's good luck in life he placed high on the list having "a wife who was willing that the laboratory should be put before everything else."

Several times Gerald shepherded Varina and "the babes" to Coronado Beach to spend a few winter weeks with Papa Hayes but aside from this Varina did no traveling. Unlike some doctors' wives she never accompanied Gerald on his trips to conventions, hospitals, and laboratories. She was a homebody by choice and felt uneasy being away from the children.

She could share her husband's journeys vicariously. Gerald was a good correspondent when away, sending her daily accounts of his doings, sometimes in long letters written before breakfast or at bedtime, at other times, when his schedule was tight or especially wearying, in a series of postcards or Western Union nightletters.

His tone in these missives was intimate, loving, sharing. Once from New York he told her, "I am so lonely when I'm away from you, dear little wife, without you to talk to, tell everything to. You give me so much, all my happiness, all my comfort, Varina Mea. Hug all the bairns for me. Lots of love from your lonesome, forever devoted Gerald."

Or he could be teasing: "Now be sure to lie down after lunch for some rest. Don't stay up reading too late. I'll be able to tell from the light bill if you've been burning the midnight oil, so look out!"

It was accepted between them that he preferred to turn in early while she liked to prolong her hours of peace and quiet after the children were asleep. He was usually in bed by eleven. For wakeful hours thereafter he kept beside his bed a dictionary, a copy of *Alice in Wonderland*, and a book of poetry. Often there too was the book he was currently reading for pleasure, usually something biographical; he seldom read fiction, either old or new.

It was his custom when away to buy a dozen or so postcards at some gallery or museum and dispatch them to the children at various later stops. To the younger ones he usually wrote some funny little message from "the King and Queen of the Fairies." Once when Varina had enclosed a tear-blotched note from five-year-old Leila that was an unhappy wail because her favorite playmate had gone off on a picnic without her, he replied at once on a postcard, "I'm sorry your little friend left you behind. When I get home you and I will go have a picnic together."

Robine too he frequently pointed forward to the day when he and she would visit New York together.

On Marka's eleventh birthday he was in Washington and took note of the day in a telegram to her followed by a "grownup" letter: "My dear big Marka: This day eleven years ago you made your mother and daddie very happy people." Then he told her about his visit the day before to "the old colored man who was your great-grandfather's body servant" and about meeting the President's daughter at dinner and riding back to his hotel in the White House limousine. "I know you enjoyed your fine party and hope you have many more happy birthdays. Your Daddie is proud of you."

His letters to Varina frequently revealed the disorganized haste in which he had set out. He was likely to discover that he had left behind some necessity which he asked her to send on at once: one time his notes for a paper, another time a set of illustrative slides, often this tie or that shirt or vest, once his entire outfit of evening wear.

And almost every letter named one or more patients or visiting relatives whom she should see or telephone or take books or flowers to. For one instance, from Chicago in 1912 he wrote her, "Do look after Mrs. Bromley. She isn't doing well and I'm worried about her. Tell Gilbert to be sure to see her every day. I'll try to write her to cheer her up."

Varina's letters, shorter and more matter-of-fact—she was not one who could lay her heart out on paper—included many reminders and requests of her own: names of friends or kinsmen, their addresses and phone numbers appended, whom she wanted him to greet for her.

Only once in the record did she ask him to go shopping for her: "Please bring home with you a puppy for Gerry, he wants one so badly." Succeeding letters spelled out suggestions as to size (medium), color (black), gender (male), and kind — she had found an illustrated advertisement for Belgian police dogs and thought one of those would be just the thing. The next day's mail brought Gerald an information sheet from the Belgian kennel in upstate New York with a note from the proprietor: "Your good wife has asked us to let you know what pups we have available now and at what prices."

This was too much. Gently Gerald put an end to it: "I don't like to disappoint you and Gerry but I really can't buy the puppy from here. What would I do with it as I zig-zag around the country on my way home? Perhaps when I get back we can ask the kennel to ship us the pup if you still want it. Tell Gerry [ten years old] I'll begin teaching him to shoot this summer."

He must have kept this promise because the next year he wrote the boy from Atlantic City that he had just bought some clay pigeons and the trap to release them and together they would practice with these when he got home.

He also bought the Belgian police dog puppy. Gerry named it Toughie.

Why Varina and Gerry wanted another dog is hard to imagine. The Webb domain was constantly overrun with animals. Varina could never turn away any homeless creature or resist the lure of a new and different pet. At one time her "menagerie" included a pedigreed Boston bulldog named Jay Lippincott, several stray mongrels she was feeding back to sleekness, two cats, a burro, a coyote named Mowry, two sheep that Gerald tagged Romulus and Remus, and two Shetland ponies called Rowena and Castanet.

The ponies had belonged to the daughters of Amelia Scudder. When her father Mr. Cupples died in 1912 she decided to move back to St. Louis permanently and offered the ponies to the Webbs. Gerald's whimsy took over. He suggested to Marka and Gerry, then seven and six, that they "plant" a pair of horseshoes and see whether these would grow into ponies.

Eagerly the two buried the steel "seeds," kept them copiously watered, and sprinted the first thing each morning to the nursery window to see if they had "sprouted." And there one morning, tethered in exactly the right place, stood Rowena and Castanet. There followed a flurry of expectant horseshoe-planting in the neighborhood.

As Marka and Gerry grew too tall for the ponies and were allowed to ride instead their father's polo mounts, Soda Pop and Lit-

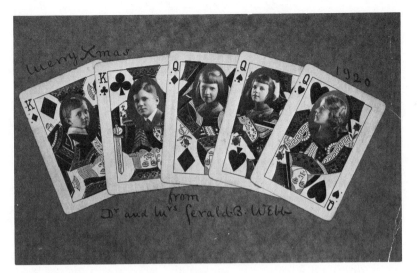

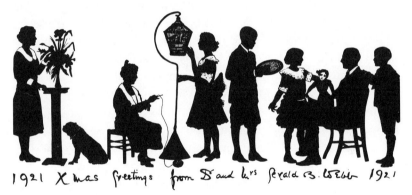

Christmas cards by Varina. *Above*, the full house; *below*, one of the
Scherenschnitte (scissor cuttings) at which she excelled

tle Steve, the Shetlands were passed down to the younger children.
By the time they came to Joel he found them "plain ornery, real
meanies." He could never find them. They had learned to escape the
incessant demands upon them by lying still among the tall grasses
to hide their spotted coats from seeking eyes.

Varina's whimsy expressed itself in nonsense verses she wrote
for the children, in the fanciful themes she elaborated for their parties and picnics, in the clever costumes and furnishings she made
for the girls' dolls and dollhouses. Long remembered were the pet-

ticoat flounces she fashioned from straw flowers, the fluted bowls she carved from mushroom caps, the tiny teacups she made from acorns.

She still found time to paint watercolors from sketches of wildflowers and birds she made during the walks at Tall Timbers. And she was a wizard at cutting out speaking likenesses in silhouettes. Gerald learned this art from her and used it to entertain restless children among his patients.

At a time when sending Christmas greetings was not the commercial custom it later became, Varina established the practice for the Webb family. Each year she devised an original design and produced, usually by her own hand, scores of copies which she and Gerald sent to their personal friends and his professional colleagues. Many of the recipients treasured and kept them, so that even today, as old homes are broken up and estates settled, complete sets of the Webb Christmas cards are sent back to Colorado Springs.

Besides reading during her night-owl hours, Varina cut and pasted to keep up to date a "baby book" for each child and a series of huge scrapbooks, one about the Jefferson Davis family, another about the history of Colorado Springs, and several full of clippings, convention programs, and similar mementos of Gerald's doings.

In this task she obviously wasted no time on organizing the accumulated items. They went into the books helter-skelter, just as they came to her hand, quite without regard to any order in either time or topic. Few of them bore any indication of date or source though occasionally Varina did add a comment. Alongside a satirical magazine piece, "What a Husband Should Do to Keep His Wife Happy," she penciled "Presented to me by my husband!"

Many of her daytime hours she gave to sewing and embroidery. She still made some of her own and the children's clothes, but rarely anymore did she apply her nimble fingers to apparel for Gerald.

He continued to buy practically all his clothes by mail orders to Thomas the Tailor in Cheltenham. In the way of English tailors, that firm kept his preferences and measurements on record and every few years he asked them to send him a new suit or two, having only to say "add an inch all around" or "take off an inch" as his weight went slightly up or down. He rarely deviated from his chosen sturdy dark blue cloth or the double-breasted style he favored.

His shoes too, requiring a special lift in the left heel, he ordered custom-made from Sharpe the Bootmaker in Cheltenham — though occasionally in an emergency he made do with a cobbler named Jones in Denver. He seldom wore a hat except when traveling.

For winter wear he added only a lightweight gabardine coat and buckskin gloves. How, so lightly clad, he could endure the cold as he went about town and stood talking to his patients on their open sleeping porches neither Varina nor the children could understand. They forgot that he had been reared in the lower temperatures and absence of central heating in England.

Although a Colorado Springs tailor once told Varina that her husband was "the best dressed man in town" and she vehemently agreed, Gerald himself felt his English clothes made him conspicuous and was often shy about them. But when he once tried buying an American-made suit it was money wasted; it just did not fit well and he was uncomfortable in it. Nor did it wear as well as the product of Thomas the Tailor; some of his Cheltenham suits remained serviceable for twenty years.

Marka once described the North Cascade house of her girlhood:

"The large livingroom faced Cascade Avenue, with a sunny diningroom next to it to the south. To the north of it a long narrow hallway led to Daddie's waiting room, office, and laboratory. Later, when he moved his offices to the Burns Building, these rooms were used for his den, his books—though there were books, books, books, everywhere!—and for mother's collections. One of these was of Dresden and Staffordshire china figurines and another was of the Pikes Peak flasks and other historical bottles. These were attractive in shapes and colors and were becoming antique treasures. Mother and her friends kept on the lookout for good specimens and she gathered an extensive collection of them.

"From the livingroom a beautiful winding staircase, with low treads and two wide landings, one two steps up and the other midway, rose to the second floor. At the front upstairs were two bedrooms belonging to our parents, both with sleeping porches. We children all lived in the corresponding 'dormitories' at the back of the house, one for the girls and one for the boys, both with sleeping porches on which we slept most nights."

The house was a busy, happy home. No matter how late Varina had stayed up the night before she was always in the diningroom ready to greet Gerald and the children when they came for breakfast at seven. And at eight she would be waiting on the lower landing of the stairs, which brought her up to Gerald's height as he stood two steps below, for his kiss and invariable "Goodbye, young'un. I'm off now on my rounds." Then he would walk out to the old barn where he garaged his car, stopping on the way to give himself a good head-clearing sneeze by looking at the sun.

When in town he tried to join the family for the evening meal, at which conversation was general and lively, with none of Pater's monologues or histrionics, though books and reading, from the girls' fairy tales and the boys' cowboy stories to the parents' biographies, plays, and poetry, were frequent topics.

When eating was done and Gerald folded his napkin, it was the cue for one of the children to jump onto his lap and perhaps finger the scars on his left arm, which fascinated them all, while they played their word game. Each evening he would make little puzzles for them out of the meanings and derivations of two or three new words, then quiz them about these the next night.

From the table, his time permitting, they all moved to the piano where he played and led them in singing songs from his favorite light operas, most often Gilbert and Sullivan, or perhaps Franz Lehar or Victor Herbert or some other on that popular level. Or they might gather around the Victrola and listen to recordings of arias from *Rigoletto*, *Carmen*, *Samson and Delila*, *Aïda*.

Then he would dispatch the younger children to sleep with a bedtime story, often of his own invention. He entertained Leila and Joel for months with the series of adventures he made up for El Joe and Lilee, ending each tale with "And then they went to bed spinning on their heads."

He found time to teach each child in turn the arts of horsemanship and the fine points of good style in tennis. In these he was a severe coach and in time the Webb family alone put on many a good show on the courts of the Cheyenne Mountain Country Club. He also introduced the children to golf, chess, and bridge—with less conspicuous success.

Varina taught them skating and dancing. She also superintended their formal schooling, conferred with their teachers, attended their special class exercises. And each week she got them all dressed in their best and saw them off to Sunday school at St. Stephen's Episcopal Church, though neither parent was a churchgoer and religion was not a matter of much concern in the home. "Everyone has a religion of some kind but mine does not depend upon a church," was Gerald's one recorded comment on the subject.

Discipline too was Varina's responsibility, though she could always call upon Gerald as backup. According to Leila, "Neither Daddie nor Mother ever laid a finger on any of us. I can't remember that Daddie ever even raised his voice to us. He didn't have to. He would just look me in the eye and say very firmly, 'Young lady, I don't want you ever to do that again. Do you understand?' That was enough. When we were naughty we would beg Mother, please don't tell Daddie."

Only rarely did Gerald participate in a polo game anymore but when he did the sportswriters were sure to lament, "If only Dr. Webb could find more time for the game he would certainly be one of the nation's best players." He continued to play a good deal of tournament tennis and was frequently a winner in both singles and doubles. He found time too for evenings of chess and bridge at the club and was a whizz at both.

A new diversion for him were the play-reading and -acting evenings of the Drama Club, of which he became a founder and director in 1910. He discovered he was a good actor, that when playing a role he could shed completely his customary decorum and reserve, become even a convincing buffoon if need be. It was a release he greatly enjoyed.

Although he and Varina took almost no part in the idle partying that consumed the time of the fashionable set, they did plenty of entertaining. Varina had no need to travel to meet Gerald's friends; they came to her. If we may judge from the number who in writing to Gerald sent their thanks to his wife for her hospitality, guests must have streamed through her house in these years.

Nor were the thanks perfunctory. The writers called her witty, merry, vivacious. "She added a lot to the pleasure of my visit," said Mazÿck Ravenel. "I still remember her clever comments and laugh at them again when I repeat them here," wrote Dr. Edwin Locke of Boston. "What a helpmeet she must be," said Dr. Crile of Cleveland.

The visitors came from abroad as well as the United States. Arnold Klebs never got out to see the Webbs at home but he sent them half a dozen travelers from Switzerland. Clemens von Pirquet's sister and her friend "Prof. Rianzi" came from Vienna, Dr. Leonard Colebrook from St. Mary's Hospital in London, Aylmer May's brother from Rhodesia, Dr. Emile Dupuy from Paris several times. Livingston Farrand was a frequent guest, once bringing his entire family to stay for several days.

Varina, quick to form decisive likes and dislikes, was not enamored of all these transients—vehemently not of the difficult Hideyo Noguchi—but she put herself to trouble for them. With Gerald or sometimes alone she took them for picnics at a mountain ranch or beside the crystal ribbon of Fountain Creek, or for rides to Manitou and Glen Eyrie and of course the Garden of the Gods. She guided so many through that scenic wonder that she must have grown weary of its spectacular shapes and colors. Her trip to the Garden with the Englishmen Haldane and Douglas was by moonlight and Haldane sent her renewed thanks for the memory a full year later.

Most exciting for Varina was the coming of Dr. Wilfred T. Grenfell, the medical missionary. She had read his book *The Labrador Doctor* and was so gripped by the story of his work among the destitute fishermen of the ice-locked north that she hero-worshipped the author. When his fund-raising lecture tour brought him to Colorado Springs in February 1909 and he took the occasion to visit Dr. Webb and his laboratory, she was thrilled to meet him and be his hostess at dinner.

She scarcely knew what to make of the Irish poet Padraic Colum when he was similarly her dinner guest during his first lecture tour in America in 1914. She found his Celtic legends and mysticism bewildering.

The Webb children were never hidden away from these visitors, nor commanded to be seen but not heard. They were often a big part of the entertainment and made friends of their own who sent them messages and gifts. Unusual among the latter were two big dolls that arrived one day from Dr. A. G. Shortle of Albuquerque: a curly-haired charmer in nurse's uniform for Marka and a black-haired imp in cowboy regalia for Gerry. At dinner with the Webbs some months earlier Dr. Shortle had asked the children the banal question, What do you want to be when you grow up? and then, with much less banality, had the dolls made and dressed to order according to their answers.

Marka became the special pet of Dr. Powers of Denver, who was often at table with the Webbs when he came to do an operation in Colorado Springs. For years he sent the child affectionate remembrances from the far places to which he traveled.

Robine was the adored one of Dr. James Hart. One of his return visits to Colorado Springs coincided with her birth and it gladdened his heart to stand as her godfather. He kept on his New York desk the successive pictures of her that Varina provided him and never failed to send her love and kisses in his letters to her father. Wistfully he kept hoping he would see "that prize baby, my Robine" again before she was grown and asked her parents to "keep mentioning my name to her so she won't forget me."

The highlight visitors in the summer of 1913 were Gerald's brother Harold and his son Rupert.

The handsome Harold, now in his fiftieth year, was even more restless than usual, worried because the brick and tile business of Webb Brothers Limited was passing from boom to slump as England turned the strange trick of combining a famine in housing with a depression in the building trades. He was a fine tennis player still and worked off his tensions by giving Gerald several good battles on the courts during his visit. He had become something of a freelance journalist on the side, writing features for the Cheltenham and London newspapers, and he brought Gerald clippings of two of these pieces, one on the origins of lawn tennis, the other on what he decried as antic arrangments and behavior in Parliament.

"Although the Houses of Parliament were designed and built by a near relative of my mother," he had written, "I think the debating chamber of the Commons combines the minimum of convenience with the maximum of ugliness."

Gerald welcomed the family news Harold brought because since Mater's death correspondence among the Webbs had grown sparse and sporadic.

Sister Nell, said Harold, was having another patch of poor health, in pain from arthritis much of the time and longing for her son Geoffrey, who had begun his career in the Royal Navy.

Gentle Ida had wholly given up her singing and was getting to be a timid, mousy little doormat. For this the brothers indignantly blamed her husband Fred, a Church of England "parson" whom they considered a domineering, browbeating boor.

But Amy, also married to an Anglican parish priest, David Edmondes-Owen by name, was as spirited and energetic as ever, busily mothering her two daughters Nancy and Robine and running a scad of diocesan affairs. Everybody was fond of her husband Daff, as they called him from the Welsh spelling of his name, Daffyd. He had many friends among the literati of England and was more than an amateur in horticulture. He kept the lawns and gardens of his and Amy's home at Llandwedd Vicarage in Builth Wells so beautiful in shrub and flower that they filled the Webb boys with nostalgia for Heimat.

Things had never been better for Wilfred. He was still with the Crossley Engine Company in Manchester where he was becoming the foremost British expert on the new diesel engine. Harold had never seen him happier. His wife Blanche had borne him a daughter six months before, their first child, whom they named Cynthia. She was a happy, lively baby and Wilfred was besotted about her.

(Three years later Gerald got a frantic cry for help from Wilfred. Cynthia had contracted tuberculosis of the spine and developed a curvature. She was immobilized in splints from neck to knee but the deformity was growing more pronounced and she was losing her cheerful spirit. Please, please, what would Gerald advise? Unwilling to prescribe a treatment he would not be present to direct, Gerald could only suggest as much sunshine and fresh air as the splinting permitted.)

Harold's news of Roland's and Lilian's only child Eric was of special interest to Gerald. Upon graduation from the Dean Close School Eric had won a scholarship to Guy's Hospital and was to begin his medical education there the coming fall. He hoped to do good enough work to win him the post of dresser for his Uncle Gerald's friend, senior surgeon L. A. Dunn. Gerald passed the word on to Mr. Dunn who replied that he would keep an eye out for the boy.

Mater had been terribly wrong, Harold said, to oppose and postpone for a year the marriage of her youngest, Frank, to his chosen Ann Robson, the smart, pretty, redhaired daughter of his landlady while he was a solicitor's clerk at Alnwick. The year apart had been hard on the young couple, especially on Frank's health. But Mater had grown fond of Ann and admitted her mistake to them all before she died. Frank and Ann were now the happy, loving parents of three sons, known in the family as the three Ds: Donald, Dick, and Denis.

Frank had come finally to enjoy his dry-as-dust profession and was acquiring a large clientele and much respect as a solicitor in the town of West Hartlepool in the north of England. He still enjoyed playing the piano, writing verses, and above all, drawing and sketching. His brothers agreed that in talent and inclination Frank was probably the most literary and artistic member of the family.

Harold was pleased with his own family. In spite of four miscarriages and a stillbirth Enid had given him four children: Rupert aged fifteen, Josephine nine, and two small sons of five and four named John and Bryan, all bright, healthy youngsters.

Rupert, his father's companion on this trip, had just finished his schooling, and Harold, thinking back to his own experience in Australia when he was eighteen, wondered if it might not be good for the boy to have a similar adventure.

The upshot was that when Harold departed for home he left Rupert behind to spend a year as a cowboy on a Colorado ranch under his Uncle Gerald's supervision. Unfortunately *Doctor* Gerald felt it necessary to cut the year short when the boy began showing signs of an allergy to alkali dust and Rupert returned to England in time to join his contemporaries in the trenches of the Great War.

That war was increasingly on Gerald's mind after the United States joined the Allies in April 1917. He wanted to be in it. But he was somewhat uneasy about his health.

Ever since the respiratory ailment that almost prevented his going to Rome in 1912 he had been bothered by sporadic touches of illness. Late that year he entered a Denver hospital for an operation by Dr. Powers, of what kind we do not know. Three years later he did the same, this time, he said, "to follow the fashion of the day and have my tonsils removed."

Actually he was trying out a more basic fad of the time: the widespread belief that many aches and pains were caused by bad tonsils or teeth acting as "foci of infection." Gerald was suffering from transient spells of "much pain" in his right hip accompanied by "twinges of pain" in his hands and feet. The tonsillectomy did not relieve him of these but they vanished in a year or two. Perhaps they were a forerunner of the arthritic gout that afflicted him in later years. Or the cause may have been emotional stress.

For this was the time when Dr. Webb was giving up his experiments with live-germ vaccination and also with lymphocytes, and the time when he was having to recognize that vaccines were not a panacea and to question his belief in phagocytosis and antibodies. He was certainly disheartened if not depressed by the failure of his quest for immunity to the tubercle bacillus. And he was more than a little bored by the repetitive problems and routines of his practice. He needed a change.

It was his continuing deep fatigue in the spring of 1917 that made Varina insist he take "a long, lazy loaf" in Atlantic City before the convention of the Association of American Physicians. Perhaps Dr. Thayer of Johns Hopkins suggested, as they hiked the boardwalk together, that something amiss with his heart might be causing his malaise, because shortly after he returned home he decided to go to Denver and see Dr. Sewall "about my heart"—and also to order a new pair of shoes from Jones the shoemaker; the boardwalk miles had worn out his old ones.

He chose to make the trip by auto in order to take Gerry along for an outing. The youngster reported from the Brown Palace Hotel: "Dear Mother   we got here safely   we didn't have any blowout or puncture. We are soon going out to play golf. We had a good hair cut. Love from Gerry."

His father penned a postscript: "Gerry seems to be having a bully good time and is a strenuous companion. Will see Sewall and Jones tomorrow. May go to Idaho Springs about 90 miles away before coming home. Will keep you posted."

Sewall's verdict must have been reassuring because a few weeks later Dr. Webb went off to serve in the war.

XIII

Over There

THE NATION was slow and clumsy in gearing up for combat after it entered the Great War in April 1917 as an associate of the Allies against the Central Powers. It had never fought a war so massive or so far away, and it took the military leaders an astonishing while to realize that more would be required of them than just defense of our own Atlantic coast.

Men, money, matériel, all were shockingly inadequate for the commitment the United States had made and efforts to increase all three many times over and in a hurry lurched forward more or less together.

The weary and dispirited Allies, their forces depleted by the long and deadly stalemate in the trenches, were clamoring for a quick infusion of fresh troops. General John J. Pershing, named to command the American Expeditionary Force, estimated that he would need one million soldiers overseas a year hence, with at least as many more to supply and serve them. But the standing army numbered barely 100,000 and the National Guard could at best muster only 400,000 more. How were all the others to be gathered in?

Among those who advocated recruiting local companies of volunteers led by community celebrities was the fiery Theodore Roosevelt. Remembering the glory of San Juan Hill, he demanded permission to reproduce his famous Rough Riders and lead them into action in France. Many scoffed at the idea and the debate was fierce. In the end, realities prevailing, Congress passed a selective service act instituting a draft as the most effective way to collect the regiments needed.

The selection and movement of men began, and with it a gigantic bustle of building camps to house them, railway cars and ships to transport them, huge depots of supplies to feed and clothe them while they were inducted, trained, and sorted into military units.

Included in the induction routine, for the Army and the National Guard as well as the draftees, were medical examinations to weed out those physically unfit to fight. Owing largely to the urgent persuasion of the NTA, special emphasis in these examinations was to be placed upon the detection of tuberculosis.

When Gerald Webb went to NTA headquarters in May 1917 to ask what he could do to help in the war effort he found everybody in the office alarmed by reports of rampant tuberculosis in France. The year before, a Harvard faculty member serving as an exchange professor at the Sorbonne had passed home to the Rockefeller Foundation the tales he kept hearing of decimating disease on the battlefields. The Foundation immediately sent Dr. Hermann Biggs to Paris to study the situation. Biggs had just returned with his report.

A scarred veteran of many a public health battle, Biggs no longer bothered to be tactful. France had always ignored her tuberculosis problem, he said, and now she was paying the high price of her negligence. Consumption was taking a huge toll everywhere among her people. Poor screening of conscripts and the stresses of combat, enormously increased by France's customary failure to provide decent care for its troops below the rank of commissioned officers, had aggravated the death rate; in 1916 alone nearly 100,000 French soldiers had either died of tuberculosis or been discharged from the army in an advanced stage of it.

Whew! The French were insulted, the Americans scared, by Biggs's blunt indictment. What kind of a pesthole were we about to send our boys into?

The Foundation immediately named a special commission to undertake an anti-tuberculosis campaign in France and summoned Livingston Farrand from the University of Colorado to head it. Farrand opened an office in Paris and, being more skilled in diplomacy than Biggs, soon assuaged the hurt feelings of the French and secured their cooperation in instituting measures of tuberculosis control.

Meanwhile the NTA officials were showering advice upon the Surgeon General of the Army, William C. Gorgas, who gave them a sympathetic hearing. After his famous exploit in eradicating yellow fever from "the white man's graveyard" in Panama, General Gorgas had become interested in controlling other infectious diseases and needed little urging to set up a Tuberculosis Section in the Army Medical Corps. To be its chief he selected Colonel George E. Bushnell, who for a decade had been in charge of the army's tuberculosis sanatorium at Fort Bayard, New Mexico.

Dr. Webb knew Colonel Bushnell well. The two men had exchanged views often during Webb's visits to New Mexico and to Bushnell's hospital at Fort Bayard and they had visited sanatoriums together during the International Congress in Rome in 1912. Each respected the other's competence.

Colonel Bushnell immediately drew up minutely detailed instructions as to proper examining procedures for detecting tuberculosis, including a long list of conditions and symptoms that would warrant rejecting a man for army service as tuberculous and an even longer list of those that would not. The Surgeon General issued these instructions as Circular No. 20 on 13 June 1917 and a few weeks later sent out a call for physicians to serve under contract on Tuberculosis Examining Boards charged with screening the draftees.

One of the first three Colorado Springs doctors to sign up as "contract surgeons" at a hundred and fifty dollars a month was Gerald B. Webb. The other two were Will Howard Swan and Henry Hoagland.

Webb was dispatched forthwith to Fort D. A. Russell, an established army post three miles from Cheyenne, Wyoming, where he arrived in his Franklin on Saturday, 21 July 1917.

He had barely unpacked his bags when a telegram arrived from Varina. His New Mexico friend had not forgot him. In a letter delivered just after he left, Colonel Bushnell offered him a captaincy in the Medical Reserve Corps and urged him to accept it.

"In order to get the raise in salary I telegraphed accepting!" he wrote Varina the next day. He did not tell her that the change of status, while not altering the work he would do, would take away his freedom of action; he would thenceforth be under army orders for the duration of the war.

The other two doctors on Fort Russell's examining board were Colorado friends of Webb's and soon the three men were each ticking off with ease the required sixty examinations a day, usually in no more than five hours.

"I see I shall learn quite a little about chests," Gerald told Varina, "if corns do not grow on my fingers from percussion and in my ears from stethoscope rub. It is a kind of rapid transit chest examination like the rapid transit chess games I saw played in New York."

His commission arrived early in August and as Captain Webb he was official chief of the examining team.

He found the new life refreshing. The examinations were strenuous while they lasted but he had plenty of time to rest. And he became aware how much the lack of involvement with patients decreased the strain on him: "The routine without grief to carry is good for me."

Fort Russell, housing five thousand men in mostly cavalry units, seemed a huge post to him. He took his meals with the officers of the 25th Cavalry, who welcomed him gleefully into their polo, tennis, and chess games when they discovered his skill in all three. They assigned him a horse for daily rides in return for the auto transportation he provided them to events in Cheyenne—even, grimacingly, to the nightly movies they wanted to see. He enjoyed much more the rodeo events of Frontier Days, Cheyenne's annual fiesta.

Not all his spare time went to play. He wrote an editorial for "Vaughan's journal" (the *Journal of Laboratory and Clinical Medicine*) about "Tuberculosis and the Army," seeking to spread more widely the word about the tuberculosis problem in France and the preventive purposes of the Tuberculosis Examining Boards. And he began collecting statistics that might settle a current argument over the effects of smoking on the incidence of tuberculosis. Many doctors thought cigarette-smoking was a significant cause of the disease and Webb was quick to see that the records of the examining boards might be a good source of figures to prove or disprove the idea.

Matters back in Colorado Springs caused him concern. His impulsive enlistment, for just a few months he had thought, had left everybody, including his patients, unsettled. Now that he was in the army perhaps for years, he must make lasting arrangements.

What was to be done about the new research series he had started? And about Cragmor? Dr. Forster was preparing to enter the Medical Reserve Corps himself. Varina and the children were clamoring to join him in Cheyenne. Would it be wise to let them do so, when diphtheria, measles, and scarlet fever were nearing epidemic proportions at Fort Russell?

When Gerald got his first weekend pass in mid-August he drove home and settled these problems in a few packed hours on Sunday morning. He made quick rounds to say goodbye to his patients, ending with those at Cragmor, where he then conferred with the doctors who would be taking charge when Forster left. After talking with Dr. Gilbert and the staff in the Burns Building office, he paid brief visits to Daddie Hayes, to console him about his son Jefferson who had impetuously enlisted in the newest and most adventurous branch of military service and was already in training as an aviator; Constance and William Elmslie, to warn the frail William off his foolhardy plan to join up; and Maria and Benjamin Allen, to reassure them about their sons Wharton and Curtis who were seeking admission to officer training camps in Philadelphia.

Dr. Gilbert gamely agreed to shoulder the burden of the practice and keep an eye on medical matters at Cragmor and experiments in the laboratory. Mr. Hayes would take charge of business matters at Cragmor. And young Dr. Ryder, with the assistance of Dr. Minnie Staines and Dr. Gilbert's wife Margaret, would maintain a pared-down research program, taking care to stretch as far as possible the six hundred dollars remaining in the budget out of last December's donation from the Allens.

The availability of Dr. Charles Tripp Ryder was a godsend. He had been working off and on with Webb and Gilbert for about two years. A graduate of the Harvard medical school, he had gone on to study research methods with the best of all teachers, Dr. Theobald Smith, and had become one of Smith's favorite assistants when he grew gravely ill with tuberculosis. He made his way out to Colorado Springs and into the orbit of Dr. Webb in 1913. When he had recovered a measure of health he wanted something to do to fill the few hours a day he felt able to work and Dr. Webb was glad to provide it, at a stipend of thirty dollars a month.

Ryder proved an exceptionally able and inspired research man who could without qualms be left to carry on Webb's and Gilbert's latest attempt to induce resistance to tuberculosis by transplanting tubercular lymph nodes into healthy guinea pigs.

His business done by early afternoon, Dr. Webb picked up his family, who refused to be left behind, and started the drive back to Fort Russell. He had to be there by midnight, when his leave expired. He made it, the Franklin and its tires cooperating.

The pleasant life at Fort Russell came to an end only two weeks later. In early September orders arrived transferring Gerald immediately as "*Major* Gerald B. Webb M.R.C." to head the Tuberculosis Examining Board at the base hospital attached to "Camp Bowie, pronounced Booey" three miles east of Fort Worth, Texas.

The change was a shock. Camp Bowie, still very much under construction, already housed 24,000 inductees and was planned to receive some 50,000 more. Fort Russell was a midget in comparison. It looked as though Webb's stay in Texas might be a long one, and he was alone again; the family had returned to Colorado Springs.

Conditions at the camp were dreadful. The drafted men were housed in pup tents set up in tight rows that seemed to stretch without end across a flat unshaded plain. The doctors were provided with makeshift quarters in a partially reconstructed but wholly undeodorized hen house furnished with rough wooden trestles to serve as tables and chairs. On the rutted roadway just outside the door noisy steamrollers rumbled past all day long. For sleeping the doctors were given narrow cots to be unfolded on top of tables in the mess hall after dinner.

Food was ample but awful. Neither electricity nor hot water was available. Work necessarily began at dawn and ended at nightfall. And for Gerald Webb the Texas heat was "simply hellish," day and night, unrelieved either by the winds that kept the air forever full of stinging sand or by the frequent rains that turned camp grounds and roads into morasses of mud. *C'est la guerre* was already the familiar shrug-off to all complaints.

Major Webb soon had his examining board and its schedule organized. The required number of examinations had been increased to one hundred a day per physician. Not too much of a load, he thought, but he quickly discovered that his fellow examiners, all doctors from Texas, knew next to nothing about diagnosing tuberculosis. Dismayingly wont to judge merely by appearance, they had to be reminded again and again that slight physique alone did not guarantee the presence of the disease.

At Fort Russell Webb had paid scant attention to Colonel Bushnell's detailed Circular No. 20; it had been primer stuff to him and his Colorado colleagues. But here in Texas the need for it was manifest. The Major had to be tactful teacher as well as examining physician.

His hours of work lengthened to match the hours of daylight. Almost. One amenity the doctors' quarters did provide was a

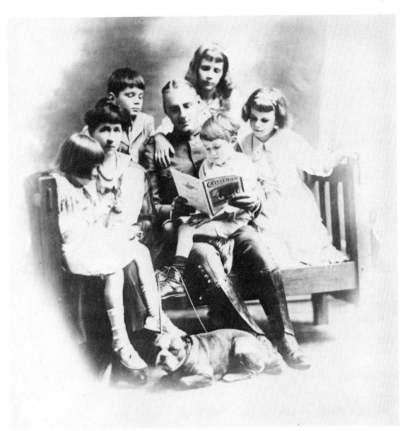

Major Webb and his family at Camp Bowie

shower of sorts, and after ten or so hours of drenching sweat in the stifling hen house Webb allowed himself enough daylight at day's end for a cold shower and half an hour of reading.

His book at the moment was a biography of Alfred, Lord Lyttleton, the Edwardian politician and Cabinet member who was Gladstone's nephew by marriage. Lyttleton's habit of reading late at night reminded him of Pasteur, Wright, Stevenson, "and other great men who burned the midnight oil to find time for all the things they wanted to do. There is no hope for this sluggard who likes to sleep."

There was no more chess, no more polo or tennis. Gerald's big treat now was a Sunday drive to Fort Worth, or perhaps the thirty miles to Dallas, where in one of the big hotels — that such splendid ones existed in these dusty cow towns on the edge of nowhere amazed and puzzled him — he would get himself and his clothes

thoroughly clean and enjoy a good meal or two in civilized surroundings.

The fretting rub of camp conditions inclined him to entertain
Varina's plea that she and the children come again to join him. Not
until the summer heat was over, he decided; "the children would
surely sicken in it, especially little Joel."

By mid-October the Webbs were together again in a home of
Varina's making, at 1712 South Adams Street in Fort Worth, and
the Major was using his nights and Sundays to complete his study
of cigarettes and tuberculosis and write it up for publication in a
new journal, the *American Review of Tuberculosis*. Reading it
there early the next year, Colonel Bushnell promptly wrote to ask
the author's permission to publish it also in the *Military Surgeon*.

Webb had found that of the draftees rejected as cases of active
tuberculosis by the examining boards many more were nonsmokers
than smokers. Dr. Allen K. Krause, editor of the new *Review*,
commented that the constant inhalation of tobacco smoke might
set up a low-grade inflammation in the lungs "that should be mildly
stimulating and tending to repair."

All the same, Gerald Webb must have had his doubts, for he
now cut his own consumption of cigarettes to five a day and presently to none at all.

Record-setting winter cold and a change of post suddenly arrived
together in mid-December. With only a few hours' notice Major
Webb had to leave his shivering family and entrain for Chicago, on
his way to the base hospital at Camp Custer in Michigan, six miles
east of Battle Creek and fifteen miles west of Kalamazoo.

As he learned when he arrived, Colonel Bushnell, suspecting
something amiss with his Tuberculosis Board at Camp Custer
because of the few and peculiar reports it was sending him, had
gone out to look it over. He found the Division Surgeon in command of the base hospital "tearing his hair out" because the slow-
ness of the tuberculosis examiners was skewing up his schedules,
and the examiners themselves were irritated and confused by
divergent instructions from their two feuding chiefs. He immediately dismissed the bickering twosome and sent for Major Webb.

Webb's way was smoothed by "a good deal of prestige" preceding
his coming. After just a week he wrote Varina, "Have at last got
order out of much disorder. Things were pretty mixed up. I reor-
ganized the whole machine, got in 12 more clerks, and the men are

now getting through 100 examinations apiece every day instead of 30. They are largely Indiana, Michigan, and Wisconsin men, a fine lot of fellows, eager to do their best, but they are not the equal of our Colorado men on tuberculosis. They all seem to like me in spite of my autocratic ways!"

It helped that a tuberculosis specialist in Kalamazoo immediately invited the entire board and his local colleagues to meet Dr. Webb and hear him speak, and that, according to the local newspaper, the officers of Camp Custer welcomed Major Webb with *two* banquets in his honor at the Holland Tea Shop in Battle Creek!

Camp Custer was an established army post like Fort Russell. Its quarters were in two-storied steam-heated barracks that provided "all the comforts of home." Gerald could again enjoy his customary cold shower in the morning and hot bath at night. The mess was excellent; "it ought to be, it costs twice what we paid at Camp Bowie."

His one irritation now was caused by the "uncomfortable and foolish" high collar of his uniform and "the absurd jewelry" that designated his rank; he was always pricking his fingers on its pins. "What with hooking one's collar and pinning on the gold oak leaves, one needs a lady's maid," he wrote Maria Allen.

The Tuberculosis Board was allotted an entire spacious ward for its work—"luxury after that hen house. They keep it so well heated that the men go about their job in light clothing. In fact it's too hot for my liking," said Gerald.

Not so outdoors. There the temperature fell to 15° below zero. "It would soon solidify your bone marrow, Varina Mea." Deep snow rounded the shapes of everything in the landscape and the skies were leaden, but the air was clean and crisp. "The country is very pretty, quite picturesque, hilly and woodsy, with a nice little lake near us. The whole atmosphere of the place is very much like a New England town."

The Major soon discovered that Camp Custer was "kind of a sorting out place," troops constantly coming and going in a regrouping of regiments. The flow of men to Webb's board was consequently erratic; "they send us 1200 men one day and less than 600 the next."

The number dwindled to a trickle as Christmas furloughs were passed out and when he learned that no new draft was scheduled until February he knew his work at Camp Custer would shortly be done. He hoped for reassignment to a post in the South where he and the family could be together for the winter. He brushed aside Varina's fear that he might be sent to France: "Be of good heart without foolish forebodings."

To finish off his batch of reports for Washington Webb went himself to the officers' barracks to examine the Division staff. Was it necessary that the commanding general be examined, asked a colonel. That was for General Parker to decide, replied the medical reserve corps major, but of course the Camp Custer records would not be complete if he was not included. Presently the colonel returned to conduct Major Webb into General Parker's office for the examination.

It was at once clear that the tall, burly general expected only a pro forma procedure. He refused to remove his jacket and shirt and went into a fuming tantrum when Webb said the required examination could not be made through his uniform. He stalked up and down the office ranting about all this medical nonsense. Webb stood silent, unyielding, his hazel eyes steady and steely. With a final burst of profanity the general dismissed him.

Fearing he might have committed some grave lèse majesté, Webb went at once to report the incident to the Division Surgeon and was relieved when that officer just chuckled and commended him for upholding the dignity of the medical profession in the face of military arrogance. It was well known that the macho brass of the army viewed its medical corps with disdain—and equally that the regular army doctors cursed the current influx of civilian medical specialists.

Webb's dinner that night was interrupted by a phone call from General Parker's aide. Would Major Webb please not send his reports to Washington until the next day? The general wished to be examined in the morning.

The big man was all smiles when Webb appeared next morning. He promptly stripped to the waist and during the examination entertained the doctor with anecdotes of his recent visit to the battlefields in France. The two men parted amiably.

In high spirits over his little victory, Gerald gave rein to his whimsy. He bundled together his examination reports and hiked into Battle Creek in search of something he heard a lot about in the camps but had never seen. He found a shopkeeper who was sure he had some of it though he couldn't remember when he had last had a call for it. Hunting around on back shelves and through jumbled drawers he finally found it. So Major Webb's reports went off to Washington neatly wrapped in slightly soiled red tape.

The approach of the Holidays made Gerald homesick. "How I shall miss those horn-blowing children on Christmas morning," he wrote Varina. "But we shall have many more such mornings together when this separation is over." The next sentence revealed the drift of his thoughts: "When registering here the clerk asked me the color of my eyes but without asking put down grey hair! My, what a jolt!!!" He was forty-six.

He began Christmas Day by opening his cards and gifts, then, "thinking it best to keep myself busy," he went into the general wards of the hospital to do rounds with the doctors on duty, "seeing lots of pneumonia, measles, meningitis, and smallpox. It wouldn't be to everyone's taste but I greatly enjoyed it."

After "a superb Xmas dinner in the mess" he took a brisk seven-mile hike through the deep snowdrifts and got back just in time to board the interurban car to Kalamazoo, where he ate another Christmas dinner at the home of one Dr. Whyte, a Scotsman from Wisconsin whose dour wit he enjoyed.

Now impatience set in. Where, where were his new orders? He began phoning Division Headquarters every three or four hours to ask whether they had arrived.

Varina wrote that she had succeeded in selling the Franklin for five hundred dollars ("A good price. Bully for you!"), that there was lots of sickness at Camp Bowie, that the children had caught the measles. "Isn't that the devil!" he replied. "Don't let them get out of bed too soon no matter what others are doing. Hold the fort, dear little wife. I'm sure they will send me south again and I can soon be there to help you."

He used his idle hours to write letters acknowledging his Christmas mail, among them a reply to Benjamin Allen who had written, "We don't want in any way to cripple your research, but at this time we want to do all we can to help in the war effort, and if you can manage without our donation this year, we would like to apply the money in that direction."

Gerald agreed that the nation's needs must come first now, that active research could wait until after the war. He described the arrangements he had made with Dr. Ryder and expressed the hope that "once the Hun is licked" he could count again on the Allens' generous support of his laboratory.

He ended the letter, "We are trying to live on my large! major's salary and thanks to Varina's gameness we have so far succeeded." His salary was two hundred dollars a month—at a time when, say the historians, two thousand dollars a year was "a moderate income."

He wrote a few more editorials for Vaughan's journal and prepared a formal address on "Tuberculosis: Immunity, Diagnosis, and Treatment" for the January meeting of the Kalamazoo Academy of Medicine. He began playing chess again with the Division officers, among them two guests from the French army who had been sent over to guide American training in trench warfare. Their tales of German successes at the front were discouraging.

He sought out a gunnery sergeant who enthusiastically agreed to take apart one of the marvelous new weapons, the machine gun, and show him how it worked. Learning that Varina's brother Jefferson had just shipped out for France to fly reconnaissance planes in the command of General William "Billy" Mitchell, he wangled an invitation from an aviation instructor to go up for his first ride in an airplane.

"It was exhilarating." It took him back to that winter in Georgia with Jenny some twenty years before when he had watched the flight of the buzzards and thought that if man was ever to fly it would be by imitating the strong curves and lifts of those huge wings. He had not imagined then that human flight would be achieved in his lifetime.

One afternoon, the talk of the French officers on his mind, he walked across the fields to the training trenches and wandered about in them for a couple of hours, following their sharp twists and turns through the woods and exploring the sandbagged walls of their dugouts. He tried to imagine what it would be like to live in them for rainy days and black nights on end, never knowing when an enemy shell might explode upon you and your buddies. And to go "over the top" from them, with sixty or so pounds of gear strapped to your back, straight into the enemy's murderous fire.

Such fighting certainly could not be much like the splendid battles of the past he had read of and seen pictured in paintings. It could provide little of their romance and heroic adventure, none of their blood-stirring pomp and panoply and fanfare. It must be instead a long terrible misery in muddy holes and ditches.

Another day he walked into town to visit the renowned Battle Creek Sanitarium, introduced himself to its superintendent Dr. John H. Kellogg, and ate "nuts and bran mashes" with him for lunch. He liked the doctor's enthusiasm but thought "his food thing extreme and faddish."

His orders arrived at last on 25 January. They startled him. He was to proceed immediately to Washington for conferences with Colonel Bushnell and from there to the army War House for senior officers at Columbia University. On 27 March he was to sail for France as Senior Tuberculosis Consultant for the American Expeditionary Force.

Loyal Varina, heavy of heart but as usual shedding no tears, took the children to New York to see Gerald off. He was glad for more than sentimental reasons. She could deal with all the telegrams and letters arriving to wish him godspeed and could buy the clothes he had no time to purchase for himself.

The Winter Night Club sent him an elegant leather valise and she went to Brooks Brothers to fill it with khaki shirts, silk underwear, woolen socks, and two pairs of shoes, which he was surprised to find as comfortable as those he got from Sharpe the Bootmaker. She added a handsome trench coat, several khaki-bound Line-a-Day diaries, and a little Corona portable typewriter that signaled her wish for lots and lots of letters from him.

Gerald took with him to France the comforting memory of his "brave little wife" standing on the dock to wave him out of sight on the Hudson River ferryboat that carried him to the pier. There the troop ship was waiting to take aboard its allotted thousands of doughboys and then move out to join its convoy of destroyers on the open sea.

Major Webb was immediately too busy to worry about the dangers implied by those bristling escorts. As the highest ranking medical officer on board he was named Transport Surgeon, charged with responsibility for the health of the troops during the ten-day crossing. "I am glad to be so occupied. It keeps me from thinking and chases away the blue devils," he wrote from "At Sea."

The paralyzing damage done to Allied shipping by German submarines earlier in the war had greatly diminished since the introduction of the convoy system in mid-1917 but the U-boats were still active and their threat was not to be ignored. The troop ship zigzagged its way forward in total darkness at night, a harrying complication for Major Webb as he made his way from deck to deck through tight ranks of sleeping soldiers to check on the enforcement of his orders.

He drew up these orders literally overnight and had a typewritten copy of them ready the first morning for each of the twelve medical lieutenants who were to carry them out. He bade the officers, among lesser chores:

—to examine each soldier on their stations every day, paying special attention to his tonsils, parotid glands, and "skin to the waist"—and be sure to ask him about the condition of his bowels and his bathing;

—to douse their stations with disinfectant twice daily, the latrines and drinking fountains more often of course—and be sure there was plenty of toilet paper and soap available at all times;

—to keep on the lookout for uneaten food and crumbs and drinking cups used in common and get rid at once of any such they found;

—to make sure all ventilators were working at all times, and that the vents were not closed by bedding or clothing hung over them;

—to enforce strictly the rule that each soldier sleep with his head opposite the feet of the man next to him (a prescription for helping to prevent the spread of respiratory diseases that Major Webb had picked up from a young lieutenant at Camp Bowie).

It was the last two of those orders that kept Webb prowling the blacked-out decks at night. The soldier boys did not like all that air blowing around and they griped about having some other guy's feet in their faces, and many of the lieutenants agreed with them, so the Major checked up for himself. As he wrote Will Otis from France, "I covered some miles night and day while crossing. In fact, I walked from Somewhere-on-the-Hudson to Some-Port-in-France. But we landed with a record clean bill of health for the thousands we brought."

He was indeed vindicated by the special commendation he received from both the ship's commander and the army medical chief in France for the record of minimum illness he had achieved.

The troop ship docked at the port of Saint Navaire at the mouth of the Loire River. Dr. William Henry Welch once witnessed such a docking and described it in his journal: "At 4:30 p.m. on a bright, balmy day a transport ship came in. The troops completely covered the decks, which seemed a mere mass of human beings. They were singing and cheering and all gay enough, the poor fellows on their way to the trenches, many to be 'cannon-fodder.'"

The high spirits did not long survive the dazing confusion of disembarkation. Gerald Webb found it exhausting—the marching thousands, the churned-up mud everywhere, the daunting disorder of a huge camp still in the early stages of construction.

No orders awaited him and he thought he deserved a spell of rest anyway. He spent several days hitching rides on trucks or horse-drawn drays—motorized trucks were a new conveyance in this war and there were not nearly enough of them yet, so horses and mules were still indispensable—to go exploring the Loire Valley and its historic chateaus.

He arrived in due course at the base camp and hospital at Savenay, a hundred or so miles upriver, across the Loire from Nantes. Feeling adrift, not knowing just what he was supposed to do, he was glad to find there his opposite number for cardiovascular diseases, Major Alfred E. Cohn of the Rockefeller Institute, who had been doing his consultant's job in France for ten months.

Webb had not grasped the scope of his responsibilities, said Cohn. Here in France he stood in the same position as Colonel Bushnell at home. He would lose a lot of time if he waited for orders from Washington. Such orders as he got here, more like advice, would come from Colonel William Thayer, the Chief of Medical Consultants (and the Johns Hopkins physician with whom Gerald had hiked the boardwalk in Atlantic City a year ago). But for the most part Webb would have to plan and carry out his task himself.

Each mid-month, said Cohn, all the medical men gathered in Paris for a day or two of discussions arranged by the joint British and American Medical Research Committee. The April meeting was to be held the following week. Perhaps it would be a good start for Major Webb to attend it.

He did so, and at last felt at ease. Present were many of his old friends, including Dr. Jim Miller who was on assignment overseas as a contract surgeon and Livingston Farrand in whose hotel apartment he lodged. The meeting, so like the familiar medical conventions at home, transformed Gerald's outlook; it lifted his spirits and dispelled his confusion. "If only you were all here, it would be perfection personified to the millionth power," he wrote home on 20 April.

From that time forward, Major Webb was a man on the go. What he called his "proper station" was at the Medical Consultants' Headquarters in Neufchâteau, a town four hundred miles southeast of Paris in the Vosges Mountains not far from the Swiss border. But he was seldom there, especially during the spring and summer months while he was shaping his program.

His overall task, Colonel Bushnell had said, was "to stop the tuberculosis leak home"—that is, to reduce to a minimum the number of soldiers lost to the army by incapacitating tuberculosis. This meant improving and standardizing the methods of diagnosing and treating the disease in American hospitals overseas. After his experience with examining boards, Webb was not surprised to discover that many, probably most, of the doctors staffing these hospitals had only vague and outmoded notions about consumption; they were as likely as not to order that any doughboy who had a cough or a wheeze or a pain in the chest be discharged and sent home as tuberculous. Webb would again have to take on the role of counselor and teacher.

He therefore began a schedule of repeated visits of inspection, advice, and instruction to all the base hospitals and to some in the field—well over one hundred and fifty of them by war's end. He crossed and recrossed and crisscrossed central and northern France and Belgium—from the Vosges to the ports the Americans were using on the Bay of Biscay (Bordeaux, Saint Navaire, Brest); along the Marne, the Seine, the estuary of the Gironde, the Loire; from the Puy de Dome across the Dordogne and up through Brittany, Normandy, Picardy, and Flanders.

After a few days of paper work at Headquarters at Neufchâteau or the monthly meeting in Paris he would be on the road from hospital to hospital for two or three weeks. On one such trip from Paris to Bordeaux and up along the coast he visited eighteen hospitals in twenty-one days, "as if I were on an Orpheum circuit."

Usually, though, he stayed for two or three days at each stop. The first day he would examine the patients on hand, making each one a demonstration of proper procedures. He wore to a nub more than one indelible pencil, the tool he found best for delineating on moist chests the proper points for percussion and auscultation. The second and third days he would lead conferences and give lectures, preaching his gospel of fresh air and absolute rest, his own "postural rest" when possible. He soon got to be known as "a crank" on the subject of keeping hospital windows wide open.

At first he had also to demonstrate and teach the proper reading of X-ray plates, at which he so often felt unsure of himself that he asked Colonel Thayer to have Washington send over a radiologist to help him.

As he became acquainted with the men staffing the hospitals— he already knew many of them, some very well—he exercised considerable authority over appointments and transfers. "It is mostly up to me to see that the right men are in charge and the wrong ones sent to where they can do the least harm."

He did not always relish that responsibility, especially when the man in question was a friend. In late July he told Varina, "They have sent over my eccentric friend 'Bully' Bullock of Silver City and he wants to assist me. Whatever shall I do with him?" He finally assigned the bubbly New Mexican to one of the disembarkation camps.

Gerald made his rounds by train, but such traveling was not smooth. Many times there was no seat for him on the train he wanted. He got used to being stranded for hours on a station bench or in a back corner of some dark and noisy provincial café, got used to reaching his destination hours, even a day or two, late. His baggage rarely arrived with him. His beautiful leather valise was soon lost or stolen and he had to replace it with a shoddy duffel bag, and a little later his handsome trench coat disappeared too. He was surprised but grateful that no one seemed to want his useful little Corona.

It was a treat when another officer was going his way and the two could travel in a motorcar with a driver. Once the fellow traveler was Colonel Thayer, on a trip all the way from Neufchâteau through Chaumont, Orleans, and Tours to Savenay. When Thayer decided to complete his journey to Calais by train, he asked Webb to take the limousine back to Neufchâteau.

"This was pure heaven," Gerald told Varina. "One couldn't ask for a better companion than Colonel Thayer, he is always kind and thoughtful, in every way a fine gentleman and scholar. And as you know, the French roads are superb. Our American chauffeurs are crazy about them and we have to watch that they don't whizz along them too fast."

Upon arrival at a destination the Major's perennial problem was finding a billet. Frequently he ended up *faut de mieux* on a folding cot in a corridor or operating room of the base hospital. He found the YMCA, Red Cross, and Salvation Army "amazingly helpful" in locating rooms, often in French homes.

"In the past two months," he wrote Fred Kissel, "I have slept in more than twenty different beds, some with sheets, some with blankets, some with mattresses, but none so far with insects."

Especially on weekends he tried to get accommodations in an inn or a chateau where he could mend and wash his underwear and socks and dry them "in the sun on the windowsill" or "over the hot water pipes that run through my room." The prospect of a comfortable bed and adequate sleep in a good hotel lured him to Paris each month as much as the medical meetings themselves.

Even in Neufchâteau he could not find a billet of his own; every cranny there was occupied and he had to bunk in the room of some other consultant who was away. In late July he wrote Varina, "I am staying in the billet of Colonel Thayer and have slept the clock around. Bedding down in a base hospital or YMCA canteen or some strange house is not conducive to sleep and I'm in need of lots of it."

It was during this stay that he ran into Shirley Putnam, a friend of Laura Gilpin's who was doing Red Cross work in Neufchâteau. She was about to return to the United States and arranged to transfer her billet to Major Webb. "It is a great relief to get settled in a place of my own. It is a good-sized room, very comfortable. Now like Napoleon I can come here and sleep for a week. Mrs. LeRoy, my landlady, is a motherly woman, eager to do all sorts of things for me"—including his washing and mending. He confessed it was a real pleasure to get into clean pajamas; "I have had to sleep in the same unwashed pair for the past 9 weeks."

He lingered longer at Headquarters after this. He felt his work was largely done at the older base hospitals and he need pay close attention only to the new ones being opened. Using the "remarkably excellent library" the Red Cross had provided for the medical consultants in Neufchâteau, he began preparing brief illustrated papers that he could distribute at the hospitals to supplement Colonel

Bushnell's famous Circular No. 20. "How I wish you were here to help me do the charts and graphs, my clever Varina."

He had also got permission to establish "salvage centers" to which those only mildly ill with tuberculosis and other pulmonary disorders could be sent for recuperation and rehabilitation, somewhat on the pattern of Forster's farm colonies. With Thayer's help he had selected three sites, one near each of the major ports, and was supervising the building, staffing, and programming for them.

He was crusading too for earlier detection of tuberculosis. "Just as the shrapnel-wounded do better if they are got to the surgeons quickly, so the tuberculosis-wounded are more likely to recover if they are spotted and sent to the doctors early," he argued.

It was this mission that took him to field hospitals in the "advanced zone" to the rear of the battlefields, and at least twice to evacuation hospitals immediately behind the fighting line—first at Chateau Thierry in early August when the Americans were helping the French to push the Germans back from their forward position on the Marne, and again east of Verdun in September when the First United States Army was "pinching out" the St. Mihiel Salient which the Germans had held since 1914.

When the St. Mihiel battle was over and the Germans had been driven back almost into Lorraine, Webb came somehow to be riding in a horse-drawn cart moving on the rails of the single-track narrow-gauge railway the Germans had been using to supply their troops. He saw the horrible devastation their demolition corps had left behind—the land was not theirs so why hesitate to destroy it?—and got a hint of why German prisoners-of-war could not believe their eyes when they saw the ample goodies and sturdy clothing their enemies enjoyed; *they* had not seen such delicacies and serviceable uniforms for more than a year and their officers had assured them the enemy was on even more spartan rations.

Looking as usual for ways to answer controversial questions, Major Webb in these autumn months intensified his efforts to persuade army pathologists to search at autopsy for healed tubercular lesions, in the hope of accumulating evidence as to whether or not childhood infections and the consequent walled-up tubercles might provide immunity to tuberculosis in later life.

He made little headway. When he got from the Central Laboratory in Orleans the names of pathologists who might help him, then made a special point of talking with these men in their hospitals, he found only three who would enlist in his project; "each of the others had some pet project of his own he wanted to pursue."

His visits to postmortem rooms dismayed him; only once did he see a thorough autopsy of the kind he thought proper. "That man studied with Ghon in Vienna. I know it. Because he's the only one who does it carefully in Ghon's way, looking for everything."

He tried to secure the help of pathology's bright lights. At Savenay he discussed the problem with Major Richard Cabot, the Harvard pathologist who was well known through his published autopsy reports, and later at Bordeaux he talked of it during an hour's walk in the rain with Major Louis B. Wilson, the Mayo Clinic pathologist who had developed frozen-tissue diagnosis and identified intestinal pouches as the source of diverticulitis. Both men were easily persuaded to endorse his cause and probably did their best to advance it.

In the end he was able to collect reports of some two thousand autopsies with virtually unanimous statements of surprise from the men who did them at the very few healed tubercular lesions they had found. He made good use of this evidence in reporting to the NTA after the war.

Little of these professional concerns appeared in Gerald's twice-a-week letters home. In the first of them he warned Varina, "It is defendu or interdit to write of our affairs, so all we can report is on the weather and our health, both extremely good. After days of weeping heavens, the sun has come out today for a few hours, enough to give me a good sneeze again."

He was not allowed to say where he was, had been, or was going but he and Varina found a way to circumvent this proscription. He quickly guessed that the censors—more likely to be "censorettes" he said—were not well acquainted with the history, biography, or even general geography of France and so began identifying his stopping places by allusive tags which Varina, thumbing through encyclopedia and atlas, could translate from his "Somewhere in France" to the names of regions and cities and so follow the routes of his journeys.

Nantes became "the place where the Edict was signed"; Dordogne "the country of the caves that contain magnificent drawings by Neanderthal men"; Rouen "the city the LePlastriers fled from";

Orleans "where the Maid was put on trial"; Vichy "the famous spa whose mineral waters are bottled for sale as those of Manitou used to be"; Dijon "where Pasteur once taught, the big city near where he was born"; Quimper on the coast in Brittany "the birthplace of Laënnec"; Neufchâteau "where Robert Koch was stationed during the Franco-Prussian war"; et cetera.

Predictably, under the restrictions of the censor reinforced by Gerald's wish to keep Varina in good cheer, he wrote more of nature than of war, more of jokes current in mess halls and canteens than of suffering at the front or in the hospitals. He wrote Varina virtually a botanical gazette of the changing seasons in France.

In early spring he was entranced by the fields of cowslips along the Loire, which reminded him of his boyhood springs in Cheltenham. He picked a few and enclosed them, along with anemone and periwinkle blossoms, in his first letters home. Next he was intrigued by the roadside carpets of a flower new to him, a fringed blue beauty the French called "ragged robins." Why "robins" when the blossom was all over the deepest of blues? Could Varina identify it?

As summer came on, his train rides were made cheerful by the view out the window of "pretty fields of a yellow-flowering turnip the French raise to feed their cattle" — rutabagas perhaps — and by the wild roses, morning glories, and white hawthorn coming into flower alongside the tracks. The red hawthorn followed the white into bloom, "as beautiful as you and I saw it in Vienna ten years ago."

By the time the blackberry hedgerows were fruiting he was traveling more often by auto and would have his chauffeur stop at the roadside to let him sample the swelling globes. At his first tries the berries were still too tart but later on "I eat lots and lots of them." It puzzled him that "the frugal French whose thriftiness outdoes the proverbial Scots never make any use at all of these delicious berries."

He waited eagerly to hear a nightingale for the first time but when at last one sang for him he was disappointed; its performance "wasn't half as good as that serenade by a catbird on our wedding night." More exciting was the summer flight and song of the lark. He would stop in his tracks to watch and listen when one began. In July he wrote from Savenay, "I watched a wonderful wheeling lark flight the other night at 9 p.m. — it doesn't get too dark to read without lights until 10 p.m. now. The bird was singing gaily all the while it soared and dipped. It seemed almost artificial, a regular orchestra bird."

The mountains around Neufchâteau and in the Puy de Dome to the southwest gave him joy and solace. Their peaks and canyons and nestling meadows reminded him of Colorado and he seized every chance to hike and climb and picnic among them. The resort atmosphere of Vichy took him home too, both to Cheltenham and to Colorado Springs. On each visit to that city he drank waters from all its springs and spent his leisure hours on its esplanade. On 1 July: "I am again at that famous spa and this sunny Sunday afternoon I am writing you with the Corona sitting on a picnic table underneath the trees in a pretty little park. People are loafing on the grass all around me."

Such letters did not please everyone he wrote to. One of them brought an acerbic reply from his brother Roland on 3 July: "I am glad your thoughts are so detached that you can be so interested in nature and scenery."

Few in England could be detached any longer. The exactions of wartime had almost ruined the Webb Brothers' brick-and-tile business and many other such enterprises. Worse, the carnage on the battlefields had left hardly a family untouched by death or injury. England had already lost well over half a million of her young men and was losing hundreds of thousands more in the German offensives of spring and early summer 1918.

In those months General Erich Ludendorf, commander of the Kaiser's forces, taking renewed heart when the Bolsheviks removed Russia from the war and thus released more German divisions for use on the Western front, launched four successive drives against Allied positions in the hope of breaking decisively through the enemy's lines and winning the war for the Central Powers before the might of the arriving Americans could become effective. Each of the drives gained ground for the Germans, the third one carrying them to within forty miles of Paris, and in each the dogged defense cost thousands upon thousands more of British and French lives.

"Everybody here is glum," reported Major Webb in May. "The sword of Damocles hangs over our heads, and it looks as if the war may go on for years."

That reference to what was happening in the war itself was exceptional. Gerald's letters were chock-full of pleasant recreations:

horseback rides and invigorating hikes; congenial fellowship, good meals, and chess games at officers' clubs; shopping, parades, the circus, and the opera in Paris; sightseeing among ancient Roman forts, mills, and amphitheaters in the north as well as in the caves of the Dordogne in the south; happy encounters everywhere with friends, former patients, and colleagues from home—"I do think the whole U.S.A. must be over here"; browsing in bookstores and stalls; searching for posters and postcards and miniature reproductions of military insignia to be sent home.

Efforts to improve his skills in French were a recurring item. When in Neufchâteau he took three French lessons a week. He read French newspapers regularly and made each billet in a French home a chance to practice conversation. On trains he tried to sit beside a native who would tell him the French names for objects they saw out the window. In Tours he went to the theater expecting that at last he would be able to follow the comedy's dialogue in French. To his chagrin he understood hardly a word of it.

"I have greatly increased my vocabulary and knowledge of the grammar," he wrote Varina, "but pronunciation—JAMAIS!" More and more he splattered his letters with French phrases, the most often repeated being "*Je t'aime.*"

In striking contrast he made scarcely a dozen passing references to the maiming and death and disruption he must have been seeing on all sides.

In March the Germans, dug in along the ridge called Chemin des Dames seventy miles north of Paris, began shelling that city with long-range guns they had engineered for this purpose. They kept up the bombardment throughout the summer into August, but only on his June visit to the capital did Major Webb refer to it: "It is warm and Big Bertha makes it hotter. The *alertes* come quite often, even at night, but I don't let them worry me. I just turn over and go back to sleep. I don't run for the cellars as others do. But I must agree with Farrand that the daytime *alertes* do take your mind off your work. In the bank this morning we were all keeping our eyes on the clock—we knew that shells would hit every ten minutes."

As he traveled through rural France during the summer he observed "the gentle shepherdesses all past 70" driving their herds and flocks along the road or tending them on the hillsides "while their elderly husbands toil in the fields and gardens raising food for the armies. Only the old people and children are to be seen at home. The young men are all in the army, the girls at work in the factories."

During a tour of "the intermediate zone" in late summer he reported, "The Boche are doing less bombing of hospitals than we expected, but whether by intention or mischance they do hit one every once in a while."

In the autumn when fighting was heavy around Chaumont, some fifty miles northwest of Neufchâteau, he wrote of hearing the distant gunfire and the troops marching past his billet windows all night long, and from Chaumont itself he said, "I see train after train unloading the wounded." Once he commented, "My job would be splendid if one didn't have to think of all the cost being paid in suffering." And after the fighting had ended, "It's a blessed relief to know there will be no more anguish."

And that was all. He did not mention his presence at Chateau Thierry and Verdun until months after the fact, and then with no description or comment.

The disproportion is puzzling; Gerald Webb was not an insensitive man. Concern for Varina's morale is not explanation enough; he knew the Colorado Springs newspapers were publishing long bulletins from the battlefield. Excessive prudence about the censors probably accounts for it. He knew, for instance, that Dr. Harvey Cushing, despite his renown and dedicated service as a surgeon, had barely escaped court-martial for too freely reporting his doings and feelings in letters to his wife.

Gerald may have righted the imbalance between pleasure and pain in his Line-a-Day diaries, which he faithfully wrote up each night to be read with Varina when he got home, but somewhere over the years these have been lost.

He did, in a letter to Dr. Gilbert, tell of going into the surgical wards of the base hospitals and wondering at the marvels wrought by the new Dakin antiseptic solution: "The large shrapnel wounds heal astonishingly fast and clean, and the wards are entirely free of odor. That solution is the most wonderful benefit of the war I have seen."

He also told Gilbert of his anger when he saw gas gangrene victims, because the doctors were not using Dr. C. G. Bull's antitoxin against the ravages of the gas bacillus that William Henry Welch had identified long ago and traced to its habitat in, among other places, open soil, of which there was certainly plenty in the battle zones.

That neglect was further evidence of the army medics' hostility to laboratory scientists, whom, along with civilian specialists, they considered pothering nuisances. Their antagonism was so intense that they persuaded General Pershing to ask Washington to stop sending to France "all these medical experts."

That attitude probably accounted for Webb's obvious satisfaction when he learned that Congress was considering legislation to meld the Medical Reserve Corps with the regular Medical Corps. He wrote his sister Amy about it in June, telling her "There are only a few hundred medics in the regular army but some 18,000 in the Medical Reserve Corps, including the best medical men in the United States." The act was passed but not until late summer could Major Webb change the M.R.C. to M.C. after his name.

His ascent in rank remained pending even longer. In June Colonel Thayer told him he had been recommended for promotion to lieutenant colonel and thereafter he kept telling Varina (and himself) not to be impatient. "These things come about slowly but they tell me it will come."

In the meantime Dr. Alexius Forster, having become a Medical Reserve Corps major in his turn, grew restive in successive camp hospitals at home. He let Webb know that he wanted to be sent overseas and Gerald requested his assignment to assist in the direction of the three salvage centers. "I hope he arrives soon; I have much for him to do." But when Webb learned that the Surgeon General was initiating the building of government sanatoriums to take care of tuberculous veterans, he immediately recommended Forster for a post in that program. "It's the perfect place for him."

A month later Varina informed Gerald that Forster had been put in command of an army sanatorium in New Haven, Connecticut, and had been promoted to lieutenant colonel.

Webb can only have been galled; *he* was still a major. When Marka asked if he would now have to salute Dr. Forster, he professed not to mind at all; "I got him that job and knew he would do well in it." But he added, "They tell me the nearer you are to Washington the faster you get promoted. Once you get overseas they tend to forget about you." He probably protested at Headquarters, for his chief, now *General* Thayer, cabled twice to Washington in the next few weeks "to remind them that my promotion has been long on the tapis."

Word of his new rank, certified in Washington on 7 September, finally reached him on 2 October and he was happy to exchange his gilt leaves for silver, "which better matches the grey at my temples, a sure sign of antiquity." His salary was now increased to $250 a month plus $25 for foreign service, of which he tried to send $200 home to Varina. She was also receiving directly from the army $70 a month for "commutation of quarters," i.e. in lieu of the quarters she and the children would be occupying were they with him in France.

There can be no doubt that Gerald Webb thoroughly enjoyed his work overseas. He said so repeatedly. For one example to Varina: "I couldn't imagine a better job. My work is interesting and not heavy, since I don't have day-to-day responsibility for the wards. I am never tired at night as I so often am at home."

And another to Dr. Gilbert: "I couldn't ask for nicer work. Colonel Thayer leaves me free and footloose. I can go and come as I please, and I get to meet the best medical brains in America. They are all here. Now that I see such a concentration of them I am learning the artistic side of medical men. It is surprising how many of them are fine musicians."

He expressed equally often the guilt he felt at having such a good time. To Varina: "I feel selfish to be feeling so fit and having it so easy here. You are having by far the harder time." And again: "I write you so often to atone for being here." And later: "Don't write of me as coming home a hero. You have been the heroic one, while I have been having an exciting and refreshing life."

Perhaps the principal source of Webb's enjoyment was meeting "the best medical brains of America" and associating with them on an equal footing, not only in the hospitals and at the Paris meetings but at the Headquarters in Neufchâteau. There he ate his meals — at a superb mess managed by "young Widener of the Philadelphia Wideners" — and spent his leisure with men like General Thayer; Colonel J. M. T. Finney, a Hopkins man who was director of surgical services in the A.E.F.; Colonel Harvey Cushing, the eminent brain surgeon who had moved from Johns Hopkins to a professorship at Harvard and the post of chief of neurosurgery at the new Peter Bent Brigham Hospital in Boston; Major George B. Crile of the Crile Clinic in Cleveland; Major Warfield T. Longcope, chief of gastrointestinal surgery at the Johns Hopkins Hospital; Major Alfred E. Cohn, chief of cardiac research at the Rockefeller Institute.

Webb took many a long hike with Thayer, whose love of wilderness and wildlife matched his own, but most memorable for him were his walks and talks with Harvey Cushing. The two men shared many friends and interests. Cushing was another who turned to bookstalls and the glories of nature for surcease from his eighteen-hour days of emergency surgery in evacuation hospitals. His wartime diaries are as full as Webb's letters of references to "roadsides abloom," the "well-groomed forests of France carpeted for miles at a stretch with a profusion of flowers," the "breath-stopping beauty of wisteria in blossom against a gray wall."

Having been in service in France for extended periods since 1915, Cushing was a man beset with memories of "the marrow of tragedy." He told Webb of watching helplessly while young Revere Osler, whom he had known and loved since babyhood, died from four shrapnel wounds in the brain, of seeing the boy's body buried hastily next morning "in just another grave," of going immediately afterward to England to break the awful news to the parents, Sir William Osler, Cushing's "professional father," and Lady Osler, the great-granddaughter of Paul Revere. He did not think Sir William would long survive the blow of this loss. (Osler died, ostensibly of pneumonia, in 1919. Cushing's biography of him is a classic in the genre.)

Cushing also told Webb how he had lost another cherished young friend in the horrible slaughter at Ypres, Dr. John McCrae, the Canadian physician who during the battle wrote the haunting verse, "In Flanders' fields the poppies blow / Between the crosses, row on row..."

Over coffee one afternoon Cushing and Webb reminisced about their mutual friend Edward Trudeau, his many foibles, sad life, and great work, which Webb said had begun with an unacknowledged suggestion from Henry Sewall. Trudeau had written Webb that he was feeling remarkably better after trying pneumothorax, only a few months before he died in 1915.

All Gerald's accounts of keeping company with the "best medical brains" carry an unmistakable undertone of his "tiny grain of sand" complex. It became more than an undertone when he told Varina how General Thayer had complimented him on the reports coming to Headquarters about the great good he was doing on his visits to the hospitals: "Considering that many of my performances had to be made among men of renown from great universities whom I approached in fear and trembling, I am mighty pleased."

That was his private face. We get a glimpse of his public face in a letter to Varina from Charlotte Touzalin, a Colorado Springs woman who was working as a clerical volunteer in a Paris hospital: "Dr. Webb is obviously a very important personage and everyone here quite kow-tows to him."

For many long weeks Gerald had no idea what was happening to his family. His constant plaint was "No letters from you yet." When at last a huge packet of mail was delivered to him in Paris on 18 July he "sat down to a feast of reading all morning long" and gave himself an extra day's stay in the capital to reread it all and type off some replies.

Varina had tried to take the children to Tall Timbers for the summer as usual but had been forced back to town when Dr. Gilbert said Marka must enter Glockner Hospital to have her tonsils removed. "Do fatten her up first, and see that she gets plenty of sun baths," prescribed her father. "And ask Sister Rose to look after her at Glockner." Sister Rose did so, taking the child into the nuns' quarters to convalesce and making such a pet of her that she did not want to go home when Varina came for her.

Then it was Joel's turn for a tonsillectomy and Daddie was glad to hear that he had been "such a brave little boy" about it. Next Varina's younger brother Bill, an invalid living on a ranch outside town, took a sudden turn for the worse and everyone, including Dr. Gilbert, thought for some weeks that he would die. The anxiety brought on an alarming attack of Daddie Hayes's asthma, but both men were slowly returning to their usual degree of health.

Throughout these times of special stress Varina insisted on doing her bit in patriotic programs on the home front. She left the knitting of socks for "soldier Daddie" to Robine and Leila but took her appointed turns at rolling bandages and serving snacks at the Red Cross canteen and sold Liberty Bonds in successive fund-raising drives. Having to cope with food rationing and the weekly "meatless" and "wheatless" days and with the impossibility of finding anyone at all to help her as housekeeper or cook, she was worn out by summer's end. "Your picture shows you are exhausted and much too thin," worried Gerald.

Daddie Hayes suggested to Gerald that he tell Varina to send Gerry out to St. Stephen's School for the coming year. "He is a very good boy but he is strong and full of energy and now that he can ride the horse Lady, he gallops adventurously off into the mountains and Daughter worries that the horse will step into a hole or shy at a rattlesnake and throw him. I believe the school would be good for him and would give Daughter some relief. I have urged the idea upon her but she will heed no one but you."

Gerald did not respond to this suggestion, perhaps because he did not think he could afford the tuition fee at this time.

A dramatic reversal in fortunes and morale began for the Allies in midsummer. General Ludendorf's desperate spring offensives failed to achieve the breakthrough he had hoped for. The Allies stalled his advances and began at last to drive the Germans back.

By 8 August, "the black day for Germany," General Ludendorf knew the Central Powers had lost the war. The governments and peoples he fought for were impoverished and exhausted, could dredge up no more resources. His armies were drained and demoralized, the men falling victim by the thousands to the spreading pandemic of Spanish influenza and in ever larger groups deserting to the enemy. Despondently he gave up and yielded management of the end to civilian authorities.

"Everything is different now," wrote Major Webb in late July. "We have the Boche on the run and can really hope to end the war this year. You can't imagine the changed spirit here. The boys coming to the hospitals with minor wounds now can't wait to get back to the front — to pick up some more souvenirs. Many of them show us proudly the watches, binoculars, etc. they have taken from the bodies of dead Germans. It is said here that Germany is fighting for a place in the sun, the French for Alsace and Lorraine, the British for freedom of the seas, and the Americans for souvenirs."

As the news from the front got better and better for the Allies and "the duration" looked correspondingly shorter, Gerald planned a trip to which he, with real self-discipline, had so far given a low priority: a visit to American base hospitals in England. His brothers and sisters had been urging him to come, especially "the girls," who had been writing him with unusual frequency to express their gratitude "that you have come over to help us out." He was overdue for his seven-month leave and so allowed himself three weeks across the Channel in late September and early October.

In London, where the streets were "swarming with Americans in khaki," he paid a duty call at military headquarters, then went to Guy's Hospital and had lunch with his nephew Eric, "a gentle, nice-mannered boy" who had just completed his turn in obstetrics and was beginning service as a demonstrator in pathology. That afternoon he went out to the base hospital in Tottenham for a heart-warming reunion with Dr. Bill Williams and a number of other Denver doctors who were on its staff.

In Cheltenham next day he went at once to Thomas the Tailor and Sharpe the Bootmaker to order for himself copies of "the snappy uniforms" he had admired on British officers in France: "separate corduroy riding breeches tucked into heavy leather field boots laced to the knee."

He found his brother Harold jumpy and ill from worry over the disastrous plight of Webb Brothers and from anxiety about his son Rupert, who for three years had been fighting as a commissioned officer with the British artillery in Belgium and France.

Enid and the younger children made Gerald homesick for his own family. He was bewitched by his niece Josephine, "a most beautiful girl. Romney would have abandoned his portrait of Lady Hamilton if he could have painted this *bonbon de rose* at sweet 14."

Uncle Gerald couldn't help swaggering a little with the boys John and Bryan. Decades later John retained a vivid memory of this visit from his glamorous American uncle, awesomely tall and handsome in his uniform, who took the boys to a huge toy shop they had never been in and airily told them to buy anything they wanted as a gift from him.

Continuing northward, he stayed with Roland and Lilian while he made the rounds of hospitals and rest camps in the vicinity, then journeyed on to Manchester where Wilfred met him in a chauffeured limousine and took him out to his and Blanche's country estate. "Wilfred is undoubtedly the most prosperous member of the family," Gerald told Varina.

Little Cynthia was better now, "a bright and active child" though her back had been permanently deformed by her tuberculosis and had to be supported by heavy braces.

From Manchester Gerald went to Liverpool and thence northeastward across England to visit Frank, Ann, and the three Ds in West Hartlepool on Tees Bay of the North Sea. Frank had been rejected for military service — "his frame was thought too lean" —

but the war had not passed him by. He had enlisted in a volunteer battalion of light infantry and was now, at 45, serving as a second lieutenant in the defense of the North Sea coast.

Uncharacteristically, Gerald shivered in the autumn chill of Frank's northland. "Now I know," he told Varina, "why the English eat so many meals in a day, including tea; they have to, to keep warm."

"Ten days are gone, time is flying." He must concentrate on his mission.

He began a succession of brief appearances at base hospitals, hopping from town to town southwestward through the midlands of England "like a vaudevillian on a tour of one-night stands," ending up at Paignton in Devonshire. There he found his Colorado Springs colleague Dr. C. F. Stough in charge of the hospital, which was housed in a marble-halled mansion "built by Paris Singer of sewing-machine fame. It's a topsy-turvy world that sees a Colorado Springs surgeon running a stately English-American country house as a hospital."

Dr. Stough was holding for him a telegram that requested his immediate return to France for the mid-October medical meeting in Paris. In spite of it he took off for Wales to pay his respects to "the three Graces," his sisters, who had congregated at Amy's home in Builth Wells. He was sorry to find Daff away and Amy's two daughters just gone back to school, where Nancy was preparing for her matriculation next year at Lady Margaret Hall at Oxford. Robine's obsession at the moment, said her mother, was a vehement dislike of all Yanks. The doughboys she met were all much too cocky and brash, she thought, still smugly superior because the Americans had defeated the English in the Revolution!

Back in London Gerald found awaiting him the news of his promotion to lieutenant colonel and also the uniforms and boots delivered from Cheltenham. "I feel very well dressed now." He decided to have the insignia of his new rank attached to his jackets in the beautiful embroidered insets used by French officers instead of fussing with those finger-pricking pins.

And then departure for Paris once more. "I have certainly quite circled this little island this time."

He was wanted at the meeting in Paris because tuberculosis had been chosen as the topic to be discussed at the November assembly and he was appointed to plan and run the program. This would take some doing, he knew, but he thought he had time first for a two-week tour of hospitals and so set off by motor for the base ports, taking in Vichy, Perigeux, Montfort, and points between on the way.

He considered the trip urgent because a new problem had arisen. The hospitals were filling up to overflowing with cases of influenza and the doctors must be warned not to confuse its symptoms with those of tuberculosis. Colonel Bushnell had written him enthusiastically that he had cut the tuberculosis leak home from 15 percent to 4 percent. If the hospital physicians were careless in differential diagnosis now, this success might be jeopardized.

Until recently maybe, the historians, for the most part myopically intent on affairs of governments and armies and blind to often equally momentous matters of medicine and disease, have paid little serious attention to "the plague of the Spanish Lady" that swept through most of the world in 1918–19, killing at least twenty-one million persons, many more than died in all the battles of the long World War, and disrupting the lives of hundreds of millions more.

Appearing first in spring 1918 in a mild form that Americans called hog flu—for instance, eleven hundred men were ill with it in March at Fort Riley in Kansas—it seemed to disappear, only to erupt in the fall as a virulent killer that spread with terrifying rapidity from place to place and country to country.

Doctors could do nothing to stop it or cure it. They were not even certain whether it was caused by a bacillus or by a virus and at this time, twenty-five years before the electron microscope made it possible to see viruses, they could only try to cope with its symptoms. The result was many months of what one student of the pandemic called "universal drenching fear."

Rumors and guesses about where the "flu" had come from produced many names for it but the one that stuck, unfairly no doubt, was Spanish influenza.

Colonel Webb, under the censor's orders probably, always referred to the disease as grippe. "We are worried more by bacilli than by bullets now," he wrote Varina from Bordeaux. "General Grippe has become as much our enemy as our ally in the war. So many are sickening that the numbers overwhelm us. We all take every precaution we know, always wearing a surgical mask when we are in the grippe and pneumonia wards. They laugh at my prescription of open windows but at Savenay where it is followed scrupulously not one case of grippe or pneumonia has occurred in the tuberculosis wards."

It was hard to concentrate on work these days because all the news suggested the war would soon be over. Negotiations for an armistice were reported in daily installments. Wilson's Fourteen Points and Germany's response to them were endlessly discussed. Bulgaria signed an armistice, then Turkey, at last Austria. "The terms of the Austrian armistice ought to chill the Hun, but he should know he is licked anyway," said Gerald.

Back in Paris, he went to the bank on the morning of 11 November to send Varina a draft for two hundred dollars with a short accompanying note: "Am about to leave for Neufchâteau by motor. Paris is impatiently awaiting the signing of the armistice and we may get news before leaving."

They did. As his chauffeur drove him away from the bank the whistles and bells and shouting began and he stopped to join the wild scramble for newspapers, then lingered for an hour to watch Paris go mad. "It was a mixture of the 4th of July, an election night, a football victory, and New Year's Eve all in one. You never saw such waving and embracing, smiles and tears. FINI! FINI! FINI! resounded in my ears all the way through Paris and along the road as I passed. Passed the graves of the brave French and Americans who turned the tide."

A punctured tire forced him to stop for the night at Chalons sur Marne. The town was full of French soldiers and not a room was to be had, until a kindly French family offered to take in the bedless colonel and his chauffeur in thanks for the help the Americans had given France. Gerald was struck by the contrast between the celebrating here and in Paris. Here the rejoicing was quiet, "apparently because there were no Yanks about to show them how to whoop it up." The best description of Chalons' mood, he later decided, was what his sister Ida called England's response to the war's end: "a sad excitement."

He now buckled down to preparation for the tuberculosis symposium in Paris on 22 November. He had arranged for some French and British authorities to read papers but felt he must brush up on the literature so as not to be outdone in the discussions. He was nervous about it. "Since Flexner of Rockefeller, Wright, and others equally famous will be present, I'm glad Farrand and his colleagues have agreed to take part. I will certainly need all the help I can get.

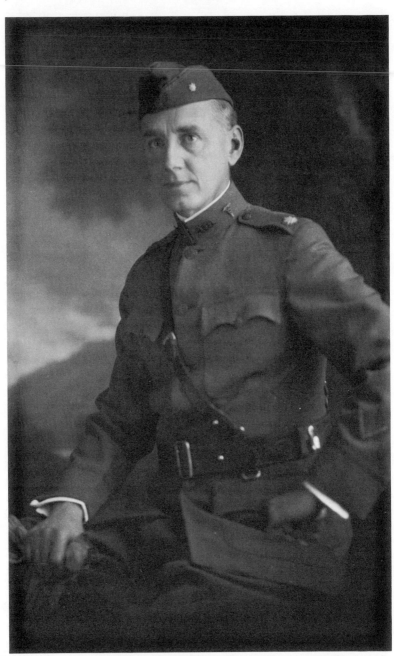

Lieutenant Colonel Webb in Paris, 1918

I've been devouring the TB literature in the library here and will go to Paris a couple of days before the meeting in order to use the Rockefeller Commission library there."

From Paris the night before the meeting he wrote, "Just a few lines tonight to get the TB cobwebs out of my head. I will be so glad when this program is over. Yesterday I lunched at Farrand's with Sir Almroth Wright. The old man is the same as ever. He plans now to take a year off from the laboratory to write a book on 'Morals.' You can imagine what it will be like from his ridiculous book on 'Suffragettes.' This new book was all he would talk about."

A postscript scribbled in haste the next night concluded the tale: "We had a packed house for the TB meeting, not even standing room left. They said it was the greatest success of all the war meetings. I have been congratulated on it from every quarter. I feel like a free man again. I may get orders to go home in a few weeks. Hurrah! Hurrah! Hurrah! without end."

His jubilance was cut short by a cry of alarm from Colonel Bushnell in Washington. Evacuation of troops was getting under way at the ports and Webb must see to it that medical screening of the homeward-bound was carefully done to make sure that only cases of genuine tuberculosis would be sent to the sanatoriums for veterans when they landed. So Webb took to the road again to institute procedures at the port hospitals for proper tagging of the truly tuberculous.

He was upset by what he found at the ports. He had been saying that the A.E.F. had grown fast like Alice in Wonderland and now must nibble something to make it shrink equally fast. He discovered that whatever it was nibbling caused dire choking and constipation.

In response to the cry everywhere of "Home and out!" soldiers by the scores of thousands were being funneled from the forward lines into the evacuation ports but there were far, far too few ships to carry them home and no decent places to put them while they waited for transport.

Said Webb, "The mental distress with so many waiting around in terrible mud camps is serious. Night falls at 4 p.m. but there are few lights anywhere and no heat, though the nights are cold and it rains and rains. The boys try to get wet sticks to burn for warmth. Beaucoup, beaucoup mud, and nothing but beans to eat. Some just sit weeping. It's too much, after all they've been through."

Returning to Neufchâteau, he found himself suddenly with

nothing much useful to do and experienced an enervating letdown. He puttered about, addressing Christmas cards Varina had made and sent him. He scouted the towns roundabout looking for pieces of French lace and embroidery to serve as Christmas gifts. He wrote for the children a tale of El Joe and Lilee on a motor trip through France. And he began smoking again, after nine months of abstinence.

He put together reports and papers about his work in France. And he drew up lists of physicians whom he could recommend for discharge. "I have sent four majors home this morning, also Dr. Bullock from Silver City. It pays to be of poor quality now — you get home sooner."

Where were his own orders? "I would be worth much more back home with my patients now."

Others were leaving. Those in service on contract had sailed weeks ago, among them such friends as Jim Miller, Charles Powers of Denver, Edward Schneider of Colorado College. Dr. Alexander "Alec" Lambert, president-elect of the American Medical Association, who had been Farrand's adviser and Webb's frequent companion in Paris, was about to accompany his wife home. Farrand himself had resigned his position with the Rockefeller Commission and would soon be departing with his family. Even General Thayer was under orders for home. "Why not me?"

Ten days in Paris in mid-December did little to ease his frustration. "It is hard to imagine the Paris of today, with its brilliant lights and swarms of people, mostly Americans, as the same place as Paris of the war, with few people and pitch darkness, when we stumbled over people and sidewalks finding our way home. A million inhabitants deserted Paris during the war and the peace and quiet except for the guns quite suited me, but now it is an abominable place with its masses of humanity and innumerable taxicabs. Dodging taxicabs in Paris is more dangerous than shellfire. I haven't experienced machine guns but should think these taxicabs are comparable."

On the fourteenth he stood on the Farrands' balcony and watched the reception given President Wilson on the Champs Elysées below. "It was interesting to see Clemenceau and Poincaré and Pershing go cantering up the avenue to fetch Wilson, then watch the fast-trotting Victorias carry the whole party back. Wilson looked well but quite bald as he swept his silk hat to and fro acknowledging the waving flags and kerchiefs and the cheers of the people. Madame Wilson and Madame Poincaré were radiant, both covered with flowers. The crowds along the street were great but I saw greater ones on Bastille Day."

That night, to wish his friends bon voyage and repay his debt to them for many social favors, he took Mrs. Farrand, her two daughters, and Dr. and Mrs. Lambert to the Opéra for a performance of *William Tell*. "Farrand does not like opera." The next afternoon, after seeing the Lamberts off: "From the Hotel Regina on the Rue de Rivoli near the Louvre I saw a gorgeous red sunset through the rain—across the Tuilleries. It ended with the old sun going west and I wished it would take me along." Instead "I took my lonesomeness to a fine performance of *Faust*."

Returning to Neufchâteau, he found the morale of the remaining consultants near zero. According to Harvey Cushing, the men were "too unhappy to talk to one another anymore."

Dr. Cushing, who had recently returned from a Paris hospital after a long convalescence from a mysterious paralyzing illness, was the gloomiest of the group. Disgusted with all the bombast about a war to end wars and make the world safe for democracy, he was certain the punitive peace terms being imposed upon the vanquished nations would only lead to more trouble and perhaps another war. Such political percipience was beyond Gerald Webb but he was susceptible to the downbeat mood of the place.

The tale of woes that arrived in a packet of delayed letters from Varina was the last straw.

Scarlet fever had come to Colorado Springs, Joel had caught it, and the family had been quarantined, she wrote. Now every hospital in town was full to the corridors with influenza patients. Her brother Bill was one of them and it was still uncertain whether he would live. More than a hundred Colorado College students were in bed with the disease and seven had already died. Gerry had broken his collarbone. Daddie Hayes was fighting for every breath and she was afraid for his life. For Ben Allen's too; he was critically ill with gallbladder disease and the doctors didn't think they could save him. Exhaustion had caught up with Dr. Gilbert and he was now too ill to look after patients. Dr. Ryder had suffered several hemorrhages and could not go on with the research.

Couldn't Gerald come home now? Daddie frets that we need you here and says your influential friends in Washington could get you released if you would ask them.

Gerald's reply revealed churning emotions: "Tell Daddie I have for weeks been pulling every wire I can think of to get me home. You have been having a terrible time and I often feel a brute to have left you. I don't deserve all your loving thoughtfulness. I think I would have been of more use at home anyway. I may have accomplished a little bit of good here, but it's not worth all you have had to bear alone. Oh Varina, I have not the pen to tell you what you mean to me. This cruel separation and these terrible trials have taught me how much I love and long for you and how my life is wrapped up in you and our children. Surely I will be under orders home by New Year's and then I will make it all up to you."

He had one bit of good news for her. He had seen her brother Jefferson and found him keen and fit. At Headquarters one day Gerald had met a guest, Colonel Whitehead, who turned out to be "our old friend 'Captain Polo' Whitehead who is in charge of aviation medicine over here." Whitehead gladly arranged for Jefferson to meet Gerald in Chaumont. Jeff and Gerald had been just missing connections with each other, once by only ten minutes, all through the year.

Jeff was a first lieutenant in the 99th Aero Squadron and, on loan to the French air force, had been flying daily reconnaissance sorties over the German lines. Many reports had come to Gerald of the lad's unfailing courage, his readiness always to volunteer for the most dangerous missions. "I swell to bursting with my brother-in-law's pride."

At the war's end Jeff was one of only three survivors from the initial eighteen in his squadron. His plane too had crashed one day but by some miracle he had walked away from it unhurt. "He is the only true hero in this war from Colorado Springs. All the others are chocolate soldiers by comparison. What we had to say to each other at lunch in Chaumont about the army's inefficiencies in aviation and medicine had better not be written here."

A few days before Christmas, notice arrived that the Headquarters office would be shut down on 1 January. Gerald cleared out his desk and packed up his belongings, presented "a big box of expensive chocolates" with thanks to his landlady Mrs. LeRoy, then after a bleak Christmas set off to await his orders in Paris.

He was in a foul temper when he wrote Varina on 30 December: "I've had a hell of a time too and am weary of everything." But five days later it was "Great joy!" He had been ordered home at last and had arranged to expedite his return and avoid "weeks of waiting in a port camp knee deep in mud and gloom" by paying his own way across the Atlantic on a commercial French liner.

He sailed from Bordeaux on 11 January and landed in Hoboken on the twenty-fourth, just three days short of ten months after he had left.

He had cabled Varina that he was on his way but she could not come to welcome him. In a desperate effort to save her father's life, she had taken him to California, in a private railway car provided by his business associate and friend, the financier Charles M. Mac-Neill. It was too late. Daddie Hayes died in Pasadena while Gerald in New York was frantically pulling wires to get himself and Jefferson mustered out immediately. "You poor girl. Another terrible trial for you to go through alone."

XIV

Mr. President

COLONEL WEBB came home to a land living in a kind of purdah. A ghostly quiet prevailed in the lobby and restaurants of the Netherlands Hotel. People, in fear of influenza, were leaving the shelter of their homes only when they must. New York's movie houses, theaters, museums, and concert halls had been ordered closed and everyone who had to be on the streets went about his business behind a surgical mask.

When Gerald was finally released and got home to Colorado Springs he found conditions there the same, plus white signs all over town marking the houses that had influenza patients within. Many were dying, some in a relapse bout of high fever and clammy chills, and those who survived were dragging through weeks of debilitation. Pallid cheeks and bald heads, their hair stripped away by fever, were common sights.

All the hospitals and sanatoriums, including Cragmor, were still full to their doors with flu victims, and Webb pitched in to help out the weary doctors and pick up the threads of his practice.

He was dismayed to learn that Sister Rose Alexius, his right hand at Glockner, she who had said the hospital ought to be called Webb Sanatorium, was leaving at the height of this crisis, transferred to a Cincinnati hospital by a new head of her order who thought it bad for a sister's soul to let her stay too long in one post. What would he do without her?

In spite of the panic and disarray everywhere, it was oh, so good to be reunited with Varina and the children, even under the shadow of Daddie Hayes's death. He was relieved to find Varina's brother Bill on the mend and Benjamin Allen recovering fretfully from the abdominal surgery he had undergone.

For all the impatience Gerald had felt in France, he was among the earlier ones sent home. Others kept drifting back throughout spring and into summer.

It was June, for instance, before William Elmslie returned. Late in the war, unable to stay out of it any longer, he had enlisted in the infantry and was among those sent to Siberia to support the White Russians against the Bolsheviks. Well informed in history and politics, he resented having to take part in an action "contrary to every principle I hold dear. We Americans are surely storing up trouble for ourselves from the hatred we are arousing in the people here by this interference against them."

It was June too before Colonel Forster returned, bringing with him a slim young Frenchwoman from Nantes as his wife. He had managed to be transferred overseas just as the war was ending. Assigned to evacuation units first at Rennes and then at Nantes, he had gone to see Webb in Paris just before Gerald sailed and "despite his weeks in those terrible mud camps, he breezed into my hotel room like a breath of fresh Colorado air."

With the veterans home again and the influenza epidemic fading into memory, Colorado Springs, like countless other towns across the United States, decided it must celebrate. Its Victory Parade was held on 26 August 1919, with Colonel Webb at its head. Impressively handsome in his "snappy uniform" inset with embroidered insignia and chevrons, sitting tall and unsmiling astride a horse he had borrowed for the occasion, he led the bands, riders, and marchers along a route of several miles ending at the Burns Theater, where the townspeople gathered for a program of patriotic speeches. Afterward he joined his proud wife and children for the community dinner and fireworks that concluded the festivities.

Dr. Webb had already resumed his annual convention and speaking rounds. The major societies all held their meetings in Atlantic City in June that year and each one was a feast of reunion and reminiscence. Gerald said he was glad "to be with all the Neufchâteau fellows again"; he knew his war service had both widened his professional acquaintance and raised his stature among his peers.

In his room at his favorite Chelsea Hotel, he "scratched off" outlines for his talks to the Association of American Physicians, the American Association of Immunologists, and the National Tuberculosis Association.

This was his first meeting as a full member of the AAP; Henry Sewall had notified him in France that he had not been made to wait the allotted five years but had been taken off probationary status at the association's meeting in 1918.

At the NTA sessions he shone. He appreciated Colonel Bushnell's public acknowledgment of his fine success in reducing that "tuberculosis leak home" but he nonetheless took firm issue with the Colonel's statement that the low incidence of tuberculosis in the army was because three quarters of the men had been made immune to the disease by mild childhood infections.

With amusing subtlety Dr. Webb drew a line between those who had observed the war from a desk in Washington and "those of us who worked with the men on the other side. During my ten months in France 300 American soldiers died of active tuberculosis and in at least half of them the disease was freshly contracted and acute." To weight his case he brought to witness those two thousand general autopsies in which the pathologists had found very few tubercular lesions.

As a cap to the kudos he was elected vice-president of the NTA for the coming year, to serve with Dr. Victor C. Vaughan as president. "Quite an honor," he said mildly. The vice-presidency frequently led to the presidency. Dr. Forster and Colonel Bushnell were elected to the board of directors.

Gerald stayed on in Atlantic City a few extra days to do what he could for Benjamin Allen, who with Maria and their son Wharton, recently mustered out of the service, was seeking convalescence at a resort hotel. Gerald arranged for a Johns Hopkins gastroenterologist to advise Allen about his postoperative regimen and diet — though, Gerald said, he doubted the advice would do much good; Ben was an irascible, unruly patient who seldom would do what the doctor said he should.

Webb then went north to Saranac Lake where he had agreed to give a lecture to physicians attending the new Edward Trudeau Tuberculosis School. He lodged as the guest of Lawrason Brown, director of this new venture in postgraduate medical education, and discussed it with him at length.

One fact above all others Webb had learned from his wartime experience: the amazing ignorance of most physicians about a disease as prevalent as tuberculosis.

This was the problem the Trudeau school was tackling and Gerald returned home infected with the idea. The next year, on 10 Sep-

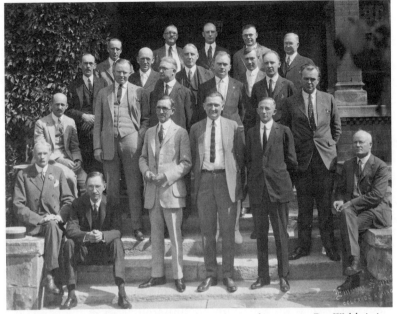

Faculty of the Colorado School for Tuberculosis, about 1925. Dr. Webb is in the center of the third row standing. Dr. Gilbert (wearing glasses) is at the left end of the first row standing. Dr. Forster (baldheaded) is the third one up of those sitting at the left. Dr. Jack Sevier (wearing glasses) stands behind and to the left of Forster. Seated below Forster are Dr. Charles T. Ryder and Dr. Charles Fox Gardiner

tember 1920, he opened the first session of the Colorado School for Tuberculosis, unmistakably on the Saranac model. He had persuaded fifteen of his Colorado Springs colleagues to donate their services as faculty members, was giving his own as president and dean, and had enrolled twenty-five doctors from outlying communities for the six weeks' course.

For more than a decade thereafter the Trudeau and Colorado schools were respected twins in postgraduate education in tuberculosis. Both were asked to train staff members for government sanatoriums until the U.S. Public Health Service could develop a school of its own for the purpose. At the Colorado school students soon outran the space and Dr. Webb had to limit enrollment to the number he could accommodate.

The training he offered included observation of patients and demonstrations of methods at Cragmor Sanatorium. Some of the patients welcomed the annual invasion. One of them wrote in July 1925, "The Colorado School for Tuberculosis is on! For the next few weeks strange doctors will overrun this place, examining, questioning, percussing, etc. All for the betterment of their education, they say. Goody!"

"Oh what a wandering one I've been of late!" Gerald exclaimed in June of that year 1920.

In early March he had sailed from San Francisco on the Matson Line's *Wilhelmina* for a month's sojourn in the Territory of Hawaii as the physician-guest of Benjamin Allen, who sought to complete his recovery in tropical climes. Gerald visited doctors, hospitals, and sanatoriums in the islands, including several leper colonies to observe the treatment of their dread affliction by the use of acidic chaulmoogra oil from India. This ancient therapy for leprosy was now of interest to specialists in tuberculosis because of the recognized likenesses between the lepra and tubercle bacilli.

But mostly Gerald was on vacation in Hawaii. He sunbathed with Ben on the beaches, went swimming in the surf, reveled in the daily array of fruit, especially the unfamiliar fresh figs, alligator pears, papaya, and sun-ripened pineapple. "I almost live on these and nuts." Dishes made from the vegetable taro he could do without.

The brilliantly colored birds and flowers excited him, and at the famous Bishop Museum he came upon "a fine semi-scientific book on the natural history of the islands. I have devoured it and learned a lot of fascinating tidbits that I use to amuse Ben when he is bored."

The highlight of the month was a thirty-mile trip by automobile along a smooth concrete road to the volcano called Kilauea on the southeastern slope of Mauna Loa. As the car made the gradual ascent to four thousand feet, Gerald remarked upon the "very clean and bright mud huts of the Japanese, the giant forests of fern, the long stretches of growing pineapple, sugar cane, rice, and coffee."

Then came their hotel, "on the edge of a vast crater extinct except for a wonderful mile-wide centre of bubbling molten lava bursting into many fire fountains and containing a lake with islands and a central river of the red hot mother earth. No pen can describe this wonder any more than it can the Grand Canyon. The sight is vivid by day but extraordinary by night. We sat on the precipitous brink of the crater entranced and silent, watching the waves and ripples of fire in this vast red hot upheaval."

When a reporter from the Honolulu *Star-Bulletin* interviewed the "distinguished tuberculosis expert," Dr. Webb eschewed the expected rapturous tribute to the beauties of the islands in favor of scolding their citizens for permitting promiscuous spitting on their streets and sidewalks. It was dangerous and should be prohibited at once, he told them sternly.

But to Varina he said, "Hawaii is all it is advertised to be, lovely, delightful. I must bring you here someday if ever we can get a real honeymoon." When he got back to San Francisco in early April and went south to spend a day in Santa Barbara, he wrote, "It all looks so drab and bedraggled here after the color and cleanness of Hawaii.... If I owned the whole of New York and Atlantic City I would sell them both and buy Hawaii."

He had only a few days at home before setting off again. By mid-April he was in St. Louis for the meeting of the NTA, and there he was elected the sixteenth president of the Association.

At age forty-nine he was the youngest man so far chosen for that position and only the second who had not been a founder and who did not come from the East.

The man elected to serve as his vice-president was his good friend Dr. James Alexander Miller.

Dr. Webb could not savor fully this honor done him by his peers. Just before the meeting he had been presented with a crossroads choice; Dean Victor C. Vaughan had offered him a professorship of medicine at the University of Michigan at $15,000 a year.

Although Gerald must have been pleased, he expressed more indecision than satisfaction in discussing the offer with Varina by letter and telegram. That it was Victor Vaughan inviting him to come was no mean tribute in itself, nor was the unanimous approval of the medical school faculty that Vaughan reported—"he says they all like me and want me."

Michigan had a long history of excellence in medical education; Gerald placed it fourth in rank, behind only Johns Hopkins, Harvard, and the University of Pennsylvania. The salary would be "about equal to our present income," but he would be on duty only eight months, would have four months a year for study and research.

Still... did he want to become a full-time teacher? What did Varina think? What did Dr. Gilbert advise? He continued to weigh his choice through the NTA meeting and the round of conventions that followed.

From St. Louis he went south to New Orleans for the "Victory Meeting" of the AMA, where he was elected a member of the House of Delegates and spoke at a dinner honoring his wartime chief, Dr. Thayer. He said all the eddyings of the four thousand members in attendance made him weary.

From New Orleans he traveled east with Dr. Thayer and other friends in the private railroad car of his Paris companion Dr. Alexander Lambert, who had just been elected president of the AMA. He was enroute to Atlantic City for the convention of the AAP and to preside over his first meeting of the Executive Committee of the NTA. On the way he discussed the Michigan offer with Dr. Thayer, who advised him "to seize this fine opportunity."

But on 4 May, from Atlantic City, he telegraphed Dean Vaughan refusing the offer.

He said it was a thought from Edward Trudeau that tipped the balance in his decision. He was reading Trudeau's posthumously published *Autobiography* while he traveled and in it came upon the analogy of a dog chasing a rabbit. If the dog stuck to the rabbit's tracks he would easily overtake his prey but if he veered off to follow alluring cross tracks he would never make his kill. The same with a man, said Trudeau; he must stay unswervingly on the road to his goal. Webb decided he too should refuse to be diverted. He would stay on the track of the tubercle bacillus.

He made the same decision and gave the same reason for it the following year when he was offered a professorship in tuberculosis in the Harvard University medical school at $17,000 a year, plus an endowment of $100,000 to support his research. Webb had been crusading for more attention to tuberculosis in medical education, and an endowed professorship in the subject was attention indeed. But he said no to Harvard too, citing again the virtue of a dog's keeping his nose fixed to the rabbit's tracks.

The illogic of this reason makes one question it. With the money and free time offered Webb, he could more easily and productively have pursued his bacillus at Michigan, certainly at Harvard, than in Colorado Springs. He expressly recognized the advantages he would have in the universities' splendid libraries and laboratories. Was he deceiving himself or only others as to his real reason?

Varina did not at all want to exchange her cherished nest and many friends in Colorado Springs for the wholly unfamiliar milieu of an academic community, which she thought would contain a lot of the women she disparaged as "mixers and movers," but she would certainly have done so if Gerald had willed it. Why did he not?

In considering both offers he listed as an advantage that "I would be always in touch with the big men in medicine." We can hear the echo there of his oft-expressed hero-worship of the "men of renown" from "distinguished universities" before whom he appeared "with fear and trembling." Is it not likely that he shrank unbearably from constant workaday relationships with his admired "giants"?

Despite his many friendships among them he did not feel truly at ease with them. He just could not, even when he was president of the foremost association in his specialty, feel himself to be one of the "big men."

This is understandable perhaps. What Gerald Webb most respected was productive success in scientific research, and as will shortly appear, he was withdrawing from that arena—not from keen interest in it and effective efforts to promote it, but from active personal participation in it. He was too intelligent and informed not to recognize that the methods and concepts of medical science were advancing swiftly beyond his time and ability to keep up, except as an observer. Contrary to his deepest desires, his role was becoming increasingly that of clinician and medical educator and statesman.

Ironically, Richard H. Shryock, professor of the history of medicine at Johns Hopkins and author of the history of the NTA published in 1957, in classifying the presidents of the NTA as either university men or sanatorium men, with intuitive good judgment placed Gerald B. Webb among those "affiliated with universities."

Gerald had planned to head homeward from Atlantic City but problems arising at the meeting of the Executive Committee sent him on to NTA headquarters in New York for conferences with the office staff. When he finally arrived home in mid-May, Varina with unflattering concern said he looked "like a sucked egg."

But it was *she* who in a few weeks was critically ill.

The family memory is that she cut herself stepping on a rusty toy left lying about in the yard. Whatever the cause, in early June she was rushed to Glockner Hospital with a raging streptococcus infection. She came as close to dying as Gerald had with the same sort of infection fifteen years before. With her the eruptions took

332 / Dr. Webb of Colorado Springs

the form of severe erysipelas and eventually a threatening abscess in the thorax. She remained in serious condition throughout the summer.

One of Webb's patients at the time was Dr. Donald C. Balfour, a brilliant young surgeon on the staff of the Mayo Clinic and the husband of Dr. William J. Mayo's older daughter Carrie. When early in 1920, to the consternation of the Clinic partners, their laboratory men found tubercle bacilli in the sputum of their prize "stomach man," Dr. Balfour and his wife were sent in haste to Colorado Springs and Dr. Webb. They rented a house at 519 East Columbia Street for a year and were living there during Varina's illness.

In mid-August Dr. Will—as the older Mayo brother was universally known to distinguish him from his brother Dr. Charlie—and his wife and younger daughter Phoebe set off on an automobile tour of the West to see the sights of the mountain states and pay a visit to Carrie and Donald in Colorado Springs.

During their stay with the Balfours Dr. Will acceded to Gerald's request that he examine Mrs. Webb. He thought she was in need of immediate surgery and telegraphed to Rochester for Dr. A. L. Lockwood, one of the Clinic's thoracic surgeons, to come to Colorado Springs to operate at once.

Dr. Lockwood successfully removed Varina's abscess in early September, stayed with her a few days to be sure she was recovering properly—and acquired her admiration for Belgian police dogs.

On 1 October Dr. Webb wrote a note of gratitude to Dr. Lockwood: "We have Mrs. Webb at home again now. Her wound is nearly healed, a great triumph for your surgical skill and care.... We will gladly send you that Police dog pup if you still want it."

Gerald was about to sail for Europe on NTA business and coaxed Varina to come with him to complete her convalescence on the ocean and in England. But she chose not to go, saying she was sure the motion of the ship would make her seasick and she would get well faster at home.

(Dr. Balfour recovered enough to return to his surgery in Rochester but presently decided his lungs were "too weak" to remain healthy under the strain and wetness of the operating room. He gave up his career in surgery and became the administrative head of the Mayo Foundation and its program of postgraduate education.)

For all these months Dr. Webb had been tending to his presiden-

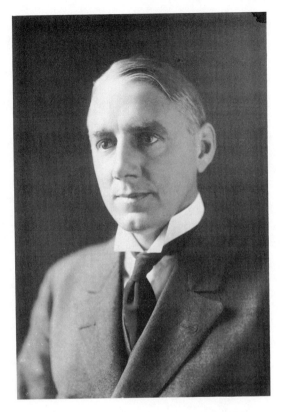

At forty-nine the youngest president of the NTA

tial duties wholly by letters and telegrams. It was time he exercised less remote control, for he could not be just a figurehead president. He knew when he took office that the year ahead would be stormy. The NTA was in turmoil. Most members were fractious on some point or other and sought the ear of the new president. The courtiers came running but so did the dissenters, whom he soon began calling "the bolsheviks."

The NTA had grown enormously in its sixteen years, to a membership in 1920 of about two thousand, plus a host more who were members of thirty-four affiliated state and municipal organizations. These local societies had been growing unhappier by the year, thinking they did all the work and contributed all the financial support but had no proper representation on the Board of Directors and so no voice in setting association policies. The directorships, they said, were passed around year after year among the same group of eastern bigshots and their chosen cronies.

That group was itself discontented. Divided between medical men and social workers of various kinds, it engaged in a continual tug-of-war with much muttering and backbiting. When the medical men returned from the war they were determined to take control away from the hygiene-minded laymen who, they agreed, had had too much to say about NTA policies and programs for too long.

President Victor Vaughan put the resolution of all this dissension squarely in the hands of Gerald Webb by appointing him chairman of a Committee on Reorganization, and Webb presented his report at the NTA meeting in 1920.

What his committee proposed was, in brief, to divide the Board of Directors into two houses. One of these would consist of fifty members elected at large to serve for one year and be eligible for reelection. The second "House of Representatives" would be made up of fifty delegates elected for two-year terms, without eligibility for reelection, by the affiliated local organizations. To elevate and maintain standards in the local chapters, each of them would be required to qualify for the right to elect a delegate to the board.

This proposal provoked a buzz of corridor discussion and side-line caucuses by the dozen. One group of affiliates threatened to withdraw from the NTA and set up a parallel organization of its own. Curiously, a leader of this group was the new vice-president, Dr. James A. Miller, who was also the head of the New York City affiliate.

Disposition of the problem was postponed by continuing the Committee on Reorganization, referring to it all contrary opinions and counterproposals, and charging it with presenting a final report accompanied by a new constitution and bylaws at the meeting in 1921.

President Webb appointed as the new chairman of the committee the highly respected Dr. David Lyman, thinking thus to rid himself of further fuss on the matter. But Dr. Lyman would not have it so: "You are an ex officio member of the committee. You must remain active on it. We MUST have you with us." So Dr. Webb continued to participate in the committee's deliberations.

These went quite smoothly in fact. The opposition calmed down and the final report and bylaws, making virtually no change from the proposal Webb had reported, were adopted with little dissent. When they went into effect in 1921–22, Dr. Webb was elected a director-at-large for one year, Dr. Alexius Forster a representative from Colorado for two years.

The underlying issue all along had been financial: How were the proceeds from the sale of Christmas seals to be divided? These, selling at a penny a seal, had provided the bulk of support for both national and local organizations for years but now the income was in doubt. Would there even be seals to sell in 1920?

Emily P. Bissell, the doughty little woman who tended the post office in Wilmington, Delaware, had really started something in 1907. Casting about for a way to secure money for the tiny tuberculosis haven of eight beds her doctor was struggling to maintain in a shack on the banks of the Brandywine, she decided to try the one-cent Christmas stamp that Jacob A. Riis said, in an article in the *Outlook*, was being used successfully in Copenhagen, Denmark. To her astonishment she collected three thousand dollars for her doctor in that first American seal campaign.

Miss Bissell thought so good a way of raising money ought to have a wider use, and as secretary of the Delaware chapter of the Red Cross she urged it upon the national organization. Working through women's clubs and its own local chapters, the Red Cross collected $135,000 from selling seals in 1908 and $200,000 in 1909.

The next year Livingston Farrand, seeking funds for the NTA, arranged a partnership with the Red Cross. That organization would act as sponsor of an annual campaign, the NTA would handle all the details of administering it, and the two societies would split the proceeds equally. The arrangement succeeded beyond the dreams of either. In a few years the annual gross from selling seals had risen into the millions of dollars.

The NTA kept about half its share of this income to support its own programs. The remainder it dribbled out to its affiliates more or less by whim of the national office staff, and this was what galled the local societies. They thought their labors in the seal sales should be rewarded according to some fixed formula so that each of them would get its fair share.

After the Christmas campaign in 1919 the Red Cross decided to withdraw from the sale of seals. The NTA could continue on its own if it wished but it could no longer use the single-barred symbol of the Red Cross. What to do had to be decided by the Executive Committee at its May meeting in Atlantic City over which Dr. Webb presided.

The logo was no problem; the NTA could easily substitute its own symbol, the double-barred red cross. But some faint-hearted members of the committee were scared at the prospect of carrying on alone. The NTA was certainly no Red Cross in the minds of the charitable, they argued; could they expect people to buy seals to support an organization they knew little about? Why risk failure? Why not just drop the sale of seals?

To Dr. Webb and eventually a majority of the committee this counsel of fear promised only disaster. Where else would the NTA find income in anything like an equal amount? Were they to risk cancellation of its programs for want of trying to keep on selling seals?

Once the decision was taken to proceed with the Christmas campaign as usual it was easy for the committee to recognize the legitimate grievance of the local societies and adopt a fair and fixed division of proceeds: the NTA would keep 5 percent of the net income and distribute 95 percent among its affiliates in proportion to their efforts.

Rebellion vanished. The local societies purred and scurried, and the 1920 seal campaign produced a gross of just under four million dollars. Three decades later, in spite of competition from copycat charities, the annual take from Christmas seals was averaging more than twenty million dollars and the national association's share had reached a million dollars.

What most alarmed the Executive Committee and sent President Webb on to NTA headquarters in New York was the budget for 1920–21 proposed by the staff. It showed an estimated deficit of $33,000. This was not to be tolerated. The NTA had always ended its year with at least a small surplus. Expenditures must be reduced.

The mimeographed copies of reports and other papers Gerald Webb collected at this meeting and in New York are covered front and back with his penciled figures—subtractions, additions, multiplications, rearrangement of sums. He did sweat over that budget. Many items were trimmed but the major reduction was in the "extension service"; the number of field secretaries and their offices and staffs were cut in half. President Webb indulged in a rare bit of boasting in public when he ended his term with a surplus of more than $100,000.

Attempts to reduce expenditures spawned two "people problems" that plagued him throughout his presidential year. One involved Dr. Charles J. Hatfield and Philip P. Jacobs of the NTA staff, the other Dr. Adolphus Knopf.

Dr. Hatfield was the Philadelphian who succeeded Livingston Farrand as executive secretary of the NTA. He was associate director of the Henry Phipps Institute when Farrand departed for the University of Colorado, and he accepted the NTA post only after six months of indecision and on condition that he be permitted to retain his Phipps position and have the NTA work brought to him in Philadelphia. As a result Mr. Jacobs, a Columbia University Ph.D. in theology who had been assistant secretary since 1910, in effect ran the New York office. Subordinate staff members complained they never knew which man was their boss.

Dr. Hatfield was an able manager who readily came up with innovative ideas, but his manner was severe and he riled many of the directors often enough to make them want to be rid of him. He was outspokenly on the side of the medical men too, saying bluntly that the policies of the social workers were ruining the anti-tuberculosis movement.

Jacobs was amiable enough but dull, preoccupied with collecting endless statistics and writing long, wordy histories and reports.

For the opponents of Dr. Hatfield the budget difficulties were heaven-sent. They rushed to urge President Webb to fire him. They said he and Jacobs had no sense of money, had multiplied and expanded NTA programs beyond reason, had increased the office staff to the ridiculous number of twenty-six professional members and thirty-two clerical assistants. Even reasonable men like Doctors Lyman and James A. Miller sought to persuade Webb that the split responsibility in the national office must end, that Hatfield must be made either to move to New York and give the NTA his full time or to resign.

All this irritated Dr. Webb. He liked and respected Dr. Hatfield and thought he and Jacobs were doing an excellent job of keeping all the NTA balls in the air.

Think how many and how complicated these were: the elaborate, nationwide Modern Health Crusade in the public schools, for instance; the extensive field service that kept specialists from the national office traveling the country to aid and advise local societies; administering and preparing materials for the Christmas seals campaigns; the famous Framingham Demonstration, a five-year program designed to show that systematic application of the latest methods of tuberculosis control in Framingham, Massachusetts, could reduce incidence and death rate in the disease—a program underwritten with one million dollars by the Metropolitan Life Insurance Company because too many of its policyholders were dying of tuberculosis.

It fazed Dr. Webb to imagine initiating a new executive secretary into the management of all these activities. "It would be a disaster to lose the services of Dr. Hatfield at this time," he wrote Dr. Lyman. "In these times of difficulty we need his ability and experience more than ever. I would not think of bringing up with him the touchy full-time question lest he quit us."

Dr. Hatfield, well aware of the agitation against him, offered to resign if Webb wanted him to. Absolutely not, said Webb. Instead he proposed to increase Dr. Hatfield's salary from $3000 to $3500 a year. Hatfield was grateful but said he thought the increase should be postponed until the financial stringency had eased.

The two men worked well together. To many a question of minor policy from Dr. Hatfield, Webb replied, "I'll rely on your judgment in this matter. Do what you think best." Webb's successor was less amiable. Dr. Hatfield resigned and the NTA staff was drastically reduced in 1922.

President Webb could not so readily cope with the prickly pride of Dr. Adolphus Knopf.

The Executive Committee of 1919–20 encouraged Knopf to prepare a history of the association and voted to publish it when he had completed it. He worked madly the following year, writing accounts of annual meetings and histories of local societies, assembling bibliographies of papers read, biographical sketches and pictures of major officers, and the like. Proudly he presented his compilation to the Executive Committee of 1920–21. Dr. Webb suggested that the cost of publishing it was an item that could be postponed to help balance the budget and the committee agreed.

Dr. Knopf yelped in anguish. He wrote Dr. Webb pages of accusation and argument. What right had Webb to renege on the pledge made by his predecessors? Did he have any idea what countless hours Knopf had spent on his manuscript, how important the history would be? He would not be soothed by Webb's plea that publication had only been put off a little until the association had more money.

Knopf poured his grievance into the ears of chosen friends, some of whom, including Mazÿck Ravenel and Hermann Biggs, wrote Webb letters of protest on his behalf. Others, more practical, sent Knopf donations toward the cost of the volume. He added a thousand dollars of his own and presented his project again to the Executive Committee, certain there could be no obstacle this time.

The committee voted to proceed with publication, but Dr. Webb and two others, one of them Dr. Biggs, secured a proviso that the biographies of all officers still living be excluded from the book.

Dr. Knopf's outrage could not be contained. What *did* Dr. Webb have against him and his book? The biographies and pictures were a vital part of the history; if living men were dropped, there would be too few left to make the section worthwhile; the book might as well not be published if it was to be so emasculated.

Gerald responded with humble apologies. "I myself shrink from such limelight and imagined others would feel the same."

The Executive Committee rescinded the offensive proviso and sought to stroke their ruffled colleague by urging him to include in the book his own biography and picture. This Dr. Knopf haughtily refused to do. The association had never seen fit to elect him to office and he would not presume to place himself among those it had so chosen. Webb and Hatfield did persuade him to add his own bibliography and it turned out to be twice-over the longest in the book.

The frustrated author's final grievance was the delay in publication caused by Webb's prolonged failure to send in his own biography, bibliography, and picture.

The book finally appeared in 1922. Although it is largely a compendium of facts and often fulsomely eulogistic, it remains a useful reference book not wholly superseded by Richard Shryock's later and more integrated history of the NTA.

Another cantankerous individual who pelted President Webb with letters was William H. Baldwin of Washington DC. He had long been a nonmedical director of the NTA but was now retired from the board and from his business as well, so that he had ample leisure in which to bother his former associates on sundry matters, including what they should do about resuming international cooperation in the anti-tuberculosis campaign.

The war had stopped all normal importation of medical books and journals and the *American Review of Tuberculosis* had been started in 1917 to provide an organ for the publication of American research. The fighting had also canceled the international congress scheduled to convene in 1918. When and where should it be held now, and equally important, who should be allowed to participate?

Dr. Gotthold Pannwitz of Berlin, secretary of the International Union when it ceased to function, raised this issue by publishing a call for the congress to convene in Berlin in 1921. "In the name of justice" he urged the physicians of the Allied Powers to attend as usual and not let "hate and shortsightedness destroy our work."

Mr. Baldwin took it upon himself to reply to Dr. Pannwitz and sent copies of his letter to the officers and directors of the NTA. He wrote:

"I think it is my duty to remind you that this work was destroyed by *German* hate and *German* shortsightedness, and to observe that your communication contains no expression of regret for this or for the greater calamities which were brought upon the world by Germany's action. When you address former associates with no reference to the suffering for which your country is plainly responsible, you show a moral deficiency which would make it impossible for other countries to accept your leadership in this work. I for one cannot and will not accept your leadership in this or any kindred matter without some expression on your part of regret for the suffering your people have caused other nations. With sincere regret that the relations of the past were shattered by Germany, I am yours very truly..."

As Dr. Hatfield commented to President Webb, "In Mr. Baldwin's attitude compromise has no place."

It was lacking too in the attitudes of French and British physicians. Dr. Léon Bourgeois of Paris, president of the defunct International Union, invited the Allied countries to send delegates to a conference in Paris in October 1920 to decide how the call from Dr. Pannwitz should be answered.

Counsels were divided in the NTA. President Webb, though he expressed disapproval of Mr. Baldwin's letter as "intemperate," had lost little of his hostility toward the Hun and saw no reason to resume relations with any of that breed. Many, probably most, agreed with him. Even the amiable Popsy Welch, who during the war refused ever to condemn the Germans, among whom he had many cherished friends, turned bitterly against them after making a postwar trip through the devastated cities and countryside of the battle zones.

But many thought otherwise, notably Dr. Edward R. Baldwin, successor to Trudeau, and his associates at Saranac Lake. They advised doing nothing for a while longer to give time a chance to cool emotions. Above all, said Dr. Baldwin, the NTA should not involve itself in the spiteful antagonism evinced by the French and the English. German physicians and scientists had contributed immeasurably to progress against tuberculosis and if their participation in international discussions was lost through a vindictive spirit, the tuberculous worldwide would be the losers.

Such wisdom did not prevail. The NTA directors named President Webb their delegate to the Paris conference. Although his departure was delayed by Varina's illness, he sailed on 12 October and arrived in Paris in time to be chosen deputy chairman of the conference and help to organize a reborn International Union against Tuberculosis from which the Central Powers were excluded. A new secretariat was to be quartered in Paris, meetings were to be held biennially, and the first of these was to take place in London in July 1921.

Dr. Baldwin had been right about the mellowing effects of time. The nations of the Central Powers were cordially welcomed into the new International Union in 1926.

Gerald Webb's most important and enduring contribution as president was to set the NTA for the first time on the path of support for scientific research.

As Shryock said, the association paid no real attention to the word *Study* in its name until after that name had been changed. The Society for the Study and Prevention of Tuberculosis became officially the National Tuberculosis Association in 1918, but until Dr. Webb came to its helm it had done nothing to stimulate or nourish research. Its energies had been consumed by matters of fund-raising, public education in hygiene, the development of sanatoriums, and other social concerns. Reports of laboratory investigations such as those read at its annual meetings by the Saranac and Hopkins men and Doctors Vaughan and Webb were listened to politely and with a measure of awed respect, but little encouragement was offered for multiplication of their kind.

The directors in 1915 set up a Committee on Research with Dr. Edward R. Baldwin as chairman but it was allotted a minuscule budget of only a thousand dollars and its program never grew beyond a kind of reference service in which the keeper of the office library looked up answers to questions from members and gathered statistics for Philip Jacobs.

Dr. Webb thought this a shameful deficiency and was determined to correct it. No matter what else had to be cut in the budget, he insisted that the funds for the Committee on Research be increased to $20,000. He changed its name to Committee on *Medical* Research and stacked it with men who could be trusted to recognize and further genuinely scientific studies.

He appointed as chairman Dr. William Charles White, medical director of the Tuberculosis League of Pittsburgh and an NTA director who had long urged just what Webb was doing. To serve with White he named Dr. Allen K. Krause, editor of the research-oriented *American Review of Tuberculosis* and a stickler for basic subjects and rigorous methods, and Dr. Paul A. Lewis, director of laboratories at the Henry Phipps Research Institute, which the philanthropic founder had surrendered to ownership and management by the University of Pennsylvania.

Webb made his ex-officio membership an active one on this committee. He took part in its deliberations and acted as its agent. His hand is visible in much it did.

The members agreed at once that their funds would be expended wholly as grants-in-aid of substantial amounts. They would not follow the usual route of choosing among applications that came to them; instead they would themselves survey the research going on in the field in order to find gaps which the NTA might effectively fill. They would select a few likely subjects and then scout around for the best men to investigate these.

For their grants in 1921 they chose five subjects: the chemistry of tuberculin, the chemistry and metabolism of the tubercle bacillus, the interpretation of X-ray examinations of the lungs, the anatomy of the lung, and the therapeutic value of chaulmoogra oil.

The study of chaulmoogra oil was not so ludicrously out of line with the others as it now seems. It reflected a deliberate policy: that a small portion of the committee's funds should be spent on official evaluations of new therapies for tuberculosis. Over succeeding decades this NTA committee issued authoritative reports on treatments from heliotherapy to antibiotics.

The other four subjects produced continuing investigations supported with renewed grants for years, even decades. Dr. William Snow Miller of the University of Wisconsin after several years published a basic book on the anatomy of the lung. By the late 1920s the committee's grants to aid study of diagnostic use of the X-ray brought standardized order out of the chaos that had marked X-ray reading.

Most farsighted of all perhaps was the grant to a twenty-year-old pathologist at the University of Chicago, Dr. Esmond R. Long, for work on the chemistry of tuberculin and the metabolism of the tubercle bacillus. He went on to a phenomenally varied and productive career. In 1929 he became himself a member of the NTA Committee on Medical Research and in 1936–37 served as the association's president.

The work of the Committee on Medical Research grew into a major activity of the NTA. Although Dr. Webb's successors were less generous than he in budget allocations to the committee, private donations kept its funds at or above the level he set. Doctors Krause and Lewis remained members of the committee until late in the 1920s and Dr. White continued as chairman for thirty years.

During that period, Richard Shryock concluded from the evidence, this NTA committee not only "supported much of the effective research done in the tuberculosis field" but became "the planning agency and clearing house for the nation's program in tuberculosis research."

It was fitting that this committee, devoted to stimulating research, should also be responsible for recognizing superior achievement. In 1924 it gave birth to the Trudeau Medal, a medallion of gold to be awarded annually to the person who had made "the most meritorious contribution on the cause, prevention, or treatment of tuberculosis."

The first Trudeau Medal was awarded in 1926 to Dr. Theobald Smith. It was soon recognized as the highest honor the NTA could confer upon a worker in the tuberculosis vineyard. The list of distinguished recipients has grown long and the Trudeau Medal is still a coveted capstone to any man's career in the field of pulmonary disease.

Dr. Webb always gave credit to Dr. White for the NTA's strong program in support of research, but he could hardly deny that it was he who brought the baby to birth and saw it off to a sound, healthy start.

And all the while President Webb traveled. He had foreseen that he would have to. When Dr. Gilbert wired him congratulations on his election he replied with condolences and said to Varina, "Poor Gilbert. He'll have to take over most of the practice again. I'll have to be away an awful lot."

Meetings of the Board of Directors and sometimes of the Executive Committee were held in or near Chicago in order to halve the distance he must go, but many a local affiliate sought a speech by the national president. Dr. Hatfield advised Webb to accept as many such invitations as he could, in order to help strengthen the local chapters. After he got back from Paris in late fall he went to speak in quick succession in Cheyenne, Phoenix, Dubuque, and Louisville.

He snatched January of the new year for himself and joined P. B. Stewart for a cougar hunt in the wilds of Montana some thirty miles out from Libby. This was his idea of living.

It made no matter to him that the only cougar they caught was a "lady lion treed for us by the guide." What he liked was sledding from ranch to ranch behind a team of frisky horses, camping out in the snow under the pines, rustling up "starlight breakfasts," tracking "a big tomcat cougar for days along the river and around the mountain and over its top," sweating while he climbed and freezing when he stopped, lunching on bouillion-cube soup and thick cheese sandwiches beside a fire while he watched scurrying squirrels and deer and twittering magpies and kingfishers and diving water ouzels and listened to the tales of Bakker the guide.

The respite made him feel fit for the quickening pace of NTA activities as the annual meeting approached. He spent all of March on the road, beginning with a day in Chicago to plan with Dr. Hatfield the agenda for a meeting of the Board of Directors in Indianapolis the next day.

He went on to Cincinnati to see Dr. Kennon Dunham, an expert in X-ray diagnosis whose advice he sought on behalf of the Committee on Medical Research. Dr. Dunham kept him on the run for several days of "a breakneck schedule" — daytime visits to hospitals and clinics, with stops at city sights on the way, and evening "dinners with the swells."

At Dunham's request he gave two lectures on tuberculosis to the medical students at the University of Cincinnati, and he enjoyed one dinner at which he sat beside Sir Philip Gibbs, president of the University, and discussed with him the good and bad points of wartime leaders like Clemenceau, Haig, and Foch.

His next stop was Pittsburgh where he was to talk over research grants with Dr. Charles White, but White had been summoned to Washington, so Webb whiled away a day hiking around the city.

He wrote the "Misses and Masters Webb" about the zoo which had begun with animals escaped from a circus and about the "idle furnaces and smokestacks" that signaled hard times in the steel center. "I see signs of great depression everywhere and am told that thousands are starving because the men can't find work. I passed a long line of them waiting for a bowl of soup at a charity mission this noon and it made me sad and angry."

Moving on to Cleveland for the conventions of the AMA and allied societies, he took the weekend off too. "The best way to save yourself, I am learning," he told Varina, "is not to let anyone know where you are, so then they will not overwhelm you. I read that Dickens' chief complaint about the United States—which led to his unpopularity here—was that people would not leave him alone. They called on him before breakfast, swarmed in on him any old time, expectorated on his overcoat, never allowed him any privacy and only a few hours to sleep. They are still a lot that way."

He added a handwritten postscript: "It is funny to be resting in these dirty cities when a corner of the Rockies and a good horse is what I would adore. But I am so deep in medical business I must go on. After my year in office is up, I'll take to the woods with you."

As usual he was reading while he rode the trains. He started off with Jack London's novel *Martin Eden* which he enjoyed because it was so largely autobiographical. Next he was absorbed in Edward Forster's two-volume biography of Charles Dickens, and when he finished that during his weekend of seclusion in Cleveland, he began H. G. Wells' *Outline of History* and got through half of that, judging it "truly splendid."

"I went for a walk last evening after reading and writing letters all day, saw many people going in for an operetta, 'Apple Blossoms' by Fritz Kreisler, and followed them. It was a tuneful show, bordering on the old Viennese light operas. The theatre was enormous but tawdry, the house common and the company common too, though it had two good voices."

Monday morning he dawdled over a late breakfast, then with a sigh "re-entered the whirlwind of modern medical life. Met Dick Dexter who was with us at Neufchâteau. Result is dinner and symphony concert tomorrow! Went out to see George Crile about research projects—result was invitation to his house for dinner and a medical meeting tonight! With 21 other doctors he has a beautiful new clinic building, with every conceivable apparatus for diagnosis—everything later than the latest. They have their own printing plant, expensive lathes and machinery for the latest in physics, electro-conductivity, radium, etc. etc. etc. After going over it all I feel very discouraged and hopeless about our small efforts."

One more stop: in Lincoln, Nebraska, to speak at a banquet of the state NTA chapter and give a lecture to medical students at the University of Nebraska. Then a telegram to Varina: "Home in time for breakfast tomorrow," 27 March. He had finished Wells's *Outline of History* and was reading a book of Kipling's verse.

Six weeks later he started off again, this time driving his new Franklin and taking with him fourteen-year-old Gerry and an adult friend, Billy Hager. As they left the graveled roads of Colorado and crossed into Kansas they began getting stuck in a succession of torrential rains that turned the unpaved roads into chasms of mud through which the auto refused to move.

"The soil here must be gumbo. When it rains there's nothing to do but wait till it dries out. The Franklin and its tires are coated with mud inches deep, and so are we. We've had to fix several punctures and the windshield wipers no longer work. We can't make more than four or five miles an hour. It would take me weeks to get across Kansas and Missouri. What am I to do?"

What he did was abandon Gerry and Billy, trusting them to make their own way across the country to their destination on Cape Cod. "Don't worry about Gerry, Varina Mea. He'll be all right with Billy, who will teach him a lot about looking after a car. Billy is a stickler about oiling the engine, cleaning the spark plugs, and all the rest of it, good habits for Gerry to learn."

He himself caught the train at Salina, Kansas, and sped on in comfort to Lenox, Massachusetts, the lovely resort town in the Berkshires where the NTA Board of Directors were holding their final meeting before the annual convention.

On 14 June, at the Waldorf-Astoria Hotel in New York City, he called to order the seventeenth annual convention of the NTA and presided over its plenary sessions for the next three days. All went smoothly. "There were still a few worries and some grumbling by a few of the bolsheviks, but they could do no harm and it was a fine meeting."

His presidential address was a forceful plea for research, noteworthy indeed for its time and audience.

He began with Seneca: "Truth lies deep, and must be fetched up at leisure." He closed with Kipling's Explorer: "Something hidden. Go and find it. Go and look beyond the Ranges. / Something lost behind the Ranges. Lost and waiting for you. Go!" And in between he called effectively to witness Roger Bacon, Leonardo da Vinci, Edward Trudeau, Theobald Smith, and H. G. Wells.

The main thesis of his remarks, he said, was "the limitations of our knowledge and the great need of increasing it." He itemized the ten "facts we know today" — one of which the many who were at the time addicted to surgery might have contested: "That of all the countless remedies proposed, REST alone has stood the test of time."

He followed with a list, "only illustrative, not exhaustive," of seventeen matters "we do not know, or know but darkly" — notable among them "the biology of the parasite"; "the physiology of the body's defense"; "the explanation of virulence and resistance, and the relative importance of the two." He emphasized that although the incidence and mortality of tuberculosis were unmistakably declining in America and Europe, "we do not know why. We can only speculate and argue about the reasons."

He urged his hearers to be proud that "for the first time in its history our association is attempting to aid and encourage a few laboratory workers whose efforts to increase our knowledge have given promise." He called it shameful that in all the world hardly a score of laboratories were doing research on tuberculosis and that few of these were investigating fundamental questions. He pled eloquently for basic research, quoting the timelessly relevant words of Wells: "As 'practical men' refuse to learn, it is only when knowledge is sought for its own sake that she gives rich and unexpected gifts in any abundance to her servants. The world today is much more disposed to spend money on technical research than on pure science."

How better could rich men spend their money than in contributions to the support of laboratory research into the hidden puzzles of this ravaging disease? Webb asked. And governments? "The nations recently engaged in the World War unhesitatingly poured out their wealth to find new methods of killing and destruction... yet not one of them has ever thoroughly encouraged any attempt to counter the terrible devastations of the tubercle bacillus, whose victims number hundreds of thousands yearly."

Gerald "jumped for joy" to have the address over. "The audience was very big," he said to Varina, "and some ex-presidents told me afterwards there had never been so scholarly and scientific an address presented to the association."

He was glad to turn the presidential reins over to his successor, Dr. James A. Miller. But he could not celebrate his release by going off to the woods with Varina as he had dreamed of doing: he had to go to Europe again instead.

The International Union against Tuberculosis was holding its first congress in Paris in late July. Gerald had appointed Colonel Bushnell as the NTA's official delegate and lined up half a dozen other members who would attend at their own expense. (Eliminating the generous ladling out of expense reimbursements was one way President Webb had cut the budget.) But Dr. Hatfield and the NTA directors insisted that Webb must also go as an official delegate "to complete the organization he had helped to initiate the preceding year."

When this decision had been made in Lenox, Gerald suggested to Varina that she and the children all go with him to Europe "if you think we should blow ourselves this way." Apparently she did not, for he took with him only Marka, aged sixteen, and Gerry, approaching fifteen. They sailed with Colonel Bushnell aboard the *S.S. Mauretania* on 14 July, after seeing Varina and the three younger children settled for a long holiday at Siasconset, a resort on Nantucket Island.

Gerald made the trip a memorable experience for his youngsters. In London he took them to see the Elgin Marbles in the British Museum and to attend a Sunday service at Westminster Abbey, then he hired a car and drove them around England and Wales to meet all their uncles and aunts and cousins before crossing the Channel and entraining for Paris.

The congress of the International Union preoccupied him for almost a week. He presided at some sessions, spoke at others, and was elected a member of the permanent governing council. Much to his gratification, Dr. Theobald Smith was elected the first president.

His mission accomplished, Gerald devoted himself to showing Marka and Gerry his own cherished spots in Paris, including the Louvre, the Opéra, and the Cathedral of Notre Dame, then motored them on a leisurely tour of France. They saw the chateaus and vineyards of the Loire Valley, the cathedrals at Rheims and Soissons, and the battlefields in Flanders and along the Marne, where he tried to describe what he had witnessed there. "He made us feel the awfulness of war," Marka remembered.

They sailed for home on 21 August. On board the *S.S. Finlandia* Gerald met in the deck chair beside his own the writer Owen Wister. Lounging in sun and sea mist the two men reminisced of their mutual friend Theodore Roosevelt, who had died two years before, not long after the World War ended.

XV

Fac et Spera

GERALD WEBB had celebrated his fiftieth birthday that September of 1921. "Your half-century husband" he called himself to Varina.

She did not think he looked much older. His face was still unlined, his cheeks still bore the English pink, his hazel eyes were still clear—warm and shining when he was having fun or feeling pity but grayed to gunmetal when he was tense or angry. The silver creeping slowly upward from his temples barely showed in his smooth blond hair.

His six-foot-two-inch frame was as straight and lean as in youth, his weight never varying more than two or three pounds from its normal one hundred and fifty-six. But his stance had taken on the solid set of maturity, which added authority to his presence, physical support to his dignified mien.

He had formed the habit of plucking a flower from Varina's bouquet or her garden as he left the house each morning and the boutonniere he made of it was becoming a familiar part of his spruce appearance.

Colorado Springs also turned fifty in 1921. Its population, which had hovered around 35,000 for a decade, began to grow again after the war. Including residents of satellite communities like Manitou, Ivywild, and Colorado City, it had reached 55,000 within two years.

The newcomers lived in the more than a thousand hastily constructed bungalows on streets to the north and west of town, or in "the big houses" along Wood Avenue and Monument Park Road and in the affluent community of Broadmoor that was sprouting on the mesa beneath Cheyenne Mountain. A number of Dr. Webb's wealthier patients had built or bought houses in Broadmoor—the Ashton Potters, Chaloner Schleys, and Benjamin Allens among them.

Spencer "Spec" Penrose, the blueblood swashbuckler who had dominated the Socialites in earlier years, was becoming the prime entrepreneur in the city's development. His daring schemes are described with gusto in *Newport in the Rockies* by Marshall Sprague, a patient of Webb's who has become the supreme teller of fascinating tales about people and events in Colorado Springs history.

Penrose had gambled the capital he acquired from Cripple Creek mining and smelting—and from betting $100,000 that McKinley would be elected president—on a highly risky venture in copper mining. It had paid off and he was now a millionaire many times over.

He had also ventured, at age forty, into marriage with Julie Villers Lewis Macmillan, the spirited, wealthy, widowed daughter of a French mayor of Detroit. After ten years of fabulous global travel the Penroses settled down again in Colorado Springs and Spec turned his flamboyance and imagination, plus his fortune, to the aid of his home town.

He began by attacking the doldrums into which its tourist business had fallen. He maneuvered the building of a twenty-mile-long automobile road to the top of Pikes Peak. Most of those who watched the road climb thought it a madcap enterprise, but when it was done Penrose, with his usual flair for promotion, organized an auto race over the steepest twelve miles of it and enlisted the name and fame of Barney Oldfield the speed king to publicize it. The Pikes Peak Hill Climb became an annual event and is still an item of national interest in the celebration of the Fourth of July.

The Pikes Peak Highway—which became a thing of joy and pecuniary importance to young Gerry Webb—along with the site of Colorado Springs at the junction of the Ocean-to-Ocean and Colorado-to-the-Gulf highways, boosted the tourist business of the region to an annual $2,500,000 by 1921.

Penrose next loosed his talents upon Broadmoor. He saw fantastic possibilities in the dusty acres on the mesa which had drained away the energies and money of the Count de Pourtales two decades before. The Count's Broadmoor Hotel and white cake of a casino had been abandoned to pigeons and vandals long since. Spec bought the site and began to build a grandly luxurious new hotel.

The townspeople jeered again. What made that fool Spec think they needed another hotel? The old Antlers Hotel, even with the big new garage it had just added, was half empty most of the time these days. And what made him think tourists would take the streetcar seven miles out from town just to get a bed for a night or two?

Spec showed them. The lavish new Broadmoor Hotel of nine stories and 350 rooms, costing more than $3,000,000, opened its doors on 1 June 1918, to the accompaniment of famous guests, grand balls, and champagne receptions—and an international advertising campaign. Major Webb saw the announcement of the opening in a glossy Paris magazine and sent a note of congratulations to his friend.

Month by month, season by season, Penrose added new attractions to his hostelry. He built a fine auto road to parallel the streetcar to Broadmoor. He put in walkways and gardens around Pourtales's hard-won lake; swimming pools and tennis courts and golf courses of professional quality; a skating rink to which Varina Webb often took the children and their friends for gaiety and exercise; two extensive polo fields with accompanying stables for four hundred mounts that resuscitated the dying sport on Cheyenne Mountain and brought wealthy sportsmen from all over to live and play in Broadmoor.

And he transferred to the hotel grounds the menagerie of wild animals he had accumulated at his Turkey Creek ranch as the nucleus of what became "one of the finest small zoos in the world"; he named Gerald Webb to its supervising board of managers.

When Penrose began building the Broadmoor he and Julie were living in what had been Julie's home at 30 West Dale Street just off North Cascade Avenue, but they soon chose to be nearer their rising hotel and bought the thirty-room Spanish villa the Ashton Potters had built on the roughed-out Lake Avenue of the Count's Broadmoor City. (Ashton and his wife Grace Goodyear had died within a few months of each other in 1916.)

The Penroses made the villa larger and dressed it up, but they kept the name the Potters had given it, El Pomar, meaning "apple orchard" in Spanish, because they had built it in the middle of a farmer's grove of apple trees.

Spec and Julie entertained constantly and lavishly at El Pomar, with the great and near-great as guests—from Paderewski and Chaliapin, Rosa Ponselle and Lily Pons, to Vice-President Charles G. Dawes and Jack Dempsey. They exploited these celebrities shamelessly, making sure to get pictures of every one of them to be used in publicizing the Broadmoor.

Spec next bought a couple thousand more of the mesa acres, divided them into outsize lots for sale, and soon had a community of conspicuous wealth filling in around his hotel.

In only a few years the Broadmoor became one of the best known hotels in the Western world, *the* place for people of wealth and importance to go for mingling with their kind and enhancing their social status. Increasingly too it became the place for the moneyed elite who contracted tuberculosis to live while they chased the cure, so much so in time that in eastern medical circles the Broadmoor was thought to be a Colorado Springs sanatorium. Dr. Webb tended many a patient at the Broadmoor.

Other movers and shakers were also changing the city. Income from the Cripple Creek mines was dwindling steadily but men who had made fortunes extracting and milling gold there were investing their capital in other ventures. A. E. Carlton, for instance, was getting his Holly Sugar Company into gear and the Wigwan Association was pumping oil south of town.

Modern methods of dry farming were turning the windswept eastern prairies into productive fields of wheat and corn, and El Paso County was leading the state in growing purebred livestock, owing in part to Spencer Penrose's herd of prize Holsteins on his Turkey Creek ranch.

The city fathers were asphalting and lighting the streets, building new schools to a total of seventeen, piping additional water down from the mountains.

Colorado College, in a worrisome period of rebuilding after a disruptive row between administration and faculty ended in the departure of President Slocum and several of the older professors, was offering vocational training to several hundred World War veterans.

A burgeoning art center was another Penrose project but this time Julie's. Gaily adding patronage of art to her chic repertoire of pastimes, she decided to donate her former West Dale Street house, complete with swimming pool, greenhouse, and spacious gymnasium, for use as an art school and exhibit hall. Although it was seven miles away from the Cheyenne Mountain mesa, she called it the Broadmoor Art Academy as a bit of additional publicity for her husband's enterprise.

At first the former gymnasium was used for such high-society merriments as Beaux Arts costume balls more than for serious students and shows. But Julie was absorbing taste and ideas from her frequent sallies into the artists' colony in Santa Fe, New Mexico, and was about to bring back with her the portraitist Randall Davey to begin informed attention to art at the Academy.

All in all, if Colorado Springs had lost the bubbling bustle of youth, it could expect to enjoy a healthy, prosperous, and pleasurable maturity.

Gerald Webb and Colorado Springs saw little of each other in their mutual fifty-first year. Gerald undertook a stupefying succession of trips back and forth across the country. He went to at least twenty states, and in the fall again to Europe.

"It seemed strange to be passing through Colorado Springs and not get to see you," he once wrote Varina from Omaha, in transit from southern California to Lima, Ohio. "But it was nice to hear your dear voice on the telephone." Without his letters from every stop, Varina would have had to feel herself a widow. He knew he was being hard on her. In September he wrote her from Georgia: "Do send a line to tell me you still love your husband. Be patient with me. After all, I shall be home for the winter, and isn't that something!"

The reason for all this journeying was the onslaught of program chairmen who had heard the past-president of the NTA was an excellent speaker and sought him to ornament their assemblies. Seldom was he allowed to get away with only one speech at a stop. In Oregon, for example, he was the banquet star for the state antituberculosis association, addressed a public health rally in a church in Portland, and the next day spoke to the state medical society.

To judge from the two addresses published in the *Journal of the Outdoor Life* and extant notes for others, he conveyed much the same message to all his audiences: the plea for more and basic research he had first made in his presidential address to the NTA. In Oregon he called it "Tuberculosis—Our Triumphs and Tasks," in Arizona "How We Are Winning against Tuberculosis." He also urged every community to follow the effective model of the Framingham Demonstration. And he consistently embellished his remarks with quotations from Voltaire, Machiavelli, Ovid, and Horace and with illustrative anecdotes from Pasteur, Laënnec, and Koch.

Dr. Webb felt free to do all this traveling and speaking because he had found another able and experienced partner to help Dr. Gilbert carry the patient load in Colorado Springs. The man was Dr. John A. "Jack" Sevier.

A native of Tennessee now in his early thirties, Sevier had taken his bachelor's degree at Vanderbilt University and his medical degree at Johns Hopkins. Like many others, he contracted tuberculosis at the Baltimore school and after graduation went to the Trudeau Sanatorium for two years, then, seeking a milder climate, to the Agnes Phipps Memorial Sanatorium in Denver for a year. In 1919 he moved to Colorado Springs and Dr. Webb.

When he arrived, Cragmor Sanatorium was just beginning to recover and refurbish after the disruption of the war and influenza years and Dr. Webb persuaded Dr. Forster to give his new patient part-time employment as a resident physician.

Jack Sevier was both a dedicated doctor and a cultivated southern gentleman after Webb's heart. When Dr. Gilbert could no longer handle the added burden during Webb's presidential year, Gerald persuaded Sevier to join the partnership in private practice from the Burns Building office, while remaining a consultant at Cragmor. Jack chose to live in the Broadmoor Hotel and so took over the resident care of the team's patients there, including Spencer Penrose.

Jack's twin brother Charles, also a doctor and also a victim of tubercle bacilli, after spending two years as patient-assistant to Rollier in Switzerland, followed Jack to Colorado Springs. From a year as Dr. Webb's patient at Cragmor he graduated to a position on the sanatorium's medical staff, where he prescribed and monitored all hours of sunbathing as well as treating tuberculous bones and joints.

Patients and employees at Cragmor had trouble telling the twins apart and often talked to one as if to the other, much to their own glee, if not the doctors', when they discovered their error. Both Sevier brothers were clinicians first and foremost; neither was inclined toward personal engagement with test tubes and microscopes.

When Dr. Webb went east "for the meetings" in the spring of 1922 he undertook a mission on the side: visiting private schools up and down the seaboard. He and Varina had decided it would be time that fall to send seventeen-year-old Marka and soon-to-be-sixteen Gerry away to school. Gerald had college in mind for both youngsters and wanted them to have a couple years of more solid preparation than he thought they were getting in Colorado Springs schools.

He made a conscientious survey of eight institutions that had been recommended to him. It was easy to settle on Lawrenceville School in New Jersey for Gerry, but the choice for Marka was more worrisome. "She is a lovely girl," he wrote Varina, "more so every year, and I fear this gift of beauty may cause her trouble. She is much more interested in flapperism than in scholarship now, so the school must be of a kind that will change this."

He finally chose Oldfields in Glencoe, Maryland. The head-mistress and teachers there seemed kindly enough "but I do not think they will stand for much nonsense or disregard of studies." He thought the buildings attractive and the surrounding woodlands beautiful; "they will permit Marka to get plenty of exercise and nature study." And not least, Glencoe was only thirty miles from Baltimore and within easy reach of Philadelphia; his friends in those two cities could keep an eye on the girl *in loco parentis.*

On his way to Europe that fall Gerald took Gerry and Marka to their respective schools and thereafter wrote them many lively letters and made occasion to visit them often. He enjoyed these interludes, especially those with Oldfields' "pretty, aristocratic jeunes filles, who are as unflapperlike a lot of girls as you'll meet these days."

His visits were exciting treats for the youngsters. "Daddy was a great hit with everyone here," Marka wrote her mother after one of them. "Everybody just adored him, thought he was a Greek god or something. Even our gym teacher has fallen for him."

He sometimes played tennis with Marka, then took her and her roommate to dine out in Baltimore. One weekend he escorted her to New York to hear a Japanese prima donna sing in "Madame Butterfly." Another time he rearranged his itinerary in order to see Gerry perform as catcher on the Lawrenceville baseball team in its big game of the season and to hear him sing in the school choir the next morning.

His medical friends came up to expectations. Marka's life at Oldfields was studded with teas and dinners, weekends and holiday recesses at the homes of the Thayers and Finneys in Baltimore and Dr. Staige Davis, a devoted former patient of Gerald's, in Philadel-phia. Dr. Hugh Young, the eminent Hopkins surgeon who was a

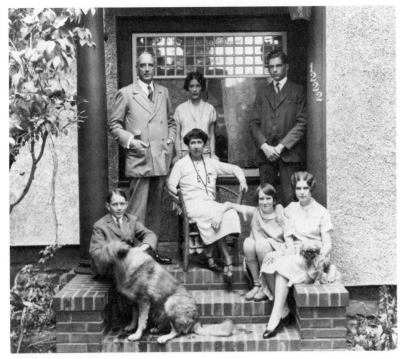

Family portrait, 1922

new friend and later a patient of Gerald's, invited young Marka to join a group of faculty members at his home for dinner and an evening at the theater afterward. He told Gerald that his adult guests thought the girl's "poise and easy mixing quite remarkable."

But none of these friends could help Gerald toward his goal for Marka. She stubbornly resisted any urging that she go on to further struggles with the likes of algebra and Latin. Dr. Finney's daughter Mary, at another school, was of like mind. "Mary balks at college too," Gerald told Varina. "I think it may be hopeless with Marka. It's too bad. She certainly has the mind for it."

He feared disappointment with Gerry too. The boy never had taken much to books; he was too full of restless energy. Now, almost as tall as his father but of stockier build, he tried conscientiously to study and did earn passing grades, but it was obvious that all he truly cared about was school sports. His short notes and postcards home reported little except the wins and losses of the Lawrenceville teams.

In his second year Gerry developed weakness and pain in first one then both knees. Dr. Charles Sevier suspected from the symptoms that the joints were tuberculous but Dr. Ryder, drawing fluid from the knees and injecting it into guinea pigs, said they were not. Dr. Webb was pragmatic; he kept the boy at home for a year of sunbathing and rest and the trouble vanished. But Gerry did not want to go back to Lawrenceville a year behind the boys of his former form, so Gerald sent him instead to Deerfield Academy in Massachusetts.

Dr. Webb's journey to Europe in 1922, his third in as many successive years, was made at the request and expense of the NTA's Committee on Medical Research. Newspapers and medical journals alike were giving much space at the time to claims and counterclaims for "the Spahlinger cure" and Chairman White asked Dr. Webb to make an official evaluation of it.

Before sailing he bought at Brentano's a Greek grammar and copies of Dante's *Inferno* and Plutarch's *Parallel Lives* to occupy him during the crossing, undoubtedly as a change from Jean Henri Fabre's volumes on mason wasps and spiders, Moore's *Life of Oliver Goldsmith*, and especially Edward Bok's autobiography, in which he had been engrossed during the preceding months.

One is reminded by contrast of the great Popsy Welch's habit of whiling away the Atlantic passage by consuming together a stack of detective novels and a box of chocolates!

Henri Spahlinger was a Swiss bacteriologist who had developed both a vaccine to prevent tuberculosis and an antitoxin serum to treat acute and chronic cases of it. He had announced these in 1914 and they had been under trial in his Geneva clinic and a few other European hospitals for eight years. Now he and a number of very vocal European backers were reporting many lasting cures even in advanced cases.

Dr. Webb spent a few days in New York collecting information and opinions about the cure, then repeated the process in London, where he was soon subjected to such heavy wooing by Spahlinger's supporters that he began to suspect commercialism was at work, and also began to fear bodily harm if he expressed an adverse opinion.

He went up to Edinburgh to talk with his admired friend Sir Robert Philip who had evaluated Spahlinger's work in Geneva for the British Red Cross. Sir Robert was inclined to dismiss it all as a hoax, but he said the British Ministry of Health was about to endorse the cure, having received an enthusiastically favorable report from its investigating agent in Geneva.

The man who seemed to be behind all the agitation on Spahlinger's behalf was a Mr. Reeves-Smith, head of the Savoy, Claridge, and Berkeley hotels. At lunch with Webb at the Savoy, Reeves-Smith assured his guest that his only motive was humanitarian, that he had no financial interest whatever in the cure, but Webb questioned this statement when he learned later that Reeves-Smith was a director of Preston Hall Colony, a popular private sanatorium for consumptives. "He is a man I do not like, and he's too intense and too intimate with Spahlinger to be disinterested I think."

Webb sought out one Dr. Cohlbeck who had personally tracked down more than a hundred of the patients supposedly cured by Spahlinger's serum, and Cohlbeck loaned him for study his thick notebooks of reports on these cases.

"He tells me that two-thirds of the cases treated some years ago are dead and while they were severe tests because advanced cases, he thinks the treatment killed them. He also tells me that when Spahlinger was in London a year ago he carried a pistol in one hand and a dagger in the other in case anyone tried to rob him of his secret! I am being cautious in everything I say, polite and admiring, especially to Reeves-Smith, and shall certainly be the same in Geneva. I am keeping Frank [his solicitor brother] informed of all my doings. You must keep all this confidential, Varina. I shall make no report, which I now think is bound to be unfavourable, till I am back in the U.S.A."

His fears were calmed when an influential friend arranged for Post Wheeler of the American Embassy to meet him in Paris and escort him to Geneva.

Wheeler and his wife made Webb think again about his verdict on Spahlinger. "They are delightful, cultivated people. Mrs. Wheeler is a novelist, writes under the name of Hallie Erminie Rives, is an interesting woman of about 50 and says she knows all the Jefferson Davis family and is probably distant kin of yours." The Post Wheelers knew Henri Spahlinger and were sure he could not be a charlatan; he might be honestly mistaken, but Webb ought to keep an open mind. "I'm sure they have no interest in his cure except for humanity's sake."

In Geneva Webb was almost swept away himself by Henri Spahlinger's urbane charm, his accents of sincerity and integrity as he talked of his work and showed the NTA investigator around his sumptuous clinic, hospital, and laboratory. "He is so different from Reeves-Smith. Maybe he has something better than we have after all. I am not sure yet."

Back in London he spent his daytime hours in half a dozen hospitals examining for himself the histories, records, and lungs of patients under treatment with Spahlinger's vaccine and serum.

Sadly he concluded that Sir Robert Philip and Dr. Cohlbeck were right: the Spahlinger cure was no cure at all. He had not found a single case in which it had made any real difference and he had seen quite a few where he judged its effects to be harmful. The rosy reports must be based on wishful thinking if not worse. He was convinced that all the promotion and pressure in London was "just a world-wide get-rich-quick scheme" — which made him angry because the newspaper publicity had "caused 45,000 tuberculous ex-service men to clamor for the cure, adding to the pressure on the government. The nice Post Wheelers are just getting their legs pulled."

He was wearied by it all. "After this give me cougar instead of TB hunts," he wrote Varina. And to Dr. Gilbert, "I suppose you think this is all a vacation, but vacations, I find, are just a change of scene in racing through life."

Still, he had found time for diversions. In Switzerland he had made a side trip to Leysin to see Rollier and his clinics again and had gone at last to visit Arnold and Harriet Klebs in Nyon for several days. In the beauty of Les Terasses on Lake Geneva he relaxed. Arnold was devoting all his time now to research and writing in medical history and to amassing a distinguished library in that subject. He had inherited his father's extensive collection of books and was enlarging it rapidly. It was well on its way to a total of 15,000 volumes.

One of these Arnold gave to Gerald as he was leaving: a copy of the seminal 1761 treatise on percussion by Leopold Auenbrugger of Vienna, who had developed the diagnostic value of thumping the chest on the basis of his childhood experience in tapping wine kegs in the cellar of his father's inn.

Arnold's enthusiasm and his enviable library enhanced Gerald's appreciation of medical history and turned his thinking and reading even more in that direction.

Concerned, as he wrote Roland, about his sister Amy whose husband Daff had died suddenly, Gerald took a weekend to motor to Wales and bring her back for a break in London. He was reassured to find her coping gamely with her loss and to learn that she would be financially able to keep her daughter Nancy at Oxford and the younger Robine in school at Reading.

It was Harold in Cheltenham who gave him real cause to worry. His brother was dangerously emaciated and half mad with pain from a stomach ulcer. No wonder; his doctor was keeping him on an exclusive diet of green apples!

Aghast at so precisely wrong a prescription, Doctor Gerald firmly intervened to forbid the apples and substitute the newly established Sippy treatment, a strict regimen on bland dairy and egg foods. This was successful and Harold was forever after humbly grateful to his brother, saying Gerald had saved not only his life but his reason.

For Gerald the big event of this trip abroad occurred in Edinburgh. His visit there coincided with an elaborate ceremonial dinner Sir Robert Philip as president of the Scottish College of Physicians was giving in honor of Jules Bordet of the Pasteur Institute in Brussels.

For years Webb had followed admiringly Bordet's innovative work on immunity and was thrilled to meet and talk with him. "I sat next to Sir Alfred Ewing, president of the University of Edinburgh, who was on Sir Robert's left, with Bordet on his right, so we all chatted together."

He was overcome by "the gorgeousness of it all," the beautiful banquet hall, the perfectly appointed tables, the finest of food and wines, the gracious decorum of hosts and guests. The latter numbered some fifty, of whom Gerald already knew more than half.

Called on to speak after dinner, he told the group that the only stories *he* knew were Scottish, hardly proper to tell on this occasion. "But I gave them all some amusement over Prohibition and your dandelion wine, Varina Mea."

He returned home in time for Christmas, to find Varina not only busy with activities of the season but full of plans for the face-lift she wanted to give 1222 North Cascade.

She thought it was time their house matched the mellowing maturity of the street, newly paved with a parkway down the middle and shaded by tall trees arching above. She was lonesome with

Marka and Gerry away and wanted something more than "my frilly little playings" to distract her. "The house is lonely. I am even depressed by the exceeding neatness of your room," she wrote Marka.

She may also have been piqued by Gerald's glowing descriptions of his eastern friends' sumptuous homes; she needed a proper setting for the "costly oriental rug" Dr. and Mrs. Staige Davis had sent them for Christmas; and she could afford to remodel. Settlement of her father's estate had brought her an immediate $2000 plus an annual income of $2400.

Gerald agreeing, she went at the task in a whirlwind of energy, standing arms akimbo on the lawn to direct the workmen in placing strips and triangles of brown siding to turn the plain exterior into a likeness of the Tudor style. She watched over the carpenters as they put down new hardwood flooring and pestered the painters as they mixed fresh colors for the walls, especially the "turkey red" she chose for the sunlit diningroom. She installed new glassed-in bookshelves from floor to ceiling in Gerald's study and matching cabinets in the livingroom to house her own collections of Dresden figurines and Pikes Peak bottles. Under all she laid the rich colors and patterns of oriental rugs in every downstairs room.

It all took months. Like most men, Gerald loathed the upheaval and disorder. He escaped it briefly when he went to Atlantic City for the convention of the Association of American Physicians, at which he heard Frederick Banting of Toronto describe how he had isolated insulin two years before.

To occupy him on the trip he took along *Don Quixote*, Cellini's autobiography, and Anatole France's *La Vie en Fleur*—the last of those because his friend Dr. Thayer said the author himself had read the novel aloud to him.

Dr. Webb confessed to "inexpressible relief" when he found his home again in polished order upon his return. Varina had finished her task just in time for the arrival of NTA members who were again stopping over for a day in Colorado Springs on the way from their convention in the East to the AMA meeting in California.

There were one hundred and eighteen in the party this time, led by Lawrason Brown, who had succeeded James A. Miller as president.

Many of the visitors sought out Dr. Webb of course, and he was embarrassed to have them see his meager laboratories and animal quarters in the Burns Building. He had repeatedly expressed to Varina and Dr. Gilbert his discouragement about these after seeing the spacious, well-equipped laboratories elsewhere. Now to have these men see for themselves how little he had to work with! He was ashamed. We may guess that he tried to gloss it over by talking about the idea he was hatching to provide himself with better resources.

His time for research, and Dr. Gilbert's too, had been scant since before the war. Work in the laboratory had to be left largely to Dr. Ryder and often he had to return to bed at Cragmor for a spell of rest. He continued to have the help of Dr. Staines, of Margaret Gilbert until she bore Burton a baby, and of transient amateurs. One of those amateurs who in time became expert was a tuberculous dentist, Dr. William Francis Drea.

Dr. Drea, "one hundred percent Irish," as he described himself to me, was born and reared in Cambridge, Massachusetts, took his degree in dentistry at Harvard, and began to practice as an oral surgeon in Back Bay, Boston. When the tubercle bacilli took hold in him he was told he had better move to Colorado.

He arrived in Colorado Springs in 1914, became a patient of Dr. Webb's, and when he felt better established a practice in dentistry. "But I had a lot of curiosity about things, particularly X-ray. Dr. Webb encouraged me to study it. So I took some courses in math and physics at Colorado College and began doing X-ray work for the Sisters at Glockner on the side." State law requiring a medical degree for such work, Dr. Drea spent his nights with medical textbooks for two years, passed the state medical examination, and was licensed to practice as doctor of medicine.

His study turned his curiosity upon medical problems and he offered his help "in the only medical research going on in town, just to see how it was done and what Webb and Ryder thought they could do to better things in tuberculosis."

The only time he could give Dr. Ryder was at night and on Sundays. "It didn't take long to get me hooked on the laboratory once I got the hang of it, and I was fed up with all the bickering, all the rivalry and competition, among the doctors at Glockner, so I asked Dr. Webb to give me a job at the same salary, $1200 a year. He did, but of course I had to keep on with my practice and did most of my work for him at night. Sometimes I cut my day short at the office in order to have more hours in the laboratory. It was rough then. I guess I was working all told, office and laboratory, about seventy hours a week."

Under such circumstances the only scientific research to come from the Webb laboratory in these years was a series of experiments with implanted tuberculous tissues in guinea pigs. Those had begun in 1916 to test out Dr. Webb's surmise that if injecting tubercle bacilli, live or dead, would not induce immunity, implanting tuberculous lymph nodes might do so. Dr. Ryder continued this investigation during the war and the first report of it was published while Dr. Webb was in France.

It was quite clear by then that such implantation did not achieve the slightest degree of immunity, but the experiments raised all sorts of questions: Might tuberculous liver or spleen tissues turn the trick? How long did the bacilli retain their virulence in the lymph nodes or other tissues, when these were untampered with and when they were covered with a film of collodion? What weakened the virulence? What killed the bacilli? And so on.

Dr. Webb said he was "gratified," when he appeared to read the second report of these investigations at the NTA meeting in 1921, to find "the hall was packed, not even standing room left, and the applause when I finished was long." He attributed this reception to interest in his subject, but we may guess it was at least equally an expression of respect and affection for the outgoing president.

By the third report of the series, in 1923, the emphasis had shifted to probing the health and longevity of the tubercle bacillus. Ryder and his aides had proved that the parasite retained its vigor longer when its host tissues were incubated in a saline solution than when these were incubated without such a surrounding bath or were kept unbathed in a refrigerator. Why? He speculated that when left to fend in putrefying tissues the bacilli might weaken and die from lack of oxygen. This called for new studies of the gas requirements of the bacillus.

Dr. Webb had been piecing out these reports of laboratory work with papers reporting, in conjunction with Doctors Gilbert and Forster, clinical observations on the effects of artificial pneumothorax, the correlation between bronchitis and sinus disorders, the way the tubercular cough could fracture ribs.

He also, feeling secure enough now to let bygones be bygones, joined with Dr. Charles Fox Gardiner in the publication of a careful

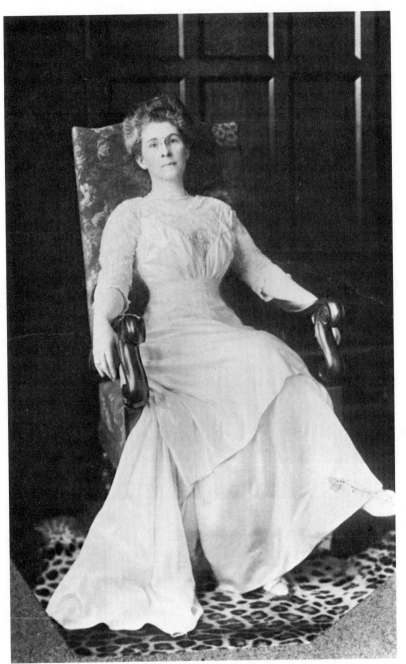

Maria McKean Allen, loyal benefactress

statistical study of how altitude affected the mortality rate in tuber-culosis. Although he no longer actively promoted high places as especially beneficial in therapy, he continued to think mountain living helped toward recovery.

But these scattered efforts simply would not do for one who was talking so widely about the need for basic scientific research. All through his peripatetics in 1922 Webb wrestled with the problem of how to upgrade and expand his research.

With five children to educate he could not afford to finance lab-oratory supplies and salaries from his own pocket, and he feared he was losing the financial support of his principal benefactors. Benjamin and Maria Allen had got a divorce and gone their separate ways, Ben to California and Maria to her McKean family in Phila-delphia, just for a long visit she said, but he was not sure she would ever return to Colorado Springs.

When he attended a meeting of the Laënnec Society at Johns Hopkins in the fall of 1922 he went to talk over his dilemma with Dr. William Henry Welch. If he were to set up something like the foundation established after Edward Trudeau's death to continue garnering support for the Saranac sanatorium and laboratory, did Welch think he too could hope to receive contributions from eastern philanthropists?

Dr. Welch sympathetically encouraged him to try the foundation route but shook his head no about the prospect of eastern money, at the start anyway. He thought Webb would have to rely upon donations from his local friends and patients to begin with. If he got a foundation going and it produced some good research, he might then get a hearing from the big givers in financial centers like New York and Philadelphia.

Gerald pondered this advice as he went on to his Spahlinger mission in Europe, and on the train homeward from New York when he returned he jotted down lists of persons from whom he might get help and money.

One of these was Ruth Davis Dangler, a patient who had come to him from Chicago and was now a wealthy young widow just getting up and around after several years in bed taking the rest cure in her home in Broadmoor.

Ruth was attractive, intelligent, talented, sparkling in personality. Early in her illness she had married a fellow patient, Henry C. Dangler, and bore him a daughter. Henry had succumbed to his bacilli but Ruth, being one of those patients who "use their heads," routed hers and achieved recovery. Now she was casting about for something to do to engage her reviving energies. She responded eagerly to Dr. Webb's idea of a research foundation and was of inestimable help to him in making plans and arrangements.

The thinking, planning, discussing, and corresponding went on throughout 1923.

That year also brought to town, providentially it must have seemed, Dr. Charles Hercules Boissevain, a footloose young man of thirty, magnetically handsome and high-spirited, who was looking for work in tuberculosis research.

Charles was a native of Holland (a nephew, incidentally, of Eugen Jan Boissevain, the husband of the poet Edna St. Vincent Millay) and a medical graduate of the University of Amsterdam, where for three years he was the country's champion sculler. Such physical fitness notwithstanding, he fell host to tubercle bacilli and after graduation spent two years in Switzerland recovering his health.

Somewhere along the way he had contracted a yen for the laboratory and now was fortunate enough to acquire the best of research skills during two years as associate on the staff of Jules Bordet at the Pasteur Institute in Brussels.

He also learned there that low levels of altitude did not agree with his asthma; he was free of that affliction only in the mountains. So he made his way to Colorado.

Who sent him to Dr. Webb we do not know. It could have been Bordet himself, after his meeting with Webb at the banquet in Edinburgh. Or it may have been someone at Johns Hopkins. Boissevain was known there, because Dr. Webb, thinking Charles might be just the trained man he needed to head the proposed foundation laboratory, wrote to ask Dr. Allen Krause's advice.

Boissevain would be a real find for Webb, said Krause. He had a brilliant mind and knew what research was all about. Just one caveat, though: Webb would have to take care to keep Boissevain on the track. He had so many ideas, so much scientific curiosity, that he might be prone to start up too many hares and not all of them in the tuberculosis field.

Dr. Webb decided to take the chance.

For new laboratory space he turned to Colorado College. The time was not propitious there. President Duniway, Slocum's successor, was leaving in 1923 and Charles C. Mierow, who had been professor of classical languages at Princeton, was coming in as acting president. Understanding of research in science was not his strong point. Dr. Edward C. Schneider was no longer on the faculty; he had moved to Wesleyan University when he returned from war service overseas.

But Webb had friends, including Phil Stewart, among the trustees of the College, and President Mierow was soon persuaded to make available to the foundation two rooms of modest size, one for the laboratory and one for animals, in the basement of Palmer Hall, and also "to give our workers the advantage of ready access to all equipment in the physical and chemical departments of the College, as well as opportunities to consult on special problems with the professors in these departments."

Meanwhile Dr. Webb, in consultation with another patient, the lawyer Victor W. Hungerford, had chosen the Rockefeller Foundation as the model for his legal structure and Mr. Hungerford was drawing up articles of incorporation and a set of bylaws accordingly. Webb advised that the purpose of the foundation be simply stated: "to search for a preventive and cure for tuberculosis."

He later ascribed the motto he chose to a passage from Sir William Osler. In fact he had found it himself in an old book one noontime during the meeting of the Association of American Physicians in the spring of 1923.

Going to join Dr. Henry Sewall for lunch, he found Sewall absorbed in a classic of science, Descartes' *Discours de la Methode* (1637). Idly picking up the book when Sewall put it down, he saw on its title page a vignette of a man digging in a garden, his face and back bent over the earth, upon which fell streams of light from the sky above. Underneath was the caption *Fac et Spera.*

Work and hope! What better prescription for research could there be? Work. Not just at the laboratory bench, but in wide reading and long thinking, to probe out the whys and therefores and dredge up some what-ifs and might-it-bes. And hope. Hope for the inspired idea and hypothesis, and maybe the winning stroke of luck.

FAC ET SPERA. That was it. That would be the motto for his foundation.

By 15 May 1924 the Colorado Foundation for Research in Tuberculosis had been registered as a not-for-profit corporation under the laws of Colorado and the fifteen local social and financial leaders who had agreed to serve as trustees met in Dr. Webb's office that day to organize it. They included, in addition to Webb himself, a number of persons we have met: Spencer Penrose, William Otis, Phil Stewart, A. E. Carlton, Victor Hungerford, Maria McKean Allen (she *had* returned to live in Colorado Springs), Constance Pulitzer Elmslie, and Ruth Davis Dangler.

Others of the same quality were Alfred Cowles III, another patient from Chicago, member of a newspaper family there and a nephew of Mrs. Philip B. Stewart; Harry P. Davison Jr., son of a partner in the banking house of Morgan; Ralph O. Giddings, owner of the principal department store in Colorado Springs; Oliver H. Shoup, Denver millionaire and former Republican governor of Colorado; Eugene P. Shove, banker and mining broker; and Benjamin Strong, governor of the Federal Reserve Bank in New York.

Scribbled lists in the files show that the trustees elected officers and other members wholly according to Dr. Webb's nominations. A. E. Carlton became president, Dr. Webb vice-president and research director, Ruth Dangler secretary, and Alfred Cowles III treasurer.

The board named as associate research directors two local doctors, F. L. Dennis and P. A. Loomis, and Webb's good young friends, Jim Waring and Bill Williams. It accepted as associate members of the Foundation twenty-seven local physicians, including Gilbert and Sevier of course; Boissevain, Ryder, Staines, and Drea; Will Howard Swan and, yes, Charles Fox Gardiner; P. O. Hanford and J. B. Hartwell, who had by turn succeeded Dr. Charles W. Powers of Denver as Webb's favorite local surgeon.

One could hardly imagine a roster with more éclat than those Dr. Webb secured to act with him and Dr. Forster as an advisory council: Theobald Smith, Victor Vaughan, Lawrason Brown, Livingston Farrand, Allen Krause, James A. Miller, and Henry Sewall. He reached wide as well as high for his corresponding advisers: Jules Bordet of Brussels, Albert Calmette of Paris, Sir Robert Philip of Edinburgh, and Sir Almroth Wright of London! That so many men of such distinction were willing to lend him their names is evidence indeed of the respect and stature he had achieved.

The trustees also voted to employ Dr. Boissevain as chief of research in the laboratory and Dr. Ryder as his associate. These two and their assistants were the only ones who were to be paid salaries.

The trustees at this first meeting also initiated the endowment of the Foundation. They wanted to set their goal at $500,000 but Dr. Webb demurred; ultimately that much perhaps, but he thought $200,000 would be enough as an immediate objective. The trustees affectionately agreed to the two-level goal and set the ball rolling toward it by raising $50,000 among themselves. Maria Allen, Ruth Dangler, Spencer Penrose, and Harry P. Davison Jr. contributed $10,000 apiece and the others made up the balance and also gave some $3000 to establish a separate "maintenance fund" for immediate operating expenses.

Gerald Webb's foundation was on its way.

It is revealing that its name was not the Webb Foundation and that Webb was not its president. He had learned from the cool reception given his early Webb Laboratory for Tuberculosis Research that he could not secure wide participation on all fronts if the new entity appeared to be just a personal venture toward his own greater glory.

Boissevain and Ryder and their assistants set to work at once and before the year was out half a dozen assorted physicians and several graduate students from the College were working with them and they badly needed larger quarters. Dr. Webb begged another room from the College, which made it available by clearing out old boxes and lumber from some adjacent storage space.

Perhaps Dean Charlie Brown Hershey is to be forgiven for strongly implying, in his history of Colorado College, that the Colorado Foundation for Research in Tuberculosis was the creation of the College, not just an adjunct to it. It may have seemed so, especially since Dr. Boissevain and others on the Foundation laboratory staff were presently given rank on the College faculty.

Dr. Webb's influence as research director is evident in the investigations set going that first year. They were mostly continuations of work he and Gilbert and Ryder had done earlier. For example: studies of the gas requirements of tubercle bacilli; of their food needs; of their variations in virulence; of attenuating them by incubation of tuberculous tissues; of producing fatal tuberculosis by inoculating attenuated strains that were thought harmless; of the physiology of postural rest; of the effects of altitude on the human organism. Dr. Gilbert contributed a clinical evaluation of Dreyer's vaccine, another touted cure of the Spahlinger kind.

But the wave of the future was also present—in Dr. Boissevain's

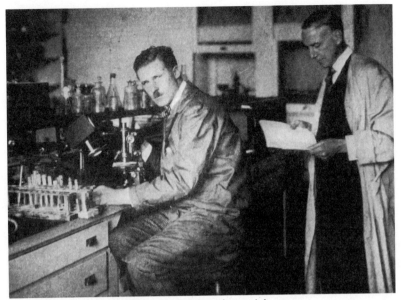

Doctors Boissevain and Webb in the Foundation laboratory

investigation of the physical properties of fatty acids and the effects of them on tubercle bacilli, in Dr. Drea's study of ultraviolet radiation within the body, and in a series of experiments on hypersensitivity and anaphylaxis.

As such biochemical and biophysical subjects took over the Foundation's agenda, Dr. Webb's participation waned. He never lost his keen interest in it, kept a supervisory eye on it, and occasionally worked in the laboratory on a project of his own, but he left direction of the Foundation's program increasingly to Dr. Boissevain and his name disappeared as co-author of published reports of the Foundation's research.

Such surrender of active involvement in laboratory research was exceedingly painful for Gerald Webb. Research had been his passion and his refreshment for more than half his lifetime. It was a wrench to give it up. But we shall see that he found compensatory solace in medical education, history, and biography.

Not all stayed serene in the laboratory. Dr. Boissevain and Dr. Drea could not get along. The Dutch and the Irish in them clashed. Also, Dr. Boissevain could not believe an untutored worker could independently produce reliable results, while Dr. Drea could not see why Webb and Ryder were less effective tutors than some bigwig in Europe. When Dr. Drea submitted a report of his work for publication, Dr. Boissevain sent Dr. Webb an adverse appraisal of it, saying heatedly that it *must* not be published under Foundation auspices.

Dr. Webb, or perhaps Dr. Ryder, must have applied some diplomatic tact, for Drea's report appeared and remains in the Foundation's bibliography. But Dr. Drea did not forget. Decades later when his reputation in tuberculosis research was secure and he had won national and international awards for his work, he still found it hard to speak kindly of Dr. Boissevain.

The study of food requirements of the tubercle bacillus was assigned that year of 1924 to Dr. Eric Webb. "Roly's boy" had finished his training at Guy's Hospital and served out residencies in several London hospitals before he came to work with his Uncle Gerald. After a year in the laboratory he decided he did not like research and went off first to Cragmor, then to Minnesota to try sanatorium doctoring. That did not please him either. He returned to England and became a medical missionary in India. Eventually he took training in theology, was ordained a clergyman, and became a vicar in Cumberland.

The struggle for funds to support the Foundation was continuous. It received many gifts of small amounts, some of as little as five dollars, and these were directed into the maintenance fund, which soon was averaging a steady six to eight thousand dollars a year. But bigger gifts to augment the endowment fund were hard to come by. By 1926 it had grown to only a little more than $70,000.

Dr. Webb seems to have taken little part in the money-raising. He talked to everyone about the Foundation and wrote articles about it, but he left the direct begging to trustees and associates who were less squeamish than he about asking for money.

Until 1927. On a trip to New York in the spring of that year he called upon a former patient, Senator Coleman T. Du Pont of Delaware, who maintained a business office in New York now that he was retired from the Senate. In the course of their conversation Webb described the Foundation and what it was doing. He was as much surprised as pleased when the Senator offered to contribute $15,000 to the endowment providing the Foundation could raise a matching sum by 1 January 1928.

In the first flurry of excitement some of the trustees who had given before gave again. Maria Allen preferred to continue her annual donation of $1000 to the maintenance fund but Spencer Penrose, Ruth Dangler, and Harry P. Davison Jr. each sent in a check for a thousand dollars to be added to the endowment. Others gave lesser amounts, including Dr. James Waring who pledged a check for five hundred dollars before the year's end. But the total of such repeat donations was less than half of what was needed.

When this remained the situation in early fall, Dr. Webb was alarmed and went to work himself, writing far and wide to friends and former patients. Several of them responded with letters outlining grandiose plans to collect thousands upon thousands for him, but their promises exceeded their performance a hundredfold. Perhaps they discovered that those who had money preferred to invest it in the stock market, which was beginning its heedless climb to giddy heights.

Webb reached back into the past with letters to Irving Bonbright and his long-ago neighbor Mrs. Verner Reed, now of Denver, whose daughter Margery he had carried as an ailing baby to her parents in Europe in 1901. Bonbright promptly sent him a check for $2000 but the only response from Denver was a holding note from Mrs. Reed's secretary saying her employer was traveling in the West Indies. Gerald wondered, would she return in time to help?

Still several thousands short of the goal in November, Dr. Webb decided he must try his hand at personal solicitation in New York.

He was ready to leave when Paul Brown, a St. Louis banker who had long been a recurrent patient, arrived again in town, this time clearly about to die. He pled with Dr. Webb to stay and take care of him till the end. When Webb gently explained why he must go, Mr. Brown said *he* would give the entire matching $15,000 if the doctor would forgo his journey.

Gerald did so and when Paul Brown died the lawyers for his estate fulfilled his pledge. The gift from Senator Du Pont was assured.

Checks in reply to Dr. Webb's letters dribbled in and the matching amount was raised without the contribution from Paul Brown. The final one thousand dollars arrived on 27 December in the form of a check from Mrs. Verner Reed.

The Foundation thus entered 1928 the richer by $45,000, its endowment thereby raised to just over $150,000. At the low rates of interest then prevailing, 2 or 3 percent at local banks and not much more on safe securities, the yield of the endowment to the maintenance fund ran about $3000 a year.

Dr. Webb had reason to be glad the Du Pont gift and the crash campaign to match it had preceded the calamitous collapse of October 1929 and the subsequent Great Depression.

It was inevitable that Ruth Dangler and Charles Boissevain, both so involved with the Foundation, should meet. When they did, in Dr. Webb's office and presence, a current crackled between them. "There it was," Gerald told Varina, "the spark between them, the glance, the leitmotif from Tristan, for anyone to see. You couldn't miss it."

He and Varina were pleased; they had grown fond of both the young people. Gerald found Charles congenial in his love for fishing and hunting and playing polo, and his fluency in several languages was a great help in translating medical literature from abroad. He took off Gerald's hands almost entirely what had been a laborious chore, the translation of books and journals in German. Varina, amused by Charles's unruly shock of dark hair and neat little moustache, his mobile face, his energetic rushing about, called him affectionately "the Flying Dutchman."

But there was an obstacle to the course of true love. Charles already had a wife. In a quixotic gesture while passing through New York he had married the Countess Marie Therese Zwetana von Hartenau, daughter of the former King Alexander of Bulgaria who was living in exile in Austria.

The two had met while seeking the cure in Switzerland. When Zwetana was refused admission to the United States because her passport was not in order and the immigration officials judged her tuberculous, Charles impulsively married her so she could get into the country. Without a further thought he then went on his way, but the Countess considered herself truly wed and eventually tracked her man to Colorado Springs.

When she turned up at Dr. Webb's office Charles shirked further encounter with her and left it to Varina Webb to take her in and explain to her that her husband-in-name-only loved another. To everyone's relief Zwetana agreed to a divorce and returned to her father's house in Austria. Ruth and Charles were married and began a life together on Fifth Street in Broadmoor.

By that time, 1928, Gerald Webb had begun his career as an author by publishing two books.

He had long felt the need for some kind of guide that he could give to patients to lure them into participation in their own recovery by telling them briefly and brightly what they ought to know about their disease. With the help of Dr. Ryder, an excellent editor and collaborator, he put together a manuscript of the kind he had in mind and added to it a selection of blank charts on which the patient could keep his own daily recored of his temperature, pulse, and weight and other manifestations of the state of his health. The whole was enlivened in Dr. Webb's inimitable way by a host of pertinent quips and quotations.

The authors called their guide "Recovery Record" and Dr. Webb took the manuscript east with him on a spring trip in that busy year of 1922.

He had just agreed to write the chapter on tuberculosis for *A Text-Book of Medicine by American Authors* (in later editions to be known as "the Cecil textbook" after its editor) which W. S. Saunders, the medical publisher in Philadelphia, was putting together. He decided to offer his guide first to that firm. Saunders thought it was more for laymen than for his professional clientele — "his salesmen just wouldn't be able to push it" — and suggested Webb submit it to the house of Lippincott, which dithered in indecision about it.

Paul B. Hoeber, whose company served as the medical department of Harper Brothers, was wiser; he accepted the manuscript for publication at first sight, on condition only that the authors agree to purchase five hundred copies of the book at $1.50 each — "to get the book off to a good start" he said, meaning, of course, to cover his manufacturing costs and reduce his risk. Dr. Webb did not hesitate; he could easily hand out that many copies among his patients and friends.

Hoeber need not have been so prudent. When the book appeared in 1923 it won enthusiastic reviews in most medical journals and some newspapers.

The *Chicago Medical Record* thought its eighty pages of text contained "the most common sense instructions we have ever read for tuberculous patients." The *Boston Medical and Surgical Journal* agreed: "This book contains more sound common sense concerning the treatment and management of tuberculosis, put into attractive form, than is to be found in any other work on the subject."

Western Medicine liked its style: "The cheerful philosophy and serenity which characterize the book make it an invaluable adjunct in the care of the tuberculous patient." *Southwestern Medicine* was breezier: "The book is worth the price for entertainment alone. The value for those who need it cannot be measured in cash. Doctors, recommend it to your patients and do them and yourself a good turn!"

And on and on.

After several reprintings of *Recovery Record* Hoeber reissued the book in a "slightly revised" second edition in 1925 under the title *Recovery Road* and in a third edition two years later with the title *Overcoming Tuberculosis: An Almanac of Recovery.*

One wonders whether it was the publisher or the authors who decided that on the successive title pages Webb and Ryder should be identified, not by their connection with Cragmor Sanatorium or the Colorado Foundation, but as president and faculty member respectively of the Colorado School for Tuberculosis.

Dr. Webb used the same identification for his second book, also published by Hoeber, in 1928.

The medical world was taking note in 1926 of the centenary of the death of the immortal Laënnec and the Denver Clinical and Pathological Society decided to make its February meeting a tribute to him and asked Dr. Webb to give the principal address.

Gerald had been interested in the great Breton physician ever since he was introduced to the Laënnec Society in Baltimore in 1912. He had visited Laënnec's birthplace in Quimper on the coast of Brittany while he was in France during the war, and had bought and read much of what Laënnec wrote. But when he began to prepare his talk he realized that while he had a lot of information about the man's work he knew virtually nothing of the man himself or his life. Nor, to his amazement, could he discover anything about these matters published in English.

The only biography he could find — probably in the private Laënnec collection assembled by Dr. Henry Barton Jacobs of Baltimore — was a two-volume work in French published by the writer Rouxeau in 1920. As he translated his way through this work, which was based on family letters and papers, he was surprised to learn that Laënnec was not just the icy intellectual of legend but was besides a truly captivating human being. The details heightened his admiration for Laënnec's tremendous achievements but in addition inspired in him a genuine affection for the little man for whom life had been so harsh.

Gerald could use in his Denver address only a smidgen of what he had learned, so he decided to expand his lecture for publication in the *Annals of Medical History*, Arnold Klebs's favorite journal. He did this, he said, "with the scholarly help of my good friend and patient W. F. C. Nelson."

The only discernible evidence of that help is a prefatory note in which Mr. Nelson skimmed the story of the Revolutionary and Napoleonic periods in which Laënnec lived and ended with a utopian suggestion: "Many illustrious men lived between the years 1781 and 1826. Who knows but that ultimately men shall judge that the most illustrious of all was the dry, meager, asthmatic, and phthisic Breton, Dr. René Théophile Hyacinthe Laënnec?"

Dr. Webb began his own "Avant-propos" with a statement that is true still: "Little is known by the layman concerning the lives of men who have advanced the art of medicine. To few outside the medical profession is the name of Laënnec known. Highly educated people have visited Quimper without noting the statue erected near the cathedral to mark his birthplace. Biographical reading is increasing today and it is hoped that students in varying pursuits may find inspiration in this sketch of the life of Laënnec, the greatest of all physicians."

It was for such laymen that he wrote his engaging "memoir," which remains worth reading if it can be found. He infused his condensation of the story from Rouxeau's two volumes with his own understanding and appreciation, bringing again to life the fun-loving, dancing, music-making hunter and farmer that lay within the pallid, hollow cheeks and short, frail body, "thin as a shadow"—the warm and tender man that paralleled the stern, uncompromising observer at bedside and autopsy table.

Webb's long walks through the countryside in Brittany let him make vivid the lush tree-and-flower-filled environs in which Théophile (so Webb called him, as his friends and family had called him) lived a happy, healthy childhood in the home of a cherishing uncle, a doctor in Nantes. Webb's familiarity with the dark, somber hospitals of Paris let him describe concretely the milieu in which the adult Laënnec worked.

Webb's memories of his own churlish, obstructing father led him to dwell on the neurotic weaknesses of Laënnec's father, who foisted his son off upon the uncle at an early age; who wanted the boy when grown to come back to Quimper to work in the fields instead of "jaunting off to the fleshpots of Paris under the pretext of studying medicine."

Webb blended effectively the role of Laënnec the clinician with that of Laënnec the scientific thinker. He retold with charm the story of Laënnec's distress when he left the bedside of an obese young female patient because his modesty and hers—and her repulsive crawling lice—had prevented him from putting his ear to her clothed chest to listen for telltale sounds from heart and lungs.

Walking shortly thereafter in the gardens of the Louvre he watched a group of boys playing near a mound of litter from which they had pried loose a long wooden log. Half of them tapped and scratched at one end while the other half giggled at the sounds they heard from the other end.

In a flash Laënnec understood the conduction of sound he was witnessing. He hurried back to the room of his adipose patient, snatched up a paperback book, rolled it into a tight cylinder, and startled those who watched by placing one end of the *cornet de papier* on the girl's chest and the other at his ear.

That was the birth of the stethoscope.

By using the new instrument, in successively refined forms, to do countless listenings to and sortings out of interior sounds, Laënnec was able to produce his epochal treatise on auscultation as an indispensable aid to diagnosis.

"His was the usual lot of the creative genius," Dr. Webb wrote. "From the competent he met with indifference, from the incompetent with ridicule. From the lesser spirits of his profession he could not expect enthusiasm or escape scorn."

Webb relished the tale of the historic joust between Laënnec and the vain and fiery Broussais, a pillar of the French medical establishment. Broussais was a fierce antagonist from the time the two men as fellow medical students differed stubbornly in public over a diagnosis and autopsy proved Laënnec to have been right.

Thereafter Broussais pursued his rival with venom, scoffing loudly at every opinion and study Laënnec published. He once devoted eighty pages of print to scornful invective, seeking to make trash of Laënnec's work piece by piece: his assertion that tubercles anywhere in the body were a sign of tuberculosis, not of discrete diseases; his conviction that tuberculosis was of specific origin, though two generations before Robert Koch he could not describe the agent; even his identification of melanomas, "black cancers" he called them.

Broussais won in the immediate end. France's physicians believed him, not Laënnec. Broussais was awarded official recognition and fawning adulation; Laënnec died almost unknown, certainly unsung. "One fought passionately for error, the other dispassionately for truth; the one who was wrong had the medical world with him, the one who was right stood almost alone," was Webb's summation.

Although Webb's memoir of Laënnec was not published in the *Annals of Medical History* until 1927 it had been submitted and accepted in mid-1926 and word of its excellence had got around. When the U.S. State Department sought advice as to whom it should name as delegates to the official Laënnec Centenary observance in Paris in December 1926, Dr. William Henry Welch and Dr. Henry Barton Jacobs both recommended Dr. William S. Thayer, now *emeritus* professor of medicine at Johns Hopkins, and Dr. Gerald B. Webb of Colorado Springs.

The two delegates crossed the Atlantic together. Dr. Thayer had been asked by the French officials to deliver a tribute to Laënnec on behalf of all the foreign delegates, and he composed his remarks on board the boat. It gave Dr. Webb quiet satisfaction to be able to contribute some significant facts Dr. Thayer had not known, and also to have Thayer accept his suggestion that the tribute be broadened to recognize the long succession of French contributions to the understanding of tuberculosis.

The daring and defiant concluding sentence in Dr. Thayer's remarks we may plausibly credit to Dr. Webb: "Perhaps it is reserved for a Frenchman, a modest yet bold investigator, Calmette, to forge the last link in the chain that will render impotent the ancient enemy."

To make that suggestion in the very year of the devastating Tragedy of Lübeck!

For more than twenty years Calmette and his colleague Guérin had been working toward a vaccine against tuberculosis. Beginning with a virulent strain of bovine bacilli they had slowly weakened it by growing it in test tube after test tube, year after year. When at last experiments all over the Western world had confirmed their finding that the strain had lost its virulence but not its immunizing power in animals, Calmette was convinced of its safety and began using it to inoculate the newborn babies of tuberculous parents.

The effects seemed good: at worst a mild lesion or two that quickly disappeared but left the infant immune to tests with tuberculin. There were of course many voluble critics and much controversy, but a few others in Europe gingerly began using the Bacillus Calmette-Guérin, BCG for short, to vaccinate children.

Then in 1926 a group of 249 babies were vaccinated in Lübeck, Germany, and 76 of them died of acute tuberculosis. The uproar of I-told-you-sos was deafening. A storm of panic-bred denunciation broke over Calmette and the Pasteur Institute.

An investigating commission composed of eminent French and German physicians and scientists proved conclusively that the inoculated material, though labeled BCG, was in fact, by mistake and not malice, an entirely different and virulent strain. But the damage was done. The widespread publicity and public fear left a scar in both medical and lay minds that has not been wholly eradicated to this day, though the usefulness of BCG is now established.

Gerald Webb had often discussed BCG with Calmette and had come to think it likely his French colleague had found something good. For several years before the Lübeck disaster he had sought to persuade Chairman White that the NTA Medical Research Committee ought to evaluate Calmette's vaccine, but Dr. White judged the statistics from European experiments to be inadequate and thought such things as the Spahlinger cure and Dreyer's antigens were more promising.

During the Lübeck panic Webb retained his faith in Calmette's integrity and scientific judgment and wrote him to express sympathy and enduring confidence. It was much more like Gerald Webb than like William Thayer without Webb to make a public declaration of support for Calmette at the height of the furor.

For several years thereafter Webb followed closely the course of research on BCG and sometimes in editorials and articles expressed his continuing hope for the vaccine. He took over a workbench and some guinea pigs in the Foundation laboratory to check for himself a couple of points at especially heated issue and in 1928 ventured to vaccinate with BCG the high-risk baby born to two of his tuberculous patients.

The following year he boldly concluded a paper on BCG he read to the American Medical Association with this declaration of confidence: "I am of the opinion after careful study of the literature and after personal investigations and experiments that BCG should be administered to infants born to parents with open pulmonary tuberculosis. With further proof of the harmlessness and efficiency of the vaccine it may be found that all new-born infants should be vaccinated against tuberculosis with BCG."

When Webb's memoir of Laënnec appeared in the *Annals of Medical History* Paul Hoeber seized upon it as a good item for a group of medical biographies he was publishing and issued it among them the next year. Dr. Webb dedicated the book "To my wife and children / and to the memory of my Huguenot mother / Frances LePlastrier Webb."

Given the low book prices—the Laënnec memoir also was priced at $1.50 per copy—and minuscule royalties of the day, neither of Gerald's books made him rich but they did add appreciably to his pocket money. His widespread acquaintance and reputation increased their sale and they in turn added to recognition of his name.

In 1928 Gerald became a Fellow of the American College of Physicians—"the highest American honor that can come to a physician, I understand" wrote his sister Amy when notified of it by postcard.

If not that, it was more of a distinction than it has since become, because the purpose of the College was to select and certify physicians of superior training and achievement, to set them apart from and above the host of nondescript practitioners who were still being granted medical degrees by inferior schools of medicine. Admission to the College may have assuaged Gerald Webb's insecurity about his medical education.

He achieved another reassurance the following year when he was elected—in his absence, since he had thought "it was Burton Gilbert's turn to go"—the forty-seventh president of the American Climatological and Clinical Association. The ghost of Edwin Solly was laid at last! Regardless of what Dr. Webb had come to think of this society, it was a pleasure to join the long line of eminent medical men who had been president of "the Climatological."

It was no coincidence that during Webb's term the discussions began that two years later produced a further change in the organization's name, to the American Clinical and Climatological Association. The group could not bring itself to give up its cherished *climatological* but at least it recognized that *clinical* should now come first.

Dr. Webb's presidential address was surely the dullest paper he ever wrote. The society's governing council suggested that he should speak at the 1930 convention on some topic in medical history. Since the gathering was to be in Quebec, Dr. Webb chose "Early Medicine in Quebec" as his subject and went to ground again in several libraries to collect his material.

Perhaps when he spoke he threw in enough asides and anecdotes to hold his audience but by the time his paper reached print in the pages of the *Transactions*, it was little more than a boring catalogue of antiquarian facts and forgotten names. Fortunately it was also brief.

In contrast, two of Webb's best efforts were an address on "The Role of the Physician in Literature" to the New York Academy of Medicine in December 1928 and one on "The Prescription of Literature" to the Association of American Physicians the following spring. Today, and perhaps even then, both seem startling choices for their respective audiences but both were sparkling hits and remained in exceptional demand as reprints for years afterward. They revealed both the range of Dr. Webb's interests and his holistic approach to his patients.

XVI

Physician Extraordinary

GERALD WEBB often called Cragmor Sanatorium "my sixth child" as with deepening satisfaction he watched it emerge from the neglect and disarray of the war and influenza years and rise rapidly to an acknowledged position among the top-notch sanatoriums of the world. Some acclaimed it as the very finest anywhere of such havens for the tuberculous.

Dr. Webb never went quite so far as that but he did brag to his friends about each new building and improvement and about Cragmor's steady 100 percent occupancy rate and its lengthening list of patients waiting for admission. He once guessed it was booked full for a year in advance.

Much of the credit for this spectacular success belonged to the resident physician-in-chief Alexius Forster. He too won increasing recognition in the national arena. He was president for some years of the NTA's affiliate society, the American Sanatorium Association; he served several terms on the board of directors of the NTA; he was chairman and prime mover on its important committee charged with promoting the welfare of convalescent patients; he was elected vice-president of the Association in 1925. His engaging bonhomie made him extremely popular at convocations in many states.

On the home scene Dr. Forster was never wanting in ambitious schemes for Cragmor. Each time the Corporation's directors authorized an expansion he produced plans for breathtaking splendors in size and style — and each time he was thwarted by having to accept the feasible instead. But what he achieved was quite grand enough.

At the beginning of the 1920s a patient arriving at Cragmor found little to enthuse him beyond the mountain view and the promise of restoration to health. In the middle years of the decade he found, said one, "a haven of great beauty," said another, "a Paradise on earth." The community had grown to more than two hundred patients, plus numerous residents and visiting relatives, including happy children at play, and some hundred and thirty staff members and employees.

The impressive group of buildings occupied nearly a thousand acres. The proximate grounds were lavishly landscaped with trees, shrubs, and beds of flowers and were laced with smooth pathways that invited strolling. One of them, laid out on laboriously leveled ground, curved through lilacs and elms and around the bluffs for more than three miles; the patients dubbed it "Happy Walk."

Main Building, which still housed the communal diningroom and recreation hall, had acquired a softening cloak of ivy on its walls, a semicircular expanse of green lawn in front of it, and a fourth floor providing additional rooms and suites for patients. It was still flanked by the renovated twin dormitories labeled the Men's Cottage and the Women's Cottage.

Off to the south stood the New Building, permanently called so because the naming of it was left to the patients and they could not choose among South Hall (too stodgy), Edwin Solly Hall, Windswept Hall, and Dr. Webb's suggestion, Laënnec Hall (probably too arcane and hard to pronounce).

Up on the hill behind Main and New stood three or four spacious houses owned by patients affluent enough to build them.

To the north ran a cement pathway overarched by trees that in its farther reaches was bordered on both sides by small stuccoed bungalows. Numbering nineteen eventually, these "cabins," as they were referred to, were used primarily to house couples or families and were collectively called Cragmor Village.

They were all that had come to be of Dr. Forster's dearest dream: a large rehabilitation colony for convalescents replete with woodworking and machine shops and surrounding fields of grain and produce to encourage a moderate amount of manual labor. Forster was responsible for the development of many such colonies in the nation but he never managed to get one going at Cragmor.

He did acquire among the patients one disciple in the cause of occupational therapy: Ishbel MacLeish, sister of Archibald MacLeish the poet and also Librarian of Congress. When Ishbel had, as she said, "slowly made the long, long climb from illness back to health," she built one of the private houses up on the hill and began encouraging her fellow convalescents to occupy themselves with weaving, embroidery, and other such crafts. With a quartet of friends she opened what she called Half Way House, first at Cragmor and later in downtown Colorado Springs, as an outlet for the sale of the patients' handiwork. It flourished so mightily that the merchants of the town finally protested its competition in sales to tourists and put it out of business.

The sanatorium had its own federal post office, located in a first-floor corner of Main Building; its own circulating library which grew by donations to more than a thousand volumes shelved along the walls of the recreation hall; its own emporium called The Shop, which sold not only candy and cigarettes, cosmetics and stationery, but the latest books, including stacks of Webb's and Ryder's *Recovery Road*, and photographs by Laura Gilpin.

Laura had returned to Colorado Springs to begin her career and as a friend of Elizabeth Forster, Dr. Forster's sister and a nurse on Cragmor's staff, often visited the sanatorium and took pictures of its people and rooms.

Cragmor also had its own greenhouse, which kept the sanatorium's rooms gay with fragrant flowers all year round; its own taxi service on call for trips into town or for leisurely sightseeing rides on fine spring and summer evenings; its own piece of the Prudential's rock in the form of a group life insurance program for staff and patients through which the sanatorium insured the lives of Dr. Forster and Dr. Webb for $50,000 each; and from 1924 on its own fortnightly magazine, managed, edited, and mostly written by the patients, whom Dr. Webb had prodded into starting it.

They were a clever lot. They named their journal *Ninety-eight-Six*, sometimes written 98.6, from that normal temperature they all relentlessly sought. The humor page they called, significantly indeed, "The Relapse"; verse, most of it quite bad, appeared under the rubric "Pin Feathers from Pegasus"; the gossip columns by "Genevieve" that ribboned through many back pages of advertising in each issue were headed "All of Us," surely in echo of the reiterated phrase in Thomas Mann's *Magic Mountain* (1924), "All of us up here."

Contributions by the patients, virtually all nonfiction despite the short story class conducted in the recreation hall by a professor from Colorado College, ranged in subject from sunbathing as an affront to modesty and reminiscences of service in the Great War to a study of women in the works of Ibsen and Strindberg and the philosophical ruminations of a reluctant atheist.

Almost every issue contained a book review or two, usually of some current bestseller—e.g. Van Vechten's *Nigger Heaven*, Sinclair Lewis's *Dodsworth*, Hemingway's *The Sun Also Rises*, Remarque's *All Quiet on the Western Front*. One such review by Dr. Charles Ryder said bluntly of a new novel, "It's too long, makes too little concession to its public, and is too obscure to bother about." A large public shared his opinion at the time, for the book was Joyce's *Ulysses*.

Each issue of *Ninety-eight-Six* featured a question-and-answer page by Dr. Forster which collectively could serve as a textbook on principles and methods of treatment in tuberculosis at the time. And it was a rare number that did not contain an article by Dr. Webb.

Gerald said he wrote these contributions on Sunday afternoons, sometimes just reshaping a favorite topic such as tuberculosis carriers, or reporting a recent event as in a long piece on the Laënnec Centenary in 1926, but many times composing fresh biographical sketches of great medical men like William Harvey or of tuberculous poets like Percy Bysshe Shelly and John Sterling. Of some of these, more presently.

Throughout the 1920s this famous and excellent sanatorium was essentially an adjunct to the private practice of Doctors Webb, Gilbert, and Sevier. During the first half of the decade they were its only medical consultants and their colleagues Dr. Boissevain and Dr. Ryder were directors of its laboratories. Later on, when full coffers permitted Dr. Forster to hire assistant physicians and add more consultants, they remained at the top of the list as consultants in diseases of the chest, their associates continued in charge of the laboratories, and they provided three of the newcomers: Dr. Eric Webb as an assistant physician, Dr. Drea as consultant in radiology, and Dr. Charles E. Sevier as consultant in orthopedics and heliotherapy.

This close medical connection, publicized in the Cragmor advertisement that appeared on the back cover of each issue of *Ninety-eight-Six*, renders startlingly incongruous the journalistic accounts of Cragmor that have recently appeared in newspapers and magazines. The authors have mined records and memories for shiny nuggets about noisy high-jinks, drunken revelries, eccentric celebrities, and scandalous escapades at Cragmor, then melded them all into sensational feature stories that make a joke of the sanatorium's pretense to healing and imply that its doctors were lax incompetents.

We need not deny the truth of the anecdotes to consider the composite portrayal a sorry distortion, false and unfair. What do the authors imagine a good sanatorium to have been? A grim prison, with the doctors as jailers?

So Cragmor's after-dinner social hours and weekly bridge games and motion pictures *did* sometimes degenerate into tipsy hilarity and ribaldry; the worst of such times were mild in comparison with the goings-on of Hans Castorp and his fellows at the authentic Davos sanatorium in *Magic Mountain*.

So some Cragmorites *did* go often to buy liquor at speakeasies in nearby Papetown; some patients left the great Trudeau Sanatorium desperately ill for want of sleep because they had been kept awake night after night by the arrival of clattering trucks come to deliver bootleg whisky.

So Cragmor Village *did* often resound with the playing of phonographs and radios; Alec Waugh came back to London from a visit to a well-known sanatorium in the German Alps with a tale of patients driven into hysterical fits by two feuding music lovers who sought for long hours every day to drown out each other's favorite recording, the Italian's "O Sole Mio" and the German's "Ride of the Valkyries."

A perennial in these sniggering tales is the Colorado Springs townsman who, driving home from Denver, passed Cragmor at three in the morning and saw Main Building ablaze with lights on all four floors. He seems not to have wondered why but just assumed it was for revelry. It may have been so, but it may equally have been for some emergency or disturbance—as on the night when a timid young woman awakened to find a field mouse nibbling at the crumbs on her writing table and screamed the house down. "My patients were fidgety all the next day," Dr. Webb told his sister Ida.

In contrast to the impression of ceaseless noise and activity is the account a Scottish patient wrote for *Ninety-eight-Six*. Shown to his room and put to bed by a nurse when he arrived, he lay for several hours without seeing another soul or hearing a sound. Certain by then that he could never endure such isolation and silence, he was preparing to leave the place when he got some reassurance from the faint sound of a radio playing softly on the floor above. A few weeks later he moved from his room in Men's Cottage to a cabin in the Village, thinking that while it might be just as quiet there he would at least see people passing on the path outside.

Not everything all day every day was wild abandon at Cragmor.

These were the "roaring twenties," remember—years when release from the tensions of war and pandemic let loose an explosion of excess in behavior, years marked by emancipation from old mores and conventions, by glorification of smashed taboos and new freedoms. Among the young and in the smart sets women left their pedestals and their kitchens, bobbed their hair and shortened their skirts, smoked in public, drank with their men in speakeasies, whirled their nights away in such frenetic new dances as the Charleston and the Black Bottom. The idols of the decade were Clara Bow the It Girl and Rudolph Valentino "the Latin lover with the bedroom eyes." Popular songs celebrated hedonism: "Ain't we got fun," "I'm running wild," "I'm sittin' on top of the world."

Men and women did not forsake such giddiness when tubercle bacilli grew in them and forced them into the hunt for health; some of them brought their new lifestyles with them and tried to go on whooping it up. Cragmor had its share of flighty playboys and flappers—made all the more so by the hectic flush, the *spes phthisica* produced by their disease.

But these were a self-indulgent few. Cragmor patients were of all kinds, in all forms and stages of their disease, some ambulatory but at least as many confined to bed or wheelchair on their open porches.

The myth born of extrapolation from the few portrays Cragmor as a carefree, happy-go-lucky, merry place in which to chase the cure. But disruption of life and career and fear of dying do not make for more than the mask of laughter. A weighing of the evidence reveals more of weeping, heartbreak, and despair than of merriment in Cragmor's rooms.

"If you can lie and not grow tired of lying / Or hearing sobs, not give way to crying / If you can bear to see the progress you have made / Twisted by relapse and made in vain" wrote one patient in an imitation of Kipling's "If."

Consider the beautiful Harriet Cowles, a niece of Mrs. P. B. Stewart's come from Spokane. When she arrived Genevieve told

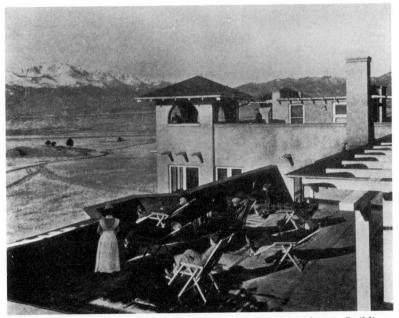

In Cragmor's heyday. The "lordly scene" from the rooftop of Main Building

her readers the newcomer requested no visitors please; she just wanted to rest and read. No further word about her appeared for two years. Then Genevieve announced that Harriet was now receiving visitors and six months later that she was getting out almost every day for an auto ride: "Her long diligent rest was well worth it." It was almost another year before Harriet was named as a guest at a bridge party. "She is a lesson to all of us. We would all be better off for some of her self-discipline and perseverance."

In almost every column Genevieve included one or more items that reported long seclusion like Harriet's:

"Maggie Mathers is now, after years in bed, able to be up and around and occasionally go calling. She has taken up the study of mathematics."

"Mrs. Nettie Cetlinski went out for her first ride last Sunday, and did she enjoy it! She has been confined to bed at Cragmor for years."

"Mrs. Wilson is at last allowed out of bed and is able sometimes to come to the movies in her wheelchair. She looks forward to some bridge games in the future."

But there were also the likes of Boyd St. Clair, one of the gadabouts, seemingly the life of every party. He was forever rounding up a quartet of "ladies and gents" to go with him in his Buick to the Antlers or the Broadmoor for dinner, to some rodeo or air show, to Denver to see a play. Then suddenly came Genevieve's sorrowful announcement that Boyd had sold his Buick; he had relapsed and must go back to rest in bed.

Half a year later he emerged anew and bought himself another Buick (for which he paid $1190 and the tank of which he filled with gasoline at 16¢ a gallon!) but he was manifestly less active, contenting himself with being the sedentary editor of *Ninety-eight-Six*.

Young Henry Chase Stone, just graduated from Cornell University, arrived at Cragmor in 1924 and stayed there for ten years. He remained so long probably because he interrupted his cure every few months to go jaunting off to New York to visit at home and to consult the brokerage house for which, when he was in residence at Cragmor, he traipsed from room to room recruiting purchasers for stocks and bonds.

Chase Stone did his clients more than financial good; they welcomed his visits as antidotes to depression. He himself prospered mightily, built himself one of the houses on the hill behind Main Building, and in time became the leading financier in Colorado Springs.

Among others who carried on their business while "resting" at Cragmor were a New Jersey merchant who was said to have doubled his fortune while at Cragmor by selling goods to the Russians via the telephone in his room and Ira A. Weaver, the inventor from Springfield, Illinois, who filled his two years of "curing" at Cragmor with dreamings and drawings that when he was well again made him a highly successful manufacturer of automotive gadgets.

Akin to these was Felix Doubleday of the prominent New York publishing family, a curmudgeon who growled himself into being left alone to polish his collection of statuettes. He so mumbled his words that when he ordered a frightened maid to bring him his nightly dose of a laxative called Food for the Gods she understood him to say "food for the dog" and presented him with a bowl of gristle. His roars of outrage probably again lighted Main Building from top to bottom.

Equally eccentric was Arthur Billing, a Cambridge University graduate and like William Elmslie a former secretary to Joseph

Pulitzer, for whom his biggest task had been designing the interior of the magnate's yacht. At Cragmor he employed his artistic talents in helping Dr. Forster dream up fairy-tale plans for new buildings and exotic renovations.

Arthur was one of the uncontrollables. He persisted in doleful drinking and wandered where and when he willed. Dr. Webb was called one winter night to help rescue him from the snowdrift into which he had sunk exhausted and coughing up blood many miles from Cragmor. Dr. Forster, a loyal friend, persuaded Arthur into abstinence and restored him to reasonably good health—only, after an urgent all night's drive to Estes Park with Dr. Webb, to watch him die of injuries received in an auto accident.

Another perverse one was the woman we know only as Goldy, rich and beautiful but doomed. She defied her consuming fever by staging elaborate parties at the Broadmoor—$35,000 worth of them in the single year before she died. The running whispers said she had been the mistress of five Chicago millionaires.

Less flamboyant was Ruth Draper, a wisp of a girl who perfected the monologues that later made her famous by performing them again and again as after-dinner divertissements for her fellow patients.

And the young black-haired, hollow-cheeked Cornelia Otis Skinner who, while "vacationing in Colorado," as she artfully told her Bryn Mawr friends, honed her thespian skills by standing high on a cliff and hurling the words of Shakespeare into the wind—all the while, contrary to the bard's advice, "sawing the air" in gestures so wild that other patients watching her from the lawn below were terrified lest she propel herself over the cliff's edge.

The idiosyncracies of these and other well-known persons spangle the story of Cragmor, giving rise to the prevailing picture of "posh Cragmor," the exclusive "West Palm Beach of sanatoriums," where the tuberculous famous and wealthy could recover in the lap of luxury and an "anything goes" atmosphere.

This legend does not survive careful scrutiny. In fact, the excessively rich now pampered themselves at the Broadmoor Hotel or in homes of their own on Monument Park Road or in the community of Broadmoor. The majority of Cragmorites were ordinary middle-class folk.

Why, otherwise, did Dr. Forster want woodworking and machine shops in part "to help those who lack money to earn their keep"?

And why did Ishbel MacLeish say her second purpose in establishing Half Way House was "to offer partial means of support to those who need such help"?

In the spring of 1927 Dr. George Dwire, a dentist who was a patient of Dr. Webb's at the time and who later became the managing director of Cragmor, published in *Ninety-eight-Six* a statistical description of Cragmor's population. He had gathered facts about one hundred patients chosen at random, roughly half the Cragmorites at the time.

The ages of his sample ranged from five to fifty. Twenty-one of them were college students, "whose careers had been wrecked before they began," and seventeen more were housewives. Not all in those two categories had rich papas or well-heeled husbands. One of them, for instance, composed an essay in praise of the rest cure, "O Boy! O Joy!"

"The patient who once was a housewife has cause to rejoice," she wrote. "When before could she dawdle in bed all day? Now she has no fire to start, no ashes to shake down, no breakfast to cook and serve, no dishes and dishes and dishes to wash. She has no kitchen to scrub, no washing to do on Monday and ironing to get through on Tuesday. All that dusting and dusting is a thing of the past and those endless meals and meals and meals can fade into memory. Now she has time to indulge in orgies of the reading she used to dream about."

No hint of money to burn in that.

Nor was there such in Dr. Dwire's further enumeration of four nurses and four schoolteachers and two each of farmers, railroad clerks, secretaries, bookkeepers, milliners, hairdressers, pharmacists, and carpenters. About the finances of six doctors and varying numbers of merchants, contractors, and executives there is no telling. The six who declared no occupation may have been leisured millionaires; they could hardly have been hoboes.

Among the cars owned by those in his group who were well enough to drive, Dr. Dwire found two Cadillacs and one Pierce Arrow, but two Chevrolets and seven Fords.

The financial state of more than a few Cragmor patients was suggested by another couplet in that patient's "If": "If you can make one heap of all your earnings / And risk it on one turn for health and joy..."

Dwire also tallied the home states of his subjects. Illinois ranked first with ten; New York and Michigan tied for second with nine each. Colorado was home to eight, Ohio to seven, Minnesota, North Dakota, and Kansas to six each, and Nebraska to five. Sixteen other states contributed varying smaller numbers. The one "foreigner" had come from Canada.

That one may have been Carol Davidson of Toronto, a niece of Sir William Osler. She was a patient of Dr. Webb's at Cragmor at about this time.

By chance Dwire's survey missed all the refugees from academia who were among Webb's favorite patients. How the Doctor loved to talk with the professors, to roam through time and the universe with them. "He knows so much about things I know nothing of," he said of Edward Mead Earle, professor of history at Columbia.

The two men began their long friendship in discussions of the late war, in which Earle had served as a second lieutenant in the field artillery. They were soon on first-name terms and kept in touch after Earle recovered, returned to his Columbia post, then moved to the Institute for Advanced Study at Princeton. During World War II when Earle was serving on various government investigating commissions he continued to write Dr. Webb sporadically and Gerald quoted him enthusiastically to his brother Frank, who sometimes disagreed sharply with "that Yank."

"But he's a super-prof, a very great intellect, an adviser to F.D.R.," Gerald protested in reply, certain that such credentials guaranteed the accuracy of Earle's statements.

Another historian Gerald liked, and pitied, was James Phinney Baxter III, a young man from Maine who was nearing his master's degree at Williams College when tuberculosis laid him low. He despaired of ever getting back on track as a scholar but Dr. Webb advised patience and reading about other things, then after a while encouraged him to send for his books and papers, finish his thesis from his wheelchair, and take his degree *in absentia*. When he was on his feet again, Dr. Webb secured for him a not-too-onerous job for one year as instructor in history at Colorado College.

Baxter returned to the East, took his doctorate degree at Harvard, and became a professor of history on the Harvard faculty. In a reminiscent mood then, he sent Dr. Webb a reprint of one of his scholarly articles with an inscription: "Without your care and encouragement I should not now be alive to pursue the study of history."

Dr. Baxter lived on to become a long-term president of Williams College.

With the astronomer Henry Norris Russell, Webb's rapport was immediate, for Russell had been born in Oyster Bay and reared in the shadow of Sagamore Hill and its larger-than-life squire Theodore Roosevelt. He had taken his doctor's degree at Princeton and when he brought his tuberculous daughter Elizabeth to Dr. Webb, he was a research associate at the Mt. Wilson Observatory in California. He came often to visit Elizabeth and converse with her doctor and soon had Gerald Webb absorbed in the mysteries of the cosmos.

Almost certainly to Russell's influence was due an abrupt right-angle turn in a long essay Dr. Webb was writing on "Heliology and Heliosis" for publication in *Ninety-eight-Six*. He started out with several installments of relevant information about "sunrayism," that is, sunlight treatment for tuberculosis, but suddenly he veered off into disquisitions on the universe of planets and stars and comets and he stayed aloft in outer space till the series petered out in its seventeenth installment, a year and a half after it began.

Dr. Charles Sevier had long since rescued the readers with a concise one-issue explanation of current theories and practices in heliotherapy, "The Sun God's Cure." But Dr. Webb had awakened a new interest in a few of those readers, whom he gathered together on clear summer nights around a telescope set up on Cragmor's lawn to search out the visible stars and constellations he was writing about. One of those patients wrote him a decade later, "Ever since that time at Cragmor the night sky has worn a friendly face for me."

Henry Russell also introduced Webb to Harlow Shapley. The two astronomers had been graduate students together at Princeton and Russell had taken Shapley's place at the Mt. Wilson Observatory when Shapley left to become director of the observatory at Harvard. Shapley never had to seek Webb's professional services but he did drop in to see the Doctor occasionally when passing through Colorado Springs. On one such visit the two joined efforts to satisfy their mutual curiosity about the ways of a colony of the peculiar honeypot ants Gerald had found and identified in the Garden of the Gods.

Princeton! Again and again. Recommendation of Dr. Webb obviously made the rounds with tuberculosis at that university. Philip Marshall Brown, another of Webb's patients, was professor of international law there. Before taking up teaching he had spent many years in the Foreign Service, as secretary at embassies from Guatemala to Constantinople, and when he recovered he began the crusade for peace among nations that dominated the remainder of his life. Marshall was too solemn, too self-important, too lacking in humor for Webb's liking; the two were never simpatico.

We cannot be certain that all these academic patients achieved their recoveries at Cragmor, for Dr. Webb was also taking care of patients at Glockner and St. Francis hospitals and in homes and boardinghouses scattered around town. But we do know that Ruth Harris, wife of the Harvard economist Seymour Harris, who brought forth books on the dismal science like rabbits, took her cure at Cragmor from 1926 to 1930. She was the militant feminist author of "The Woman Question," a study of the mistreatment of women by Ibsen and Strindberg published in *Ninety-eight-Six*.

Ruth's fierce opinions amused Dr. Webb; she was so positive that the recent Nineteenth Amendment granting the national vote to women was long overdue and only a first step. Her knowledge and insistence on logical argument awed him a little too. "Mrs. Harris surely belongs to your strong-minded women," he told Varina, who was inclined to shy away from that kind.

Dr. Forster had a difficult time walking the line between commonsense discipline and his "no rules—keep them cheerful" philosophy of sanatorium management. He did sometimes inveigh against the "restless, querulous, whining patients who want to shift from pillar to post." And when a patient asked him, "Is there a special chasing regime for ambulating patients like _____, _____, and _____?" he replied tartly:

"I would not call the patients you mention ambulatory. They do not walk as befits their condition; they hop, skip, dance, and run. They have all been talked to, admonished, reasoned with, advised, and preached at. They have reached a stage of recovery where a certain amount of activity combined with adequate rest is deemed safe and advisable. By what reasoning they justify their lapses from that course I do not know. They seem to have lost the moral tone that is so necessary in the recovery game."

But when it came to the point Dr. Forster could not bring himself to refuse permission for a party in a patient's room or a trip to town in search of fun.

Dr. Webb also lamented, in public and in private, the lack of cooperation and self-discipline he encountered in patients, but he was less tolerant than Forster of senseless antics at Cragmor. He often remonstrated with the permissive physician-in-chief and secured brief intervals of stricter rules about merrymaking and gadding about in town.

By this time Dr. Webb had lost faith in all forms of treatment other than the rest cure. Contrary to the prevailing trend in therapy he considered surgical procedures a drastic last resort and rarely prescribed them.

Reports of the explosion of tuberculosis in Europe following the widespread deprivation and hunger after the war led him to urge closer attention to good nutrition and he still looked with favor on sunbathing—though by the late 1920s he was beginning to have some doubts about that, thinking a large part of its benefit probably came just from exposing the unclothed skin to the air. He began prescribing the air bath, especially for patients confined to bed on their own porches.

He made this the subject of a piece in *Ninety-eight-Six* in February 1927. "Man is by nature a naked animal," he said, and the piling on of clothes and decorations (all this powder and rouge and lip salve, for a modern example) is a barbaric custom. "Women have become far more sensible than men in their current costumes, with bare necks and arms and short skirts, giving them greater exposure to the air."

He thought Benjamin Franklin was the first advocate of air-bathing, in a letter written to a French doctor in 1750. Franklin said he found the shock of cold water too violent and preferred to bathe more gently in cold air. Every morning upon arising he would sit for an hour of reading or writing without clothes on and with the window open, whatever the outdoor temperature. This was highly agreeable, he told the doctor, and beneficial to his health he was sure.

After explaining that the dry air of Colorado made the air bath pleasant and refreshing even in winter and describing ways of getting used to it, Dr. Webb ended with a passage so characteristic of his loosely integrated style it is worth quoting.

"Many patients will find the depression of the morning disappear as they become accustomed to the air bath. Have not suicides been reported among those weary of clothes! When I called my little boy [Joel, ill at the time with threatened tuberculosis of the spine] to get up one morning, he exclaimed, 'Oh Daddie! I'm so tired of dressing and undressing. Look at Toughie (the police dog). He just itches hisself and he's all dressed.' Robert Burton in *The Anatomy of Melancholy* tells us that vitiated air can cause melancholy but rectified air can cure it. What air is more vitiated than that enclosed by clothes?

"It has been written that 'The worst of all our ills is to make the doctor swallow his own pills.' Laënnec, the discoverer of the unity of tuberculosis, enjoyed air baths, finding them beneficial to his acrimonious sweats. A medical student once asked me if Laënnec discovered osculation!* I have practiced air bathing, in addition to cold water bathing, for many years."

That remark conjures up a jolting, corrective picture: the dignified and decorous Dr. Webb writing his learned books and articles while sitting naked with the window open! Writing from his New York hotel in 1928, he told Varina he had typed his notes into "The Role of the Physician in Literature" on two successive mornings "while enjoying a long and refreshing air bath."

But rest, rest, absolute rest, in bed and in the open air, for a long period was the only regimen Dr. Webb had come to trust to get a patient safely back into "the freedom of the world" again. He was now saying and writing that full recovery from tuberculosis without risk of relapse could not be expected short of four years in bed, with gradually increasing activity only toward the end of that period.

He therefore came to see and to call himself merely a "guide" for his tuberculous patients. They must get themselves well; he could only advise, support, and encourage them on their way. "Did not Hippocrates say, 'It is nature that cures us'?"

Dr. Forster was not ready to depart so far from common practice. He favored more and quicker resort to surgical intervention, at least the use of artificial pneumothorax. And whether from expediency or principle, he would not scare patients away with the threat of more than a few months of inactivity. To a question about the need for absolute rest he replied that such rest was helpful but that how long it should last depended on the doctor's judgment

*Webb's readers would have understood the joke. What Laënnec developed was the art of auscultation, of listening to sounds from within the body as an aid to diagnosis.

and the patient's willpower; "If the doctor could sting you as the wasp does the grub and suspend animation in you for six months or so, we could guarantee you a cure at the end of that time."

This considerable divergence between Webb and Forster did not become an acute problem until the great days of Cragmor approached their end late in the decade.

The decline began—or more probably, became visible—with the collapse of the nation's economy beginning in the winter of 1929–30. Two patients killed themselves when the October crash of the stock market wiped out their wealth and others went worriedly home to cope with their diminishing funds. Since few new patients arrived in the worsening Depression, more and more suites and cabins stood vacant.

At the same time Cragmor's newest building and its most pretentious—costing some sixty thousand dollars—a four-story Nurses Home built high on a cliff south of Main Building, was undermined by sinking ground beneath it and began sliding down the slope in progressive ruin. It had to be evacuated before it was wholly occupied. Some of the nurses left the sanatorium, among them Dr. Forster's sister Elizabeth, who went to begin her long life of selfless service as a visiting nurse among the Navaho Indians.

Dr. Forster began to look worried, distraught. His personal life was falling apart too. He and his wife lost a baby to crib death and, unable to avoid mutual recriminations, separated. His customary good cheer gave way to irritability. For the first time he issued stringent rules to govern the behavior of Cragmor's patients and enforced them by threats of expulsion for noncompliance.

A former patient returning for a visit found Cragmor incredibly gloomy and quiet. "Where have all the parties gone?" she asked in dismay.

The final calamity was a lawsuit and the sorry state of affairs it uncovered.

A newly arrived patient, Mrs. Winifred J. Ackley, a schoolteacher from Ohio, opened a wrong door in the back regions of Main Building one day in late 1929 and fell down a flight of stairs into the basement. She fractured her back and broke an ankle. When she was able to limp into a courtroom two years later, she charged the three doctors who had picked her up and carried her to the operating room—Alexius Forster was one of them—with making her injuries worse by mishandling her.

Mrs. Ackley was awarded a mere one hundred dollars for her pains but the questioning in court brought to light extensive financial mismanagement at Cragmor. Dr. Webb bluntly called it fraud.

Precise details of what had happened and who was responsible remain a mystery, but the general facts are known. Insurance premiums collected from the group policyholders had not been forwarded to Prudential. Bond obligations for the defunct Nurses Home had not been met. Substantial funds were missing. The sanatorium owed more than half a million dollars it could not pay. Cragmor was bankrupt.

Dr. Webb was staggered by this discovery. "I have lost my life insurance and $10,000 besides," he told his brother Frank, who was going through a similar devastation caused by an embezzling law clerk. "But I'm sure you will agree with me that the most painful part is learning how terribly you have been deceived by a man you trusted."

He immediately severed his connection with Cragmor, moved his patients to Glockner and other hospitals, and of course took with him the backbone of Cragmor's medical staff. All except Dr. Charles Sevier, who chose to move to Denver and begin practice there as an orthopedic surgeon.

For Cragmor this loss was irreparable. The patients liked Dr. Forster but they revered Dr. Webb. They recognized that it was his presence that spread the tone of reassurance and hope through Cragmor. Agnes Erickson, one of those who stayed behind, wrote him, "We always felt something comforting was missing when you were away on a long journey. We waited anxiously for your return, and felt relief and support again when you got back, but now you won't be coming anymore at all, ever."

Benefactors came forward to discharge Cragmor's debts, a new board of directors was organized, and Dr. Forster tried to carry on. But nothing was the same. The road was swiftly downhill.

Medical care and personal service grew slack. Dust and litter, even filth, accumulated. Repairs were neglected. The grounds went untended into rank growth. Soon rumors were flying of sexual promiscuity at the "san," doctors in bed with nurses and both huddled under blankets with patients. It was also said, apparently with substantial truth, that Cragmor had become an abortion mill to which many a Colorado Springs doctor took his unwillingly pregnant patients for quick in-and-out operations.

Dr. Forster sank into degradation with the sanatorium. He suffered recurrent mental breakdowns that required periods of hospitalization for psychiatric care. He constantly drank himself into stupor and became a shabby derelict whom former friends and admirers shamefacedly crossed the street to avoid in Colorado Springs. He had to be forbidden any attempt to treat patients at Cragmor but was allowed to go on living there and ended his life as a pitiable gray ghost shuffling around the domain of which he had been king. His story is the stuff of tragedy.

The able and energetic Dr. George Dwire took over the helm at Cragmor, cleaned up the place, and piloted it through several reincarnations. It became in turn a refuge for tuberculous veterans on overflow from Fitzsimons Hospital in Denver, a rowdy and destructive lot; a charity home for tuberculous old people, mostly women; a shining place of healing and training for tuberculous Navaho Indians. At the end of its road in the 1960s it was sold to the state and reconstructed into the Colorado Springs Campus of the University of Colorado. Its days of glory, even its name, were soon forgotten on the land where it had flourished.

Dr. Webb was truly shaken by the loss of the sanatorium he had been so proud of, done so much to develop, been so well served by in building his practice to national scope. He was lucky to have the Broadmoor at hand for his more affluent patients, especially with Jack Sevier on tap there as a kind of resident physician. For others Glockner was a superior hospital well versed in sanatorium ways and needs. Also, Sister Rose Alexius had returned and though in retirement now, she could do much unofficially to help with his patients.

Still, neither the hotel nor the hospital could really take the place of Cragmor.

The need for readjustments could hardly have come at a worse time. As the Depression deepened, the flow of patients almost dried up and more than ever the doctor's bill was the last to be paid; sometimes it was never paid. Dr. Webb and his partners had been earning a good income but not a spectacularly handsome one, in part because they were all careless about collecting fees. The billing chore seems to have been left largely to Dr. Gilbert and in the hurried comings and goings the partners often failed to report their visits to patients, so the fees to be charged went unrecorded. Dr. Webb at least had scant savings to fall back upon.

He had once more to pare and pinch. He stretched out the years of service from his suits and boots, reduced largesse to his children at school, cut down on his traveling, bought fewer books, canceled some subscriptions and memberships—among the latter that in the American Association of Immunologists, in which he had lost interest because he could not see that it was doing much to advance its science.

He also at this time accepted a salaried position as medical chief-of-staff at the Union Printers Home in Colorado Springs, said to be the largest institution of its kind in the world. Operated by the International Typographical Union as a home and hospital for aged and sick union members, it was also called the Childs-Drexel Home after two Philadelphia newspaper owners who had started it off in 1886 with a joint personal check for ten thousand dollars.

Tuberculous invalids had always made up a large proportion of the Home's residents because the printing trades were a special nest for tuberculosis. Printing was considered light work, not overly strenuous, and men suffering or recovering from the tubercle disease sought employment in it. Also, son was likely to follow father for generations in it, so the disease was passed down and spread around in printing plants. "Selective recruitment and concentration" scholars call the process.

Off and on Dr. Webb had been summoned to the Home to advise about some aspect of treatment there. Now he took on medical supervision of all its two-hundred-odd residents. The duties were not onerous; he had plenty of assistants to provide the purely custodial care required. Mostly he need concern himself only with the tuberculous who might still have some chance of recovery or those who needed comfort and cheer.

Introducing himself to one of these new charges, an old man sitting alone in a wheelchair by the window in the common room, Dr. Webb asked if he was often lonely.

"Lonely? No, I'm never lonely," the old man said. "I never have been lonely. I've been able to live countless lives. I have this," and he reached for an open book lying on the table beside him. "There's a world of interesting people here in Dickens."

He could hardly have said anything more likely to endear him to Dr. Webb. If only more patients could live contentedly in the world of interesting people to be found in books. Since so few could, Dr. Webb made it an essential part of his task to lure them into it.

He used to tell the tale of an eighteenth-century physician who was called to attend a young man with a broken leg lying among strangers in a wayside inn. "He's been blooded, splinted, and strapped. Everything has been done. You need not worry more about him," the doctor told mine host.

But *had* everything been done? asked Webb. "Did the doctor just leave the patient to curse his luck? Did he make no effort to ease the patient's mind as well as his tibia? There are times when it is incumbent on the wise physician to prescribe, not a posset or a purgative, but an essay or a poem."

He had long known that a bored and restless mind could retard, even prevent, recovery of the body. We remember how he prescribed poetry for those two hyperthyroid landladies in the early years of his practice. He was still quoting Dryden, "A mind at rest is a mind distressed," and he still considered it the physician's duty not to leave the mind idle, a vacant room for self-pity, gloom, and despair to occupy.

As the prescribed term for the rest cure in tuberculosis grew longer he felt himself increasingly challenged to persuade his patients into worthwhile and enduring pursuits. In this he was at times very much the preacher and the missionary, urging that the months and years of the rest cure be seized upon as an opportunity for learning and enrichment.

He cited the example of Thomas Huxley "who wished for release from distraction and freedom from those lethal agencies which are commonly known as the pleasures of society, and who exclaimed to a friend, 'If only I could break a leg, what a lot of scientific work I could do.'" And of Alexander Borodin, professor of chemistry at the Petrograd Academy of Medicine and Surgery, "who could only find time to compose music when indisposed, so that friends meeting him expressed the wish, not that he was well, but that he was ill!"

The Doctor had an easy way with children. For them on his first visit he would sit down on the bed, take out a small square of white paper, and make a puzzle-game of showing them how to fold it origami-like into a neat little sputum cup with a circle of petals at its top, on which he sketched a smiling face to greet them when they had used the cup and closed it.

He often entertained them by cutting out amusing silhouettes of

children and animals. Or he might draw pictures for them, then
ask them to draw some to show him the next time he came.

He might tell them about the rainbow he had seen that morning
when one of his own youngsters called him to come see "the pretty
ribbon in the sky." Or he might spin the child a tale in the continuing
saga of El Joe and Lilee and suggest he make up an adventure of
his own for the pair and tell *him* the story next time. These two im-
aginary little vagabonds became members of many a patient's
family as well as his own.

With children and adults alike he probed and watched for any
spark of interest he might encourage. If the patient noticed the
flower he wore he took it apart and showed how it was made and
did its work—to the annoyance of nurses and maids when he left
the petals, stamens, and pollen strewn over the coverlet. On the
next visit he was likely to bring along a book of flower pictures or a
beginner's manual of botany.

He had a patient at Cragmor whose persisting apathy distressed
him. What *would* arouse her interest? One morning he found her
idly watching a garden spider spinning its web. Did she know the
spider spun two such webs a day? he asked. And that some spider
mothers give their babies daily sun baths? And that the females of
some species devour their mates after the nuptials?

"Just like life in New York," she said bitterly.

The flash of spirit delighted him. He brought her his copy of
Fabre's volume on spiders. She read it all and asked for more.

In a similar case the method backfired. He had persuaded a self-
pitying beauty at the Broadmoor to watch the nesting of birds in a
tree outside her window but one spring day she suddenly hurled
her binoculars out the window, saying petulantly, "I'm damned
tired of watching those birds make love when I can't do it myself!"

The two hundred and more species of birds that flitted through
gardens, yards, and fields in and around Colorado Springs were a
tremendous resource that Dr. Webb used to the hilt. He found that
many patients, if he could get them started in birdwatching, sometimes by presenting them with a pair of binoculars or a field guide
to birds, would catch his love for it and spend countless hours at
their windows or on their porches, or if they were ambulatory,
on their walks, learning to identify the birds they saw, memorizing
their songs and calls, searching for new kinds to add to their personal logs.

At Cragmor Dr. Webb had an effective lieutenant in one of the patients, Myrtle K. Low, a graduate of the University of Chicago and an enthusiastic amateur ornithologist. She and Dr. Webb persuaded the gardener to put up large feeding trays around the grounds and taught the patients to carry bread crumbs or grains in their pockets to attract the birds.

Mrs. Low never hesitated to miss a meal or to get lost among the bluffs in pursuit of some rara avis. Once when she returned to the sanatorium madly excited over having seen a mockingbird and a white robin and announced her finds at dinner, half the diners stood up and cheered. At one time fifty-two Cragmorites belonged to the birding club.

The habit of birdwatching once acquired is seldom lost and Dr. Webb sent many a patient home with not only healed lungs but a lifetime hobby. His own keen interest in natural history and his fund of nature lore made him a seductive guide into several such interests that could be pursued anywhere with enduring satisfaction.

He welcomed the coming of the radio. He liked listening to it himself — had one installed in his Stutz coupé and found it relaxing to listen to the news, concerts, and sports events while he made his daily rounds — and he recognized it as a boon for bedridden patients. But he discouraged use of it as an opiate, as when a patient lay passively listening hour after hour to whatever the broadcaster fed him, and equally as an overstimulant, as when a patient got too excited by the World Series, say, or stayed up too late feverishly twirling the dials in search of faint signals from foreign stations.

Dr. Webb's task was easy when his patient enjoyed chess or was willing to learn it. It was bound to consume hours in quiet concentration over the board and chessmen. With some he would exchange a move or two each time he came; with others he played the game by postcard.

One time, just after he won a prize for playing the best game among twenty-seven against the former world champion Emanuel Lasker in an exhibition at the El Paso Club, he was conducting thirteen games by mail simultaneously. He kept small chess boards set up in his study and decided upon his moves before going to bed, then posted his cards as he left the house next morning. A couple of times he kept a few games going in his head while he was away on a trip.

He usually found time between convention sessions and clinic visits to send picture postcards to his patients from some museum or gallery, then shared with them the events of his journey when he returned. However pressed for time he felt, he took care not to show his hurry to a patient; he would talk for an hour or more at the bedside if necessary.

The conversation was usually about some book or the meaning of some poem, for it was "the prescription of literature" Dr. Webb relied on most. He refused to accept the argument that most Americans were at the mental level of twelve-year-olds and could not be interested in anything more taxing than the trashy magazines and moronic films produced for that level. He thought almost anyone would read, if only you chose the right subject and the right book for him.

He cited the businessman who had never read a book in his life but as a patient found himself enjoying the account of his own kind in a history of the East India Company and was easily led on to intent reading of Feuchtwanger's historical novel *Power*.

Of course, Webb said, to prescribe books successfully the physician must be a reader himself, must be widely at home in the vast treasury of books preserved in libraries. He stated a dramatic new definition of the doctor of the future:

"He will be a humanist, with the widest possible understanding of human motives; a cultured man with outstanding sympathy; a lover of the arts as well as a student of the sciences. The time will come when the practice of medicine will include within its scope every influence of known power over the human spirit and when the practitioner will look on his work and see, not disease and death, but the glowing lineaments of life. As Clifford Albutt asked, 'What are the most scientific physicians if they know all things save the human heart?'"

Dr. Webb did not foresee the overwhelming surge of medical science and technology that lay only a little way ahead, or the progressive segmenting of the human whole that had already begun. He did not foresee the mad rush toward a method of doctoring that would be neither humanistic nor holistic but instead, in the words of the wise man Dr. Lewis Thomas, an aloof and impersonal "reading of signals from machines."

The range of Webb's own prescriptions for reading was marvelously wide but he clearly preferred natural history, poetry, and biography. Biography above all—along with letters and memoirs by persons of worth, which he thought were much too little appreciated as reading matter of engrossing interest.

In poetry his taste was purely Victorian, for the sentimental and the inspirational, for the likes of Tennyson and Longfellow, not at all for the later obscure symbolists who required *explications de texte* to be intelligible.

Lamenting that he could entice so few into enjoying poetry, he conceded that "for those whose fare must be prose" informal essays would serve as well as poems to calm and reassure and he recommended the essays of Lamb, Aubrey, Browne, and Stevenson for their "sanity of outlook."

In fiction he was no sure guide beyond "the classic writers who have stood the test of time," though he read an occasional contemporary novel and recommended Somerset Maugham's *Of Human Bondage* and Norman Douglas's *South Wind* as great fiction. He thought it better to involve a patient with novels rather than with short stories, "which grow monotonous if read one after another without relief."

One category of popular reading he was blind to: the detective story. He had never found a whodunit he thought worth finishing, though he admitted that "many great intellects have found relief in them." If a patient must have these, Poe's tales, A.A. Milne's *Red House Mystery*, and Chesterton's Father Brown stories would do, "but if he insists on a sheer thriller, let him pick his own!"

Dr. Webb was not a reader of the Bible either but a good many of his patients were and he did not discourage them, seeing that for the believer it provided real solace. One of them, though, grew critical about the story of human beginnings in Genesis and impaled him with a couple of sharp questions: Where did the wife Cain "knew" come from? And why did Cain build a city when there were only five persons on earth?

Dr. Webb was reading at the time about the great twelfth-century Jewish rabbi and physician Maimonides and quickly decided, he said, to take that wise man's advice to his students: "Never be afraid to say, I do not know."

For the patient who needed the direct medicine of laughter Dr. Webb had several standbys: *Alice in Wonderland*, *The Hunting of the Snark*, stories by P. G. Wodehouse "that funniest of men," and Jerome K. Jerome's *Three Men in a Boat*.

One conviction he had to modify. Aware of the human propensity to acquire any symptoms read or heard about, he was certain it could only worry a patient to read about suffering and death from tuberculosis. The lives of such as Voltaire and Ruskin who lived to ripe old age despite their tuberculosis he would endorse as perhaps encouraging, but never anything like Mrs. Gaskell's *The Brontë Family*; it was too sad a tale, bound to be depressing with its scary descriptions of the deaths of six children from phthisis.

Then by chance he learned he was wrong, that for some patients nothing was more fascinating than to read about sufferers like themselves. They would even read poetry with their symptoms as bait!

The chance occurrence was this. Webb got a postcard one day from Henry Sewall saying a patient of his had been reading Shelley's poetry and was sure from it that the poet was tuberculous. Did Webb know, was she right?

Dr. Webb chose "a brilliant young woman" from among his Cragmor patients, gave her Sewall's card along with his own volume of Shelley's poetry, and suggested she try to find what had given Sewall's patient her idea. When he came next time the young woman handed back his book open at "Stanzas Written in Dejection Near Naples" in which she had marked some lines she said so eloquently described her own feelings that she too was sure the poet had known tuberculosis:

> Alas! I have nor hope nor health,
> Nor peace within nor calm around...
> Others I see whom these surround—
> Smiling they live, and call life pleasure;
> To me the cup has been dealt in other measure....
>
> I could lie down like a tired child,
> And weep away the life of care
> Which I have born and still must bear
> Till death like sleep might steal on me.

In the interval Dr. Webb had been looking up the life of Shelley and learned that the poet was indeed tuberculous and had gone to Italy in search of health. He wrote it all up in a charming essay on Shelley for publication in *Ninety-eight-Six*.

Presently a dozen or more Cragmorites were playing the game, keeping a sharp eye out for signs of tuberculosis in the authors they read. The merest hint would do.

One of them found in the letters of Thomas Carlyle an admonition to his friend John Sterling the poet that he must learn to practice idleness: "Do you call the wheatfield idle on all days except when men are reaping wheat from it? Learn to sit still, I tell you; how often must I tell you?" She showed the passage to Dr. Webb and he got hold of Carlyle's *Life of John Sterling* and found material for another essay in *Ninety-eight-Six*.

Sterling did suffer from tuberculosis, severely so for a long time. Carlyle introduced him as a corresponding friend to another consumptive, Ralph Waldo Emerson, who wrote him long chatty letters. In reply to Sterling's description of a hemorrhage he had just survived — "It was strange to see the thick crimson blood pouring from one's own mouth while feeling hardly any pain; expecting to be dead in five minutes and noticing the pattern of the room-paper and of the Doctor's waistcoat as composedly as if the whole were a dream" — Emerson wrote:

"Please God, you are better now. But truly I think it a false standard to estimate health, as the world does, by some fat man instead of by our power to do our work. If I should lie in whenever people tell me I grow thin and puny, I should lose all my best days. Task these bad bodies and they will serve us, and will be just as well a year hence, if they do grumble today. But this is safer in this country, for we are a nation of invalids. You English are ruddy and robust, and sickness with you is a more serious matter."

For Dr. Webb the choicest find made by a patient, through an intimation in one of Lamb's essays, was Lamb's good friend Thomas Hood, the Scottish writer of comic verse who has been credited with making the pun respectable in literature. "Impugn I dare not thee / For I am of puny brood" he once wrote, and indeed he was. His mother died of tuberculosis, all his siblings had the disease, and he suffered grievously from "the consumption" all his life, spent largely in one or another of the printing trades.

Gerald Webb delighted in Hood's "word-gambols," so that his two-installment essay on Hood in *Ninety-eight-Six* was as much quotation of the poet as writing of his own.

He was all the while carrying on his own search game, in Shakespeare.

When working up material for an essay on "William Harvey and the Circulation" to mark the three-hundredth anniversary of the publication of Harvey's epochal treatise *De Motu Cordis* (1628) which described for the first time how the blood circulates and the heart functions as a pump, he learned that the Elizabethan philosopher Francis Bacon was a patient of Harvey's and thought it likely the doctor had shared his revolutionary discovery with so intellectual a patient.

Knowing of the controversial theory that Bacon was the author of Shakespeare's plays, Webb wondered whether those plays might reveal the author's acquaintance with Harvey's idea and began hunting through them for the answer.

He never found it for himself, because in *The Tempest* he came upon some lines that sent him haring off on quite a different quest. In Act I, scene ii Prospero says to Caliban: "For this [curse], be sure, tonight thou shalt have cramps, / Side stitches that shall pen thy breath up."

To Gerald those lines were proof positive that Shakespeare suffered from tuberculous pleurisy. "A man *must* have had personal experience with pleurisy to describe it so exactly. An ordinary stitch in the side eases off quickly but one that pens up your breath is certainly pleurisy. Huxley had it and described it as feeling as though a bird of prey had its claws through you."

He began reading everything he could find about the life of Shakespeare, hunting confirmation of his idea, and he speculated rashly from what he learned. Why did William retire from the theater and return to Avon so early and die so young if not from such fatigue and malaise as tuberculosis induces? Was it not William's own exhaustion and consuming disease that showed up in his graphic portrayal of Lear? And so forth.

Unable to find a copy of J. C. Bucknill's *Medical Knowledge of Shakespeare* he wrote to ask his brother Frank to hunt one up for him in England and explained why he wanted it.

For a decade correspondence between the two brothers had been sparse, often no more than an exchange of good wishes as a new year began, but now it revived in a discursive dialogue about Shakespeare that continued for more than two years. Their correspondence never again subsided; it brought them close in a relationship both cherished.

Frank as a lawyer was highly skeptical of Gerald's notions. He thought his brother's imagination was leaping much too far ahead of his meager evidence and voiced a resounding Whoa!

Presently the two drifted away from the initial argument into a general discussion of the plays and sonnets themselves, the controversies among scholars about them, alternative interpretations of *Hamlet*, *Macbeth*, and *King Lear*, and so forth. Both men searched catalogues and bookstores for writings old and new about the man of Avon, and Gerald was jubilant when at last, in a small rare-book shop in New York, he found two copies of Bucknill's book and sent one to Frank, who returned the favor in due time with a copy of Dover Wilson's latest book, *The Essential Shakespeare*.

This prolonged excursion into Shakespeare undoubtedly afforded both men surcease from their concurrent troubles, Gerald's with Dr. Forster and Cragmor, Frank's with his embezzling clerk.

It was a physician-patient who eventually found the answer to Gerald's original question about the circulation of the blood, in *King John* Act II, scene iii: "Or if that surly spirit, melancholy, / Had baked thy blood, and made it heavy, thick / Which, else, runs trickling up and down the veins." Clearly the author of those lines thought with Galen still, not with Harvey.

Inevitably Dr. Webb encountered patients whose attention span was too short for anything more than newspapers and magazines. For these he prescribed the scrapbook. Let them clip and paste to put together their own books out of bits and pieces that pleased them. He thought there was enough of the child left in every adult to make him enjoy the process.

One of his patients, an athletic young woman, arrived at Cragmor encumbered with tennis racquets and golf clubs and boxes of balls for both. Her first question was, "Where are the courts and greens?"

"No, no," he told her. "You are going to bed and stay there."

She was appalled. "But what on earth shall I do?"

"You can keep a scrap-book."

"My God!"

He suggested she keep a book on each of her sports—the scores in matches, reports of tournaments, profiles of players, and the like. After a period of sullen rebellion she began such records, and twenty years after she had recovered and returned home she told him she was still compiling a scrapbook each year for tennis and another for golf.

The scrapbook-making got out of hand with young Laura Jones (later stage name Laura La Tille) who took to clipping from the *books* she read; in one winter at Cragmor she cut her way through an entire set of Balzac and most of Kipling. Dr. Webb did not mind. He thought the person more important than the book; one could always buy another copy of the book.

He said he had worn to shreds several copies of *The Romance of Isabel, Lady Burton*, which he used to wean readers from light romances into a biography of Sir Richard Burton, the English explorer who translated sixteen volumes of *Arabian Nights*, and on to Burton's own *Pilgrimage to Mecca*. When he loaned his last copy of *Isabel* to "a lady from New York" with its binding in tatters, she returned it to him elegantly rebound in fine red leather!

He quite upset the custodian-minded tenders of the library at Cragmor by telling his patients to keep for themselves any of its books they especially liked.

He was equally free with his own library. Friends called his Stutz coupé "Parnassus on Wheels" after Christopher Morley's title for his story of migratory book-peddling, because the Stutz's back seat was always full of books Gerald had pulled from his shelves to be taken to his patients.

He did not choose these hastily or at random. He gave an hour or more each morning to selecting them, picking this book for a certain patient, then deciding that one would be better, before he went out with his arms full to start his day's rounds. He usually left his shelves a shambles of vacant spaces and rejected volumes. The perpetual chaos in his study was the despair of Varina and her housekeeper.

Gerald could laugh at his persistent untidiness. He once clipped a cartoon from *Punch* picturing an elderly bibliophile in his library. From floor to ceiling the shelves were all empty save for one last book at the very end of the topmost shelf, which the old man, teetering high on a ladder, was stretching to reach. The floor below was piled knee-deep all around with the books he had flung down in his frenzied search. Across the bottom of the cartoon Gerald wrote: "Marka says this is me!"

His family often teased him about his addiction to books—

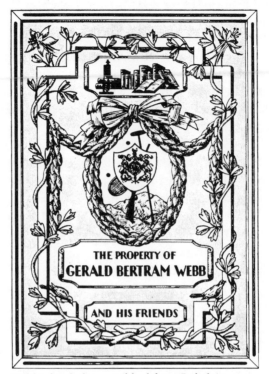

Webb's bookplate—cribbed from Rabelais

sometimes with a tinge of resentment. His adolescents wanted
many things and thought they could put to better use the money
Daddie spent on books. Once when he was leaving for New York
young Joel asked him to bring back something or other the boy
wanted, then with a resigned shrug offered to bet him twenty dollars
he would buy books instead. Gerald took the bet with a solemn
pledge that this time he would stay away from bookstores.

Two weeks later he wrote Varina: "Tell Joel I'll pay him that
$20. I passed Brentano's on the way back from lunch and found
some books I must have. When I got the package to my hotel room
I unwrapped it and thought I'd just dip into them a minute. The
next thing I knew it was getting dark and I was late for my appointment with Reggie Fitz [Reginald Fitz, the originator of appendec-
tomy], so I'm writing you later today than I meant to."

No one ever had to think twice about what to give Gerald as a
present; they just bought him a book. He gave thanks to them in

the conclusion of "The Prescription of Literature": "I joyfully dedicate this address to the many friends and patients who in return for my literary ministrations have showered me with wonderful books."

He insisted, contrary to most of humankind, that the books he loaned were always returned to him sooner or later. But the time came when two grateful patients, Mr. and Mrs. R. Clifford Black of New York, decided he should have a bookplate to identify his circulating volumes and commissioned a New York commercial artist to design it. Thinking it ought to represent Gerald's many interests, Varina asked that it include the Guy's Hospital coat of arms, a tennis racket, a polo mallet, a microscope, books and mountains of course, and some twining Colorado columbine with birds perched thereon to suggest his love of wildflowers and feathered songsters.

The artist worked all these elements into an attractive design atop the inscription Gerald himself requested, cribbing it from François Rabelais, the first physician to prescribe reading for his patients as well as the creator of Gargantua and Pantagruel. The inscription read: "The property of Gerald Bertram Webb and his friends."

Scores of those friends and patients wrote him out of the blue in later years to tell him what his "literary ministrations" had done for them. Typical is Hope Allen Ryan, Maria Allen's only daughter who had married an English army officer. When emerging from a long personal bad patch just before World War II she sent Dr. Webb a letter from London: "I've been thinking how your interest and influence on my reading during those days of my youth when I was laid up opened up vast treasure houses for me. I could never have got through the past two years if I hadn't been able to lose myself in good books as you taught me to do."

Dr. Webb's concern for his patients intensified when they recovered and were trying to find a way back into normal life. As we know, he was surrounded by physicians whose careers he had salvaged: Gilbert, the Sevier twins, Ryder, Drea, even to a degree Boissevain. W. F. C. Nelson, the frail scholar he credited with help on his memoir of Laënnec, was enlisted on the project more to further his rehabilitation than because his aid was necessary. He went on to become a professor of literature at Yale. And James Phinney Baxter III declared himself to be on the list.

Two others joined it in the late 1920s: Dr. Edward Norton Chapman and Dr. William Corr Service.

Dr. Chapman was a handsome, engaging young man, but quite a sick one, when he arrived in Dr. Webb's office fresh from his medical courses at Yale. He was determined to have a career in medical research but he was almost equally interested in economics and finance. When he was well again, Dr. Webb put him in the way of careers in both fields. He took him onto the Foundation laboratory staff, where he soon became associate research director, and he introduced him to Alfred Cowles III, whom he helped to elaborate the science of econometrics.

In record time Dr. Chapman became an active trustee of the Foundation, succeeded Ruth Boissevain as its secretary-treasurer, was elected its vice-president, and after he retired became its indispensable financial consultant.

Dr. Webb received almost simultaneously in the fall of 1929 two letters from physician friends in the East, Dr. Francis Rackemann of Boston and Dr. Robert Cooke of New York. Both men asked for his help with a promising young protégé of theirs, Dr. William C. Service, who had contracted tuberculosis just as he was about to begin an Eli Lilly Research Fellowship in Medicine. He had spent six months at Saranac Lake and then, still too ill to work, had wandered west to Colorado. Would Webb please track him down and do what he could for him?

Dr. Webb found him, lost and despairing, in Boulder and invited him to come look around in Colorado Springs.

"I remember he took me to Cragmor and the Foundation laboratory and introduced me to Forster, Boissevain, and Drea," Dr. Service wrote me. "When my health improved, I didn't know what I wanted to do. Dr. Webb told me I could join the staff in the laboratory and he talked to me frequently about immunology and allergy, which he felt was a growing field. I felt at that time that very little was understood about allergic disease and that it would be a nebulous field to go into.

"While we were talking one day, Dr. Webb picked up the phone and called Dr. George Piness in Los Angeles. [Dr. Piness was a pioneer specialist in the treatment of allergies.] He told Dr. Piness he had with him a young research man who was skeptical of the future of allergy and asked if he could send me out to learn about it. Dr. Piness said yes and I went out and worked with him for about a year. He showed me the great potential in the allergy field and when I came back to Colorado Springs I decided to go into practice in allergy instead of research."

Dr. Service made the right decision at the right time. He achieved gratifying success as an allergist. In time he had five physicians working with him in his allergy clinic in Colorado Springs, opened a second clinic in Pueblo, and when he retired, established the William Corr Service Foundation for research in his specialty. "I could never repay what I owe to Dr. Webb," he said.

Dr. Webb did not limit his help to those already on their way to careers. It was he who got the Cragmorite Maggie Mathers to take up the study of mathematics by enrolling in a correspondence course, looking toward work later as an accountant. In fact, he persuaded so many to take such courses that I.C.S. for International Correspondence Schools was a common abbreviation at Cragmor.

One of Webb's patients there was a young woman from Brooklyn, Fanny Wolf by name. Her parents scrimped to support her through years of up-and-down progress on the road to recovery. She married a fellow patient, Henry Robbins, but Henry died and Fanny was alone again when she faced return to the workaday world. What was she to do to earn her living?

Dr. Webb looked over the offerings of the I.C.S. and suggested she take the course in candy-making so that when she was able she could open her own business. He promised to get orders for her confections from his friends. More, when the time came he persuaded Mrs. Philip B. Stewart to lend Fanny the money she needed to get started.

Fanny rented an old house in downtown Colorado Springs, made the upstairs into her living quarters, and turned the downstairs into kitchens and a salesroom. In no time the delicious, daintily decorated Fanny Robbins Candies were in demand everywhere in town and Fanny was shipping them all over the United States and abroad to erstwhile tourists and patients who had sampled them in Colorado Springs.

To this day, though Fanny and her shop are gone, letters come to Colorado Springs asking for that wonderful Fanny Robbins candy.

A similar case was Maxine Lewis. To her Dr. Webb suggested

that she learn and practice calligraphy. She became so skilled at it that she got more orders than she could execute, because she remained in fragile health.

Dr. Webb himself gave her much work to do. Whenever he was asked to send a congratulatory message to be presented at a commemorative dinner for one of his doctor friends, he scribbled it out on a prescription blank and gave it to Maxine to engross and embellish on fine paper. These "Webb specials" became well known in medical circles and requests for them got so numerous they were an annoyance.

Maxine was grateful to her doctor and as a gift to him scripted on parchment one of his favorite quotations from Tennyson:

> When thou art worn and hard beset
> With sorrow that thou wouldst forget—
> If thou will learn a lesson that will keep
> Thy heart from fainting and thy soul from sleep,
> Go to the Woods. There no tears can
> Dim the sweet look Nature wears.

Varina hung the scroll on the outside of Gerald's study door, where it fixed itself in the memory of his children, especially Robine.

A long-term unmanageable problem came to Dr. Webb with the arrival of Vincent Youmans, one of the best of the popular songwriters of the day. The Doctor recognized at once that this slim exquisitely attired young man from Tin Pan Alley, a darling of the show biz world on both coasts, was not a likely prospect for the rest cure he badly needed.

Vincent was a flitter, one of the world's bright-hued butterflies, quite unable to alight anywhere for long—not even in his Larchmont home with the mother he adored, or in the Connecticut mansion he built for his wife. Except for brief stays he left her—and the two children she bore him—in the bower he had made for her and moved himself into a hotel suite in New York, from which he telephoned her several times a day and sent her masses of flowers and expensive presents.

At the height of the fame and fortune he won with *No, No, Nanette*, *Hit the Deck*, and *Flying Down to Rio*, with "Tea for Two," "Time on My Hands," "Without a Song," and a long string of other sterling hits, Vincent must have subconsciously feared he was seriously ill, for he had a dream one night while on the Atlantic crossing to Europe in midsummer 1934. His mother stood beside his bed saying sadly, "Vincent is dying of tuberculosis." He woke in a panic and half an hour later suffered his first pulmonary hemorrhage.

He made his way to Colorado and Dr. Webb later that same year, but his stay was short. He would not hear of going to bed in a hospital; he could not endure the restraints imposed in such regimented places.

He returned to the Springs the next year with a new wife, a pretty nurse née Mildred Boots whom he had met when she was a chorus girl in one of his shows. He established her in a house in Colorado Springs and for the next dozen years spent prolonged periods off and on in the mountain town. But almost never in his home. He preferred again to live in hotel suites, from which, after a few hours of rest in the daytime, he would emerge at night to drink, be merry, play the piano, and sing his songs for one or another delighted hostess and her friends.

Sometimes he chose Dr. Webb's home for his evening of music and talk. "He comes in and plays his compositions by the hour," Gerald told his brother Frank. "I feel guilty to allow this for he ought to be in bed—he is a very sick man." But Gerald enjoyed these evenings enormously. Youmans's songs were the sprightly, tuneful kind he liked and he was fascinated by Vincent's stories of his friends: F. Scott Fitzgerald and Ring Lardner, George and Ira Gerschwin and Irving Berlin, Fritz Kreisler, Lawrence Tibbett, Gladys Swarthout, Mary Chase the author of *Harvey*, and a legion more.

But as Vincent talked, Dr. Webb, a practiced listener, began to hear undertones that led him to suspect something more than precarious health was troubling the man. He eased it out into the open. Underneath all that quicksilver wit and gaiety, Youmans was deeply unhappy about his work. He thought his songs and show tunes came too trippingly from his mind and fingers. He longed instead to be a serious composer of serious music. He had ideas for symphonies and operas he was sure would be good, but he lacked enough technical knowledge of music to write them.

The solution seemed simple to Dr. Webb. Why did Vincent not use his time in Colorado to study composition? He, Gerald, had often seen art students at work in galleries copying the paintings of the masters as a way of learning their craft. Could Vincent not make similar use of musical masterworks?

The suggestion rooted. For a time Vincent Youmans spent hours, by fits and starts, sitting in his hotel suite copying orchestral scores. But the process was too slow, too sedentary, too lonesome. He was presently up and away to New Orleans to attend classes in harmony and orchestration at Tulane University. But again, not for long.

Back in New York he exhausted himself and his bank account by producing a gigantic "Cuban Revue." The critics called it "a colossal bore" and its run was short.

At such times Vincent wrote back to Dr. Webb, on the surface taking the setback humorously in stride but between the lines seeking reassurance. Once he wrote how torn apart he felt by his mother's death. Dr. Webb replied with sympathy: "I know how you must feel. I remember how I felt when the same thing happened to me while I was studying medicine in Vienna thirty years ago."

A few months later Gerald wrote Frank: "I was in court in New York last week, as a witness for Vincent Youmans, the song writer. He is a patient of mine—who, alas, will not recover. It makes me sad. But I was glad he won his case, for $11,000."

Vincent became a good friend of the Webb family. He designed their Christmas card for them in 1935 and showered them with telegrams and notes of cheery greeting on holidays, birthdays, and other such occasions.

His last return to Colorado Springs was in the fall of 1945. He was then so weak that Dr. Webb was able to keep him in a hospital bed for a month. But when a little strength returned he was away again to a suite in the Park Lane Hotel in Denver and another round of hectic nights on the town. He spent his last month in bed at his hotel, strumming tunes on the coverlet, whispering the words he could no longer sing, and giving instructions for the staging of his funeral in New York. He died in April 1946.

It was from Dr. Webb that Vincent got the idea of establishing a Vincent Youmans Memorial Foundation to support the fight against tuberculosis; he had been a generous contributor to both the endowment and the maintenance fund for Webb's Colorado Foundation. He instructed his lawyer to set up his own and willed to it his entire estate, including a trunkful of more than a hundred songs he had written while he was ill.

Unfortunately Mildred contested the will in court, although she had divorced Vincent and become the wife of the millionaire music publisher Gustave Schirmer. She won; the foundation to fight tuberculosis lost. None of those later Vincent Youmans songs was ever published.

The outcome was much happier for Marshall Sprague, another urban sophisticate, a journalist, who sought out Dr. Webb in 1941. After graduating from Princeton in the class of 1930 and learning his craft as a reporter on the *North China Star* in Tientsin, China, and then on the prestigious *Paris Herald*, Sprague joined the staff of the *New York Times*.

"I had been moving around the South doing some travel pieces," he told me, "and wasn't feeling well when I got back to New York, so I went to see Dr. Oswald Jones, a partner of Dr. James Alexander Miller. The diagnosis was tuberculosis, and Dr. Jones advised me to go out to Dr. Webb because that's where Dr. Miller sent everybody. 'Webb's the best there is for what you've got,' Jones said.

"Dr. Webb met me at the train, looking very handsome and distinguished in a tailored blue suit with a carnation in his buttonhole. I assumed I was going to Broadmoor 'Sanatorium'—that's what Dr. Jones called it—but Dr. Webb said no, he was taking me to Glockner."

When it became clear that Sprague was facing years of convalescence, his devoted wife Edna Jane—"my bonanza" he called her—moved west with their baby, rented the former Chester Alan Arthur house on Wood Avenue, and fixed up a sunny, first-floor room so Marshall could take his rest cure at home.

Dr. Webb introduced him to birdwatching. At first there was just one large feeding tray set up outside the window of Marshall's room, but in a short while this had multiplied to seven trays scattered around the commodious yard. "Watching the birds, their many colors and myriad varieties, helped me pass the long hours."

Nor did Webb forget books. "It still gives me joy," Sprague said years later in what he called "a gabble" to an afternoon club meeting, "just to think of Dr. Webb, that tall, beautiful, smiling man, full of warmth and humor, coming into my room all hunched over with the weight of the books he used to bring me. He brought every conceivable subject to me."

Having learned that resting for recovery need not mean extended boredom, Marshall wrote an article about it which was published in *Good Housekeeping*. It brought him hundreds of letters and the attention of Robert Cromwell the New York publisher. The result was a successful book, *The Business of Getting Well*. As his health returned Sprague nosed out countless stories about his new home town and its colorful past and became a lively teller of its tales in several books.

Sprague was affectionately amused by Dr. Webb's "painful refinement." "The dirtiest joke I ever heard him tell was about the male Monarch butterfly. 'He has a black wife,' he would whisper, not wanting others to know he was capable of such vulgarity. He would blush violently when I asked how long it would be before sexual intercourse could return to my life. Saying even that term—to say nothing of four-letter words for it—was utterly beyond him. He would reply, 'You are out of the woods now. But be—uh—moderate about that—uh—uh—ten-mile hike'!"

Once in Marka's presence Sprague said of Dr. Webb, "He was a real glamour boy, and I'll bet half his female patients fell in love with him."

"Maybe so," Marka responded, "but he was armored against them because he missed most of the romantic nuances. When he was examining a patient at Cragmor one time he looked up to see several nurses standing in the doorway. He was mystified and told them to go back to their work because there was nothing special about this case for them to see. The patient thought it was laughable that he did not know the nurses were there to see *him*.

"But yet, maybe he did know. He used to take me with him when he went to see women patients at the Broadmoor. They were always togged out and coiffed for his visit, wearing fancy see-through negligees and swathed in maribou. He said he took me along for my education—but perhaps it was for his protection too."

In a more serious vein from Marshall Sprague comes a moving testament to what Dr. Webb's care meant to his patients: "Dr. Webb stood between me and the dark. He made me well, but besides that it was his gift to pass his own love of life on to me; to make me want to live as passionately as he himself wanted to live. And he did that for thousands."

XVII

Affaires de Coeur

As THE TWENTIES rolled on into the thirties Dr. Webb continued to shuttle around the country for six or more weeks a year but he did so with diminishing drive, diminishing zest. "I am getting fed up with all these tedious meetings," he told Varina during his spring round in 1928. "I have been to too many of them. The crowds are getting bigger, with more young men, and it all seems less rewarding."

He let himself relax more, occasionally skipping a convention entirely and often whiling away an afternoon playing poker with Jim Waring, Jim Miller, and Alec Lambert instead of rushing off to see what new was developing at some hospital or clinic.

In October 1928 the New York Academy of Medicine sponsored a symposium on aging and Webb was asked to speak on "Climate and the Aged." He arrived a few days ahead of time in order to gather material in the Academy's library but on the second day decided to play hooky and go to an international soccer match at Meadowbrook Field, "thinking I'd surely not see anyone I knew in the midst of the 42,000 who would be there. But who should I meet before I even found my seat but Bob McKay!"

Robert G. McKay was a Colorado Springs friend whose wife was the daughter of Henry Fairfield Osborne, the longtime president of the American Museum of Natural History in New York. The McKays were spending this spring and summer in a guest house on the three-hundred-acre estate of Marshall Field on Long Island near Oyster Bay. Bob insisted that Dr. Webb come home with him for the weekend to play tennis.

Gerald's best matches that weekend were against McKay's neighbor Kermit Roosevelt, Theodore's second son, with whom he struck up a lasting friendship. They usually had lunch together whenever Gerald was in New York after that and Kermit often persuaded him to come to Oyster Bay for more tennis.

The McKays were also entertaining at the time their vivacious, flirtatious friend Lucrezia Bori, popular diva of the Metropolitan Opera, and she was delighted to find herself in the company of a gallant who could gossip with her about opera and opera houses in Europe. Gerald was her escort to a formal dinner party at "the big house" where the Marshall Fields had assembled "most of New York's 400." He and Lucrezia resumed their merry persiflage whenever she visited the McKays and other friends in Colorado Springs.

"It was a splendid weekend," Gerald told Varina, "but I got no work done and the symposium is tomorrow night. I'll have to spend the day putting something together tomorrow."

He was trying to keep free of social engagements by not letting his friends know he was in town. But in "putting together" his paper—it turned out to be a disjointed hodgepodge of anecdotes, quotations, and a few statistics—he threw in his hobbyhorse of the moment, the benefit to women of their minimal clothing: "It is just such scant clothing that men need. Nothing can be more detrimental to health than the climate which men carry beneath their unhealthy garments. Many college students and schoolboys have already discarded hats, and we can at least hope that collars and coats will next disappear."

The newspapers seized on those comments for their headlines and stories the next day. "So now everybody knows I am in town and this morning has been full of telephone calls and telegrams from people wanting to see me. Such is notoriety! What am I to do about them all?"

What he did was leave town for a journey through the southern states west to California—speaking at Memphis, New Orleans, and San Francisco—and postpone further engagements in Gotham until the Academy of Medicine summoned him back in December to participate in another symposium, this one on the contributions of doctors to culture.

This time Gerald truly prepared his paper, on "The Role of the Physician in Literature." He called the roll of scores of men of medicine who had also been writers of poetry, essays, fiction—from Imhotep of Egypt, Luke the Physician, and Avicenna of Persia down to Oliver Wendell Holmes, S. Weir Mitchell, and Robert Bridges the English poet laureate. Physicians, he asserted in paraphrase of Horace Walpole, had left lawyers and clergymen far behind, "wrangling at the gates to Parnassus."

He was pleased that William Henry Welch and Arnold Klebs were in his audience and that both took the trouble to telephone him next day to applaud his paper. It was published as a featured article in *Medical Life*, the official organ of the American Society of Medical History, and it became one of his most frequently requested reprints. Henry Sewall wrote him that "it would have gladdened the heart of William Osler."

The "ordeal of my paper" over, Gerald surrendered himself to his friends and their Christmastime round of luncheon and dinner parties and afternoons and evenings at the theater. He saw eight shows in six days, mostly musical comedies—*Show Boat*, *The Desert Song*, *An American in Paris*. "I wish someone would want to see something besides Show Boat," he complained to Varina. "George Arliss in The Merchant was a relief—Peggy Wood made a brilliant Portia. 'Porgy' is too vulgar for my liking.* The pace is killing. Such a blurring rush of things and people. I feel dazed and dazzled by the big city. Oh for a cougar hunt! Or someplace in the sun with just you and some books."

As good a rest for him in these years was a trip to Cambridge, Massachusetts, to visit his first grandson!

Marka had stayed firm in her resolve to quit the classroom and she returned from Oldfields to become her father's secretary, bringing noticeably efficient order into his correspondence. Resuming her social life at the Cheyenne Mountain Country Club, she fell in love with its rising tennis star, Gerald Webb Bennett, who had been named for her father twenty-six years before because his parents were so grateful to young Dr. Webb for the day-and-night care he gave their sickly firstborn, Jimmy.

For the first time in her life, Marka said, she was afraid to confide in her father, to tell him she was engaged to Gerry. She left it to her young man to seek his approval. This was not in doubt; Gerald thought very well of his namesake. But he played the stern father and said he would give Marka's hand in marriage only if Bennett

---

*This *Porgy* was the play by Dorothy and DuBose Heyward. The George Gershwin opera based on it appeared seven years later. The actress Peggy Wood was the wife of one of Dr. Webb's patients, the poet John V. A. Weaver, who in 1937, a year before he died, inscribed a copy of his book *Trail Balance* "To Dr. Gerald B. Webb, whose erudition is equaled only by his humanity."

could beat him in tennis. Both families gathered to watch the match. It was a battle for every point but Gerry won it.

"Marka is simply radiant," Gerald told Frank.

The wedding took place 7 January 1926 and the young couple went off to live in Cambridge. Bennett, an honors graduate of Brown University, was enrolled in the Harvard law school. Their first son, born the following year, was named Gerald Webb Bennett Jr.

The Geralds and Gerrys were getting confusingly numerous in the family! The baby was referred to for a time as Gerald IV and Marka began to spell her husband's nickname Jerry.

Grandpa Gerald went often to visit the Bennetts. He could relax there, sitting with Marka in the pretty park across the street from the apartment while the baby played on a blanket in the grass, or at another season pulling the joyful tot on a toboggan through the snow. "It is so peaceful and cozy," he wrote Varina, "to sit reading by the fire while Marka goes about her housewifely chores and Gerry is busy with his case books at the table. It reminds me of you and I with the baby Marka in Vienna twenty-three years ago."

Gerald Bennett urged his father-in-law to come as often as he could. "You give me the encouragement I need. I just hope I can live up to your expectations."

Perhaps he tried too hard. He developed a duodenal ulcer so painful and debilitating that he had to give up his studies and Dr. Webb went east to bring Marka and the baby home and take Jerry to the Mayo Clinic for an operation.

There was no possibility of the young man's returning to Harvard. He took his law degree at the University of Denver and established his practice in Colorado Springs. Marka bore him a second son in 1932, this one named Charles Francis after his paternal grandfather but quickly "Chuck" to them all.

With the Bennetts back in town the family resumed their dominance of tennis matches at the Country Club—of which Dr. Webb was vice-president in 1926–27 and president from 1929 through 1931. In 1929 the mixed doubles championship match in the summer tournament pitted him and Leila against Marka and Jerry. A reporter called it "a brilliant, hard-fought game," which Gerald and Leila won 7–5, 2–6, 6–4. Then Webb and Bennett teamed up to win the men's double championship in two sets.

The young people hardly knew whether to be exasperated or

worried about Varina. They had to prod her into any participation at all in social activities. "Oh, do I have to get dressed up and go out?" she would say.

She had found a gem of a housekeeper in Opal Moss, a small but sturdy girl with a mass of flaming red hair and a sunny disposition. The whole family doted on Opal and held their breath when she married a townsman Henry Wojtacha; would they lose her? But she stayed with them and Varina made a companion of her. "Let's go to the woods, Opal," she would say on a balmy morning and off they would go with a picnic basket to spend the day among the trees.

Gerald understood Varina's inclination to withdraw. He knew she often was not feeling well and several times wrote Dr. A. L. Lockwood, her surgeon in 1920 who was now in charge of a clinic of his own in Toronto, about her repeated spells of soreness in her chest. The two doctors agreed that the streptococcal infection she had suffered does not produce protective antibodies but instead leaves the patient susceptible to recurrence. Still, Gerald told Varina, "I marvel at how you can carry on all your duties with so little diversion."

Varina often worried about her children's ups and downs in health, schooling, and love affairs. Gerald Jr. once sent her into real panic. He was in his last year at Deerfield Academy when Charles A. Lindbergh made his historic solo flight across the Atlantic and as for millions of others the Lone Eagle became his hero. Without warning in the spring of 1928 he wrote home that he planned to go into training as a pilot as soon as he graduated.

Gerald was in New York when the letter arrived. Varina sent it on to him with a frantic note:

"Gerald darling—You must distract Gerry from this idea of aviation. I just can't enter into it. It is so terrible that I am speechless. To me it offers about as much future as standing a man up and taking a shot at him. It would be just a horror for us all for a time and then the end. I suppose there must be the sacrifice of pioneers in all new ventures but I don't want to be the mother of one, helpless to save him. In ten years flying may be of some use but now it is just an experiment—each life lost just a lesson in what to try to avert. You must give Gerry some time on this, darling—advise and help him just like you do a "*Patient.*" Please go and see him and talk it all over with him. I feel so helpless and far away."

Whatever Gerald did, it worked. In the fall of 1928 Gerry enrolled at the University of Virginia along with his best Deerfield friend Hubert Phipps of Westbury, Long Island, a nephew of Lawrence Phipps the Denver millionaire.

Hubert took Gerry with him to spend the Thanksgiving vacation at his family's second home in the hunt country near Middleburg, Virginia. When Hubert's father heard that although Gerry had never done any jumping on a horse he had done a lot of riding and his father "was said to have a fine hand, sir," he loaned the young man a mount and let him ride in the hunt that was taking place that weekend.

"Just by luck, mother, because I really didn't know what I was doing," Gerry put on a fine show on two successive days, outriding and outjumping much older hands at the sport. Mr. Phipps congratulated him and invited him to come back any time he liked. Gerry was ecstatic. Aviation was forgotten. He had found what was to become his niche in life.

Perhaps Gerald's method of dissuasion from flying had been a promise to buy the boy an automobile of his own. Gerry had become an expert auto mechanic, so much so that when the garage men did not tune up Gerald's Stutz to his satisfaction he would say, "Never mind. I'll get Gerry to fix it when he gets home." So Gerald gave his university freshman a Model T Ford, which Gerry drove back and forth across the country—so exuberantly that he did not stop at home when he got to Colorado Springs but drove straight on up Spencer Penrose's highway to the top of Pikes Peak and back. The Ford Motor Company learned of this feat, thought it a good advertisement for their product, and paid young Webb to keep on doing it.

"Gerry never enthuses his teachers of scholastic subjects but he is good-looking and has a delightful personality that makes him popular," Gerald once told his brother Frank. Whether those scholastic subjects were too taxing or too dull for Gerry, or whether the Depression made his tuition fees and other expenses too taxing on his father's budget, Gerry dropped out of the University of Virginia, spent a year in his grandfather Hayes's bank where his uncle Jefferson Hayes-Davis was now in charge, and then in 1933 went to Chicago to take a job in the steel business.

By that time Robine had flown even farther from the nest. She had grown into a pretty young woman of independent spirit, inclined more to communion with nature than to sports and social whirlings. Her temperament may have been shaped by her having been "the middle child" between the older twosome of Marka and Gerry and the younger duo of Leila and Joel. She was mature enough at sixteen to accompany her father on occasions when Varina preferred to stay at home. For instance, when the visiting Queen Marie of Roumania was honored at a formal banquet in Denver, Varina refused "to waste time at such dull nonsense" and Gerald escorted Robine to the gala dinner in her place.

He also took Robine with him when he went over for the Laënnec Centenary in 1926. Her quiet poise struck their fellow traveler Dr. Thayer as "extraordinary in so young a lady." Before the Centenary celebration Gerald whirled her around England to meet her relatives and see where he had lived, then in Paris took her along to the opening reception in the great hall of the Sorbonne and to a midnight mass at Notre Dame. The great cathedral and the pageantry of the mass thrilled her but the building was without heat and "we nearly froze to death." After a short tour of the French countryside following the ceremonies in Paris, father and daughter spent Christmas alone together on the boat returning home.

Robine succeeded Marka as her father's secretary. On a vacation visit to Gerry in Virginia that included a side trip to Washington DC she met Frederick Edward Farnsworth, a graduate of Harvard in the class of 1929 who, after a year on an archeological dig in Albania, was beginning a career in the Foreign Service. They were married in Colorado Springs on 16 January 1932 and Robine became a traveled woman of the world, bearing and rearing her three children in a succession of alien places and cultures in which her husband, "Vevy" they called him, served as secretary or consul in U.S. legations and embassies: Mexico, Sicily, Turkey, Canada, Egypt, Singapore.

It was Leila's turn to come home from Oldfields and take Robine's place as secretary in the Burns Building offices. Her irrepressible high spirits brought life and fun to the place. She often forgot the decorum expected of her in those precincts and bemused the patients — undoubtedly easing their tensions too — by addressing their dignified doctors as "Sweetie," "Gilly," and "Uncle Jack."

Her typing sometimes slipped too. Dr. Webb often told how in making a copy of a paper in which he said the falling incidence of tuberculosis was due in part to improvement in living conditions, Leila typed it "loving conditions."

"Maybe she was right at that," he would say.

Leila was an enchanting hostess when the NTA came again to Colorado Springs for a day of their convention in June 1932, but Varina could not escape the visitors entirely; too many of them remembered her from previous visits and insisted on seeing her again.

Dr. Webb spoke to the group this time on the life of Robert Koch, to mark the jubilee of Koch's discovery of the tubercle bacillus. As published in the *Annals of Medical History* his paper was a fascinating biographical sketch, scrupulously fair to its subject, though in summing up the story of the German Koch's savage attacks on the work of the Frenchman Pasteur, he made clear how he ranked the two: "Pasteur was a master architect of scientific medicine, Koch was a master builder in it."

He retold briefly his own experience with Koch and the man's offensive behavior at the International Congress in 1908 but dismissed it tolerantly: "Such incidents as this indicate human frailty, which is common to us all, and which in no way lessens the scientific stature of the man or the debt of humanity to his discoveries."

In September Gerald asked Leila to drive him to Estes Park for the annual meeting of the Colorado State Medical Society. He wanted some time alone with the girl because her light-hearted entanglements with the young men in her life were making Varina uneasy. Father and daughter talked as they hiked each morning, beginning at six o'clock, along the trails through the wooded ravines of the Park. Leila took his admonitions all the more to heart because she was this year, for the first time, witnessing directly her father's stature in his profession. She had seen it at the NTA meeting in the spring; now she watched while he was elected the sixty-third president of the state society.

His presidential address the next year was unusual for him in its attention to current affairs in the society at large: "Instead of a joyous contribution for your amusement, I must deal with serious matters for your consideration. The time is out of joint and one is reminded of a very sick man in a hospital who is going to get well in time anyway but on whom young physicians are trying out every remedy, while the older ones just hope that convalescence may not be thereby delayed.... All of us would like to have the best motor cars but the majority make do with cheaper models. In medical service all should have the best. Unfortunately, the cost of medical service due to the great advances in medicine has now reached a figure that few can afford."

He deplored the marked increase in malnutrition in children which a study in Denver had shown was in direct ratio to the rise in unemployment. "This must be of great concern to doctors. It cannot be excused in a country which has an over-abundance of food supplies."

In commenting on the current furor over socialization versus individualism in medicine, he was moderate indeed, pointing out how well socialized medicine had worked during the Great War and was working now in England and even under the despised Communists in the Soviet Union. The achievements of the latter he called "a challenge to American medicine."

He shamed his hearers for tolerating the sorry state of public health in Colorado, and for permitting the pollution of the state's air and water. "Our rivers are simply open sewers. Would that some of the money being spent on improvement of road surfaces might be diverted to improvement of our dairies and our water supplies, and to planting our roadsides with sunflowers and bee-plants instead of letting hay-fever weeds grow rampant along them."

Great changes were taking place in America, he said; physicians should be in the forefront, "not lamenting but guiding the transformation. As the genius Bacon expressed it, 'They that reverence too much old times are but a scorn to the new.'"

It was a surprising address to come from the politically conservative Dr. Webb, and it probably failed to please most of the doctors who heard it.

We can only wonder what Gerald said to his younger audience in his commencement address on a spring day in 1932 when his son Joel graduated from the Fountain Valley School for Boys.

Joel had lost a year of schooling to the sunbathing and brace-wearing prescribed by Dr. Charles Sevier to pull him through tuberculosis of the spine without deforming effects. Now at nineteen he was tall and straight, so like his handsome father in appearance and manner, even in voice and speech inflections, that all who met him were amazed by the uncanny resemblance. He excelled in skiing and was improving fast in tennis.

"I beat Joel at tennis this morning, but for the last time, I think," Gerald told Frank; "he is definitely on the upgrade and I'm on the downgrade." As Joel remembers it, though, it was another six years and his father was sixty-seven before he could take a set from him.

The class of 1932 was the first to graduate from the Fountain Valley School. Dr. Webb was a founding trustee of the new academy, had given it its name, and was the physician in charge of its health program.

The dynamo behind it, though, was Elizabeth Sage Hare, the wife of Meredith Hare, a New York corporation lawyer who was one of Webb's patients. Betty, a daughter of the Russell Sage family, was a whirlwind of energy and ideas and Colorado Springs was never quite the same after she blew into town. Her overpowering enthusiasm and honeyed tongue persuaded men and women alike into philanthropic projects they had little real interest in and never meant to contribute to.

Betty had five sons by a previous marriage, every one of them a problem boy that eastern academies seemed unable to accommodate. She was determined they should get an education and decided to establish a private school from which, their mother being its founder, they would not be expelled.

She assembled a group of trustees—including Dr. Webb, Spencer Penrose, A. E. Carlton, and her wealthy friend Ruth Hanna McCormick who was Republican congresswoman from Illinois at the time but later came to live in Colorado Springs—went east to tap her New York friends for endowment funds, and shanghaied the most talented faculty members at Avon Academy in Connecticut to come and teach at her Colorado school.

In one thing Betty miscalculated. She trusted the promise of Ruth McCormick to make secure the future of the Fountain Valley School by leaving it amply endowed in her will. But in time Ruth moved to New Mexico, married Albert Simms, and left her money to him and their several sons by former spouses. Spencer Penrose took her place as benefactor and the Fountain Valley School still flourishes.

Betty Hare, Ruth McCormick, and Gerald Webb became mutually admiring and mutually entertaining friends. Gerald welcomed the stimulus he got from Betty's lively wit and imagination and from Ruth's flow of stories about the newspaper and political worlds she had lived in.

Varina and Meredith left the three to their stratagems and amused each other. Varina spent many an hour at Meredith's bedside reading aloud to him books of their common choice.

Under Dr. Francis Froelicher and his successors as headmaster the Fountain Valley School offered the sons—and eventually the daughters—of affluent parents a truly superior education. Except, to Dr. Webb's mind, in one thing. Gerald was perpetually upset that its curriculum did not contain more of natural history, for which the school's wild and beautiful setting offered an incomparable resource. Till the day he died he kept urging that the masters put more emphasis on this vital subject.

The school's attention to music and drama enlivened the community and provided Gerald Webb with the opportunity for a cherished triumph. Each year it staged an ambitious production of some play or light opera, usually in its own auditorium or a small church hall. In 1933 it ventured to produce Gilbert and Sullivan's *Iolanthe* on the stage of the Burns Theater and chose Gerald Webb to act and sing the role of the Lord Chancellor.

Much ado turned the performance into a major social event; dinner parties were arranged for before and after the show all over town; the theater was packed. And those who knew Dr. Webb only in his professional persona could not believe what they saw and heard from him that night.

Hidden within the long white wig and billowing black robes of the Chancellor he let himself go. The boy of those parlor shows at Heimat came out; the impish, antic self he customarily repressed now emerged—along with the fine singing voice few outside his family knew he possessed. "Dr. Webb stole the show" was the unanimous cry in newspaper reviews and the talk of the town for days.

Gerald relished all the limelight and tried a couple of times later to induce it again but could not spare the time for rehearsals and had to drop out of the cast each time. Telling Frank how much fun he had had, he said, "Maybe I missed my calling. But it's too late now. I must stick to my knitting."

For years thereafter virtually every review of a theatrical show in Colorado Springs compared it unfavorably with Dr. Webb's performance in *Iolanthe* and a decade after he was gone some old-

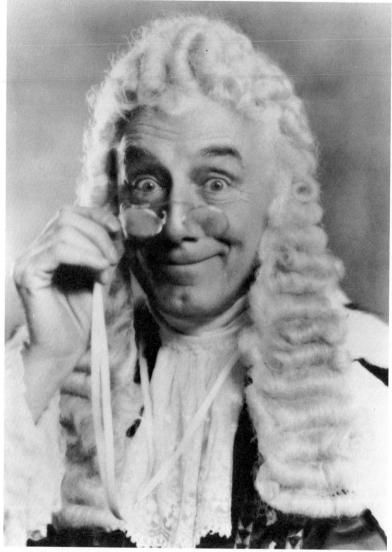

Dr. Webb as the Lord Chancellor in *Iolanthe*

timers were still harking back to "that great Lord Chancellor of Dr. Webb's."

After that sparkling high came the dark depths.

Jerry Bennett's ulcer was wearing him out again that fall and in early January 1934 Gerald ordered him to Florida with Marka for six weeks of complete rest. They left their two boys in the care of a housekeeper under Varina's watchful eye.

Six-year-old Gerry caught a cold that turned into a strep throat and put him to bed in early February and Varina went over every day to help keep him amused. As she was putting on her hat to leave one day she scratched the back of her head with her hatpin. Ten days later bloodpoisoning was raging in her veins again.

Gerald took her to Glockner Hospital and stood anxiously by while Doctors Gilbert and Sevier worked to reduce her fever and delirium. The sulfa drugs and penicillin that might have helped them sat waiting in laboratories across the ocean, still kept unavailable by commercial greed and bureaucratic indifference.

From Varina's bedside Gerald would drive home in the evening for a quick dinner with Leila, leaving his car parked in front of the house in order to save time on his return trip to the hospital for the night. On 23 February Leila, watching out the front window for his coming so as to tell Opal to get dinner on the table, saw him drive on past the house and into the garage. She knew her mother had died. Just three weeks before her fifty-sixth birthday.

Again Gerald kept the family's grief private. Gathered in the livingroom for the rector's words of farewell were only Gerald, Leila, Gerry who had sat up all night on the train from Chicago to get home in time, Uncle Jeff, Leila Shields, and Opal Wojtacha. Marka, Robine, and Joel were all too far away to be able to join them. Interment too was private, in Evergreen Cemetery, not far from Jenny's grave.

Again the black-edged stationery lay on Gerald's desk while he tried to acknowledge the many, many messages of condolence. The only one of his notes we have is the one he wrote in response to Frank's cable and letter on behalf of the family in England: "I am sad and lonely. Only Leila is here with me now. I miss Varina terribly. I was edgy and nervous as a colt until she taught me how to rest and be calm. She made life for me. But she of all people would not have wanted us to grieve our days away. Work must be my medicine and fortunately I have much to do."

But he could not escape further losses by death and winced at them often now. His sister Nell and his brother Roland died within a year of Varina and of each other. And as he said to Arnold Klebs, "It is sad so many leaves among our contemporaries are falling." Colonel Bushnell and Dr. William S. Thayer were already gone;

two men Gerald revered, Theobald Smith and William Henry Welch, died in the same year as Varina; and the jolt of Henry Sewall's death at age eighty-one came in July 1936.

This was as if Gerald had lost a father. Dr. Sewall had long been his mentor, adviser, sponsor, responsible in one way or another for many of the opportunities and honors that had come to him. He consoled himself with the thought that he had repaid a little of his debt to Sewall by many companionable visits and by what he had done for him five years before.

The medical fraternity of Denver decided in 1931 it was time they paid tribute to the dean of them all and commissioned J. I. McClymont of Colorado Springs to paint a portrait of Sewall to be hung in the library of the city's medical society. The portrait was to be unveiled at a banquet in Sewall's honor and Dr. Webb was asked to deliver the address. By great good luck he was able to arrange a surprise unveiling of his own.

In preparing his remarks he went to the society's library to look up Sewall's historic article, "Experiments on the Preventive Inocuation of Snake Venom," in the *Journal of Physiology* for the year 1887. From among the crumbling pages of that volume III dropped out a folded letter.

It was addressed to Dr. Sewall from The Hague, dated 1905, and signed by Dr. Roger Morris, the University of Michigan physiologist. (Morris later moved to the University of Cincinnati and became Webb's colleague on the editorial board of the *Journal of Laboratory and Clinical Medicine*.) In it Morris told of his visit to an eminent German professor of pharmacology who danced in excitement at meeting a man who knew Henry Sewall and showed Morris the proof of a book he was publishing which said, "The foundation of all the work that has been done on animal toxins is to be found in the work of Sewall at Ann Arbor, Michigan, in 1887, the great significance of which has not been recognized."

Here was the long-lost testimony to Sewall as the unacknowledged precursor of Von Behring and Roux, their diphtheria antitoxin, and much that followed in immunology. Obviously, receipt of the letter had sent Sewall to the old journal to reread his article and he had absentmindedly left the letter behind in the book.

Gerald was elated. He had the letter framed, read it to the three hundred doctors assembled at the dinner, and presented it to Dr. Sewall, who confessed himself touched and grateful. The memory of that occasion was a comfort to Gerald now that Sewall was dead.

There was little comfort for a sorrow closer to home that came in that same month of July 1936. Jerry Bennett's ulcer perforated and Gerald rushed him to Glockner Hospital for another operation. This time the young lawyer was too weak to recover. Marka was left a widow at the age of thirty-one. She moved with her two small sons back into her father's house, bringing him the solace of romping children and a bevy of pets in his home once more.

Leila had recently left that home, for marriage on 30 March 1936 to a dashing commercial airline pilot, Charles Harold Collins Jr., whom she had known since they were children in school together. She and "Tim," as Charles was known to all the Webbs, were married in New York, lived there awhile, then moved to California and later to Montana.

Joel, though, was soon living at home again. He said goodbye to the college work that bored him and returned to learn the banking business under his Uncle Jeff.

"I am resigned to it that neither of my boys will follow me in science and medicine. They are both inclined to go into business," Gerald told Frank. It is a plausible guess that he was not inconsolable about it. He repeatedly called doctoring "a dog's life" and for him it was not notably rich-making. It irked him that some of his friends in the NTA could give a thousand or more dollars at a time to fund the work of the Research Committee he had started, while he could spare so few dollars that he thought it less shaming to give nothing.

He expressed surprise that in these years of continuing financial stringency there were some who had money to spare for his Colorado Foundation for Research in Tuberculosis. Its funds grew slowly but they grew. By 1935 the endowment fund had crossed $150,000 and was earning $5,000 a year for the maintenance fund, which with regular donations from devoted angels amounted to between $8,000 and $11,000 annually.

When A. E. Carlton found it necessary to resign, Dr. Webb added the office of president to his own as research director. Ishbel MacLeish became a trustee and joined Alfred Cowles III as vice-president. Dr. Edward N. Chapman succeeded Cowles as secretary-treasurer. Other new members of the board were Webb's friends Robert G. McKay and Eugene P. Shove, a wealthy financier and philanthropist in Colorado Springs.

The deaths of William Thayer and Theobald Smith, the resignation of Dr. Forster, and the preoccupation of Livingston Farrand with university administration at Cornell left vacancies on the advisory council that Dr. Webb was pleased to fill with Doctors Allen K. Krause, Esmond R. Long, and Florence R. Sabin. Dr. Sabin in particular became Webb's staunch ally.

Of Huguenot ancestry and the daughter of a mine superintendent in Central City, Colorado, Florence Sabin was just a few months younger than Gerald Webb. After graduating from Smith College she stubbornly insisted against all advice in enrolling as one of the first few women students in the newly opened Johns Hopkins medical school. Her exceptional work—she ranked third in her class of 1900—singlehandedly dispelled the initial contempt of the faculty members for their "hen-medics."

Appointed to the Hopkins faculty, she proved herself a superb diagnostician and an equally fine teacher, but her passion, her only romance, was research. Spending countless hours night after night at her dissecting table and microscope she was able, among other achievements, to elucidate the ages-old mystery of the lymphatic system—its origin, organization, and function of cleansing the blood.

Dr. Sabin was induced to move to the Rockefeller Institute in 1925 when Dr. Simon Flexner decided it was time to admit tuberculosis once more to the Institute's agenda and invited her to head a concentrated attack on that disease. Almost immediately the NTA Committee on Research that Dr. Webb had initiated asked her also to coordinate the mélange of studies in tuberculosis going on at scattered universities, research institutes, and pharmaceutical houses. Making this the biggest cooperative venture in medical research up to that time, Florence accomplished wonders in fitting together innumerable bits of the puzzle, her own with others', to learn at last the chemical composition of the tubercle bacillus and the effects on tissue and blood of several components of the whole.

By the time the 65-and-out rule at the Institute forced her retirement she was bemedalled with honor the world over. And all the while, a shy, plain, dumpy woman, she wore the air, said an Institute colleague, "of a grandmother who had just put some cookies in the oven." Cooking was one of her hobbies in fact; others were going to the opera and the Dodger baseball games and camping out in wilderness areas.

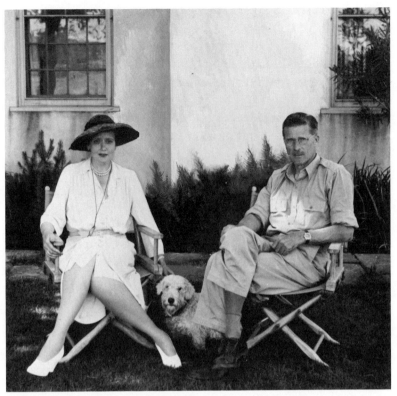

Ruth and Charles Boissevain at home

When she returned to live with an ailing, lonely sister in Denver and began a whole new career in public health, Gerald Webb lost no time in securing her participation and advice for his Colorado Foundation.

By this time Doctors Chapman and Ryder had joined James Waring as Webb's associate directors of research, leaving Dr. Boissevain in charge of the laboratory with Dr. Drea, working part time still, as his associate to carry on the experimental work with the assistance of a revolving staff of five or six younger doctors who came and went year by year.

Dr. Boissevain was sometimes a problem for Dr. Webb, justifying that early warning from Dr. Krause that the Dutchman's agile curiosity might lead him off the main track. He spent a season investigating intestinal bacteria instead of the tubercle bacillus; he gave myriad hours to a study of desert cactuses which, with the aid of Carol Davidson, the Osler niece who was Dr. Webb's patient, he made into a useful book, *Colorado Cacti*; and he, not Dr. Drea the dentist, swerved off into an investigation of tooth enamel.

For many years it had been a troubling question why the teeth of so many children brought up in Colorado Springs were mottled in color and later acquired an ugly brown stain. Concerned for his own children, Menso and Marie, Boissevain came to point when he read that a doctor in New York had found the discolored enamel in some communities in that state and thought it was somehow related to their water supply.

Charles immediately began collecting and analyzing samples of water from various places in Colorado and eventually concluded the mottled tooth enamel was caused by an excess of fluoride in the water supply of Colorado Springs.

According to Ruth Boissevain, before her husband could publish his study word of its conclusion got to the ears of the Chamber of Commerce and big guns therein came asking Dr. Webb to hush up Boissevain's facts lest they drive tourists and new residents away.

Before Dr. Webb could solve the problem, H. V. Churchill, a chemist working for the Aluminum Company of America, had reached the same conclusion about the cause of stained teeth and published it. Dr. Boissevain was left to report his study quietly in *Colorado Medicine*.

"So Charles never got proper credit for his discovery," said Ruth resentfully.

In the annual report of the Foundation Dr. Webb said, "Mr. Churchill completed his work one month before Dr. Boissevain, so that priority for the discovery rightly belongs to him." Gerald's own experience with the lymphocytosis-altitude correlation had made him unbending on this principle of credit for prior discovery.

Despite these distractions experimentation in the laboratory proceeded apace, following the trend of the times in emphasizing biochemistry. One line of investigation was aimed at determining the causes of natural immunity. Did resistance depend on the amount of ammonia in the blood? or on the amount of cholesterol? A second line tried out individual components of the tubercle bacillus to find out which of them caused the devastation it produced. Were its lipids to blame? or one of its proteins? or its carbohydrates? A third series tested allergic reactions to various substances including tuberculins.

Dr. Drea also went on trying to kill the bacilli or weaken their virulence by doses of X-ray and he searched for improvements in the mediums used to grow them.

By the mid-1930s the Foundation had published fifty-odd reports of its research, representing a highly respectable amount of work, especially considering conditions in the laboratory.

Its quarters were cramped beyond enduring. Rabbits, guinea pigs, and monkeys had to be caged and tended, a library and much equipment to be shelved, glassware and instruments to be sterilized, all in a jostle with experiments and experimenters in two small rooms. Workbenches were so few that some experiments had to be postponed or suspended to let others go forward. Priorities were argued about and sometimes tempers flared.

Dr. Webb kept hunting for larger quarters. Two successive years he tried in vain to persuade the city fathers to let the Foundation use a school building they were boarding shut. Then Colorado College, wanting the basement space in Palmer Hall for its own uses, offered to give the Foundation in exchange for it a former engineering and machine shop that stood abandoned west of Cutler Hall.

Despite the dilapidated, vandalized condition of the old building, Dr. Webb accepted the offer gladly. Since the Foundation could allocate only $9,000 for renovation, barely enough to buy the necessary materials, he argued the city council into endorsing his application to President Roosevelt's Works Progress Administration for free labor to do the job.

In May 1936 the Foundation laboratory was moved into its commodious new home, comprising three thousand square feet of floor space divided into twelve rooms: separate quarters for the animals, an X-ray room, a spectographic laboratory, a photographic dark room, an equipment and sterilizing room, and a library, in addition to five small individual laboratories and an office for Dr. Boissevain.

The motto FAC ET SPERA was retained and Webb added to it a graphic symbol executed by the noted New York book designer Warren Chappel: a guinea pig with an inoculating syringe for a tail.

From this time forward the Foundation's letterhead and its published reports carried a new line in its address: "At Colorado College."

At commencement a month later the college returned this favor by conferring upon Dr. Webb an honorary degree of doctor of science. Dean Charlie Brown Hershey made the presentation in a laudatory summation of the recipient's achievements and Dr. Webb was all sober dignity as he stooped to have the doctoral hood in college colors placed over the shoulders of his black academic robes, but the diploma given him stirred his risibilities. Scripted in formal Latin it conferred the degree upon Geraldum Bertramum Webb. He whispered to Dean Hershey he was glad they hadn't made it Webb-bum!

Honored with Gerald at this commencement were two good friends: John Gaw Meem, the Santa Fe architect noted especially for his adaptation of Pueblo Indian adobe forms into a distinctive southwestern style, and Boardman "Mike" Robinson, director of the new Fine Arts Center in Colorado Springs.

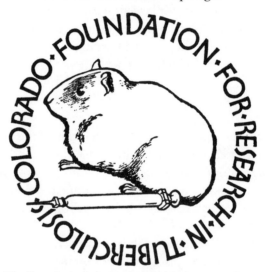

The Foundation's logo, designed by Warren Chappell

That Center was Julie Penrose's Broadmoor Art Academy reborn out of intricate scheming by Betty Hare. Her New Yorker's taste bored to revulsion by the old-style realism that adorned the Academy's walls, Betty thought Colorado Springs needed jerking into the twentieth century in the arts. She persuaded Julie Penrose to tear down the Dale Street house used by the Academy and donate the land for a new arts center. Then she took aim at the vast fortune of Alice Bemis Taylor, the widowed daughter of Judson Bemis of the Bemis Bag Company.

Mrs. Taylor was a woman of regal presence that hid a shy and malleable psyche. Behind her back everyone called her "Aunt Alice."

Her ideas for suitable philanthropy ran toward such things as a new library for Colorado College, toward which she pledged a gift of $400,000.

This sum became Betty Hare's target. She was abetted by John Gaw Meem, who was married to Mrs. Taylor's niece and who had built a dormitory for Mrs. Hare at the Fountain Valley School, and by Boardman Robinson, the Socialist head of the New York Art Students League and a WPA muralist in Washington DC whom Betty had brought out to teach art at her school. The three had an exhilarating time drawing up plans for the new center, tossing in multiple exhibition halls and studio wings and drama stages with glee. Then they descended upon Mrs. Taylor.

She was no match for them, certainly not for Betty's practiced blandishments. She withdrew her pledge to Colorado College and gave her $400,000 to the Fine Arts Center instead, plus an equal sum more before Meem's building was finished in the spring of 1936.

The week of avant-garde divertissements imported from New York by Betty Hare to mark the opening of the new Center—all of them paid for by a thoroughly bewildered Aunt Alice—left the citizens of Colorado Springs stunned and aghast, among them Dr. Gerald Webb.

Once upon viewing a painting by Gauguin in the home of Robert McKay, Gerald commented dryly, "I have not yet caught up with Gauguin's style." He never did catch up with it, certainly not with the explosively innovative works of Matisse and Picasso, nor with the "modern art" displayed in the opening exhibition put together by Betty Hare. After a long look at Brancusi's "Bird in Flight" he turned away muttering, "Where's the bird? It looks like a glycerine suppository to me."

The dancer that Betty Hare with elation secured to grace the opening was young Martha Graham and one of the numbers on her program was the now classic "Lamentation." Marka thought it expressive and moving, but her father was disgusted: "They call that dancing? It's nothing but a woman writhing in labor on an obstetrical chair."

The honorary degree from Colorado College was all the more timely because Dr. Webb had just published another book, a scholarly history of tuberculosis.

Since the Great War the library had almost wholly replaced the laboratory in Webb's personal research. He continued to keep up meticulously with new findings reported in medical books and journals and summarized them in his papers and speeches and his editorials for the *Journal of Laboratory and Clinical Medicine.* But his own attention focused increasingly on medical history.

This interest, sparked by Arnold Klebs, was fanned to heat when Webb in October 1929 attended the dedicatory ceremonies for the Institute of Medical History which Dr. William Henry Welch had planned as his last project for Johns Hopkins University. Webb's last meeting with Welch was when the tottering old man and Arnold Klebs, who had been Welch's chief adviser in purchasing the initial collection of books for the Institute's library and who planned to will his own great library to it, personally showed him through the Institute's fine new building. Their acquaintance with medical incunabula overwhelmed him. "It was an awesome feast of knowledge just to hear them talk."

He was equally awed to hear and meet the eminent medical historian Karl Sudhoff, whose Institute of Medical History at Leipzig had been Welch's model and whom Klebs persuaded to come from Germany to give the dedicatory address. "What a monumental knowledge of our medical yesterdays that man has!"

When Sudhoff's pupil and disciple, Dr. Henry E. Sigerist, succeeded Welch as director of the Hopkins Institute, Webb got to know him and his American counterpart in medical history, Fielding H. Garrison, and consulted them both frequently.

Dr. James Waring, himself a medical history buff since his student days under Osler, decided in 1933, when he became chairman of the department of medicine at the University of Colorado, that his fledgling medics ought to have a regular dose of information about their profession's past and invited Dr. Webb to administer it. Gerald eagerly accepted.

For five years, one morning each week Leila, later Marka and occasionally Joel, would drive Dr. Webb to Denver. After his lecture he would meet Dr. Waring in the cafeteria for lunch, always a merry respite for both men, then return to Colorado Springs in time to make the rounds of his patients as the sun set.

He doted on this weekly change of pace and his lectures made a hit with the students. Some of the notes from which he spoke are still in his files. He pegged the history he taught to the lives of great men and at first spoke only of the microbe hunters from Jenner down, but each year he extended his information farther back in time and included more about early pathologists, anatomists, and chemists. He illustrated his lectures with slides, many of which he made himself, copying illustrations from old books.

Inescapable is his constant emphasis on the way many of medicine's great achievers took off on their careers from a consuming interest in natural history.

In view of this experience and his previous books for Paul Hoeber, Webb was bound to be among the chosen authors when Hoeber decided to publish a series of "handbooks" on medical history under the editorship of Dr. E. B. Krumbhaar, professor of pathology at the University of Pennsylvania. The Clio Medica series they christened it, after the Muse of history. Dr. Webb was asked, in 1934 when he sought absorbing work after Varina's death, to write the volume on tuberculosis.

He might have tossed it off from his head, one would think. Instead he turned scrupulous scholar and spent innumerable hours, often for two weeks at a time, in libraries, especially the Surgeon General's Library in Washington and the library of the New York Academy of Medicine, bent over books and articles in four languages, taking notes with his trusty Corona portable on his knees.

From these notes, arranged under such chapter headings as Pathology, Contagion, Immunity, Sanatoria, Diagnosis, and Treatment, Webb produced a book that at first skimming seems "more typing than writing" (to adapt a capsule criticism from Truman Capote)—more a catalogue of names and notions than a narrative, allotting more space to the weird ideas and practices of ancient India and Egypt, of classical Greece and medieval Europe, than to developments during his own lifetime.

But a second reading arouses admiration for the amount of information Webb packed into his handbook, the fascinating facts and quotations he chose to present the history, the illuminating way he carried each subject from remote past to immediate present, making clear over and over again the theme he stated for the whole, that "there is nothing truly new under the sun." Even the infecting microbes discovered in the late 1800s were only a sharpened definition of the *seminaria* of Frascatorius in the 1500s and of "the little seeds that fly about to cause disease" of Lucretius in the century before Christ.

Webb's completed manuscript of some 50,000 words plus a bibliography of 138 items was mailed to Hoeber in the fall of 1935 and published in early spring 1936. The book was dedicated "with affection to the brave victims of tuberculosis who have been guided by the author."

At a convention two years later Dr. Webb encountered Editor Krumbhaar who congratulated him on the excellent reception given his *Tuberculosis* and told him it was on the press for its third printing of one thousand copies and that it was by far the best seller in the Clio Medica series.

Webb expressed surprise. He had thought the book was not selling at all since he had received no royalties from it. Dr. Krumbhaar, a proper and fussy man, twittered his dismay. He would check up with Hoeber at once.

It turned out that Hoeber had been sending all the Clio Medica royalties to Dr. Krumbhaar, expecting him to divide them with his authors according to their respective contracts. The poor man was embarrassed beyond bearing and apologized elaborately. He scrupulously set down the dollars and cents he had received for *Tuberculosis* and said he would send Webb a check for his half of the amount. Since the sum due Gerald was less than a hundred dollars he told Krumbhaar to keep the money "for your editorial labors."

So Webb's history of tuberculosis earned him not one cent. Paul Hoeber seems to have got the best of this deal.

That November of 1936 Gerald set off on the most exciting trip of his life. His reading for *Tuberculosis*, added to letters from Robine while she was on vacation in Cairo, made him eager to see Egypt but he thought he could only dream of going there; he certainly could not afford it. Hearing him talk of it, Maria McKean Allen sent him a generous check to pay for the trip as an early Christmas gift.

One of his patients at Glockner, a man from Baltimore, learning that Dr. Webb would be going first to England, gave him an enthusiastic letter of introduction to Wallis Warfield Simpson. Gerald left the letter behind; he had no desire to meet that woman. He and Frank had been exchanging disappointments about Edward VIII's letting them all down and agreed that, in Frank's words, "the woman is the stuff of which tarts are made."

He went first to England and the visit was depressing. Amy and dinner one night was introduced to Howard Carter the discoverer of King Tut's tomb and Maestro Arturo Toscanini, whose look of "ascetic remoteness" was belied, Gerald thought, by "the fiery intensity of his black deepset eyes."

These devoirs paid, Gerald took a slow boat up the Nile some five hundred miles to Luxor and Karnak to see the famous temples on the site of ancient Thebes. He remarked in particular upon the mix of Egyptian gods, Christian church, and Moslem shrine he saw in the great long temple at Luxor.

All the way he kept clicking his camera as an aide-memoire and searching for medical mementos in museums and shops. He picked up a few shards of ancient pottery that retained painted figures he admired, a copper statuette of Imhotep the half-legendary father of Egyptian medicine, and several old medical pictures and sketches. Two of these especially took his fancy because they demonstrated how commonplaces of later medical practice had developed from mistaken interpretations of observed animal behavior. One showed a hippopotamus with bloody sweat pouring down its flanks is said to have given rise to blood-letting in the treatment of disease, and another depicting an ibis preening its anal feathers was described as the origin of the enema.

He returned home in early May 1937 in high spirits, which soared higher when he found awaiting him a certificate of qualification, dated 1 December 1936, from the newly established Internal Medicine Board. Let anyone like Dr. Charles Fox Gardiner question his credentials now!

During the following summer the flow of patients to Colorado Springs picked up again "in a remarkable way" and Webb's practice was worryingly heavy throughout the succeeding winter. The depression still hung on for the nation but for some citizens times were getting better.

As Webb traveled his convention and speaking rounds in the winter of 1938 strain and weariness must have been showing in his face. Frank R. Spencer, a physician practicing in Boulder, met him on the train from New York to New Orleans in March and immediately on getting home wrote to President George Norlin of the University of Colorado, Spencer's alma mater, to suggest that Dr. Webb be considered for an honorary doctor of science at commencement that year. His accomplishments certainly made him worth it, said Spencer, and if it was to be given him it should be

Harold seemed acceptably well but Ida's husband Fre
and Ida herself was becoming so confused mentally tha
soon require custodial care in a nursing home. Wilfr
retiring at age sixty-two from the Crossley Works,
distressingly senile. And Frank and Ann were a pa
she with crippling arthritis, he with an injury to his
him double.

When Frank said he was also worried about his
sistently at about 46, Gerald was reassuring: "N
that. It's a family trait, probably from Mater. ?
low pulse, mine is seldom much above 60, and
the same. It's a good thing—it will see us all ir

He had an embarrassing time with Lilian
Amy, much concerned, wrote Frank about it:
cap for Gerald. She is pleading with him to
States with him and let her be his housekee₁
all a joke, but it isn't. She means to marry ₁
good husbands the Webb men make, and sʰ
her trap before he knows it. I've warned ₁
You must tell him to watch out."

Gerald was not so blind as Amy thou₁
Frank, "I'm taking care not to be alone v
when Eric is present." And he purposelʸ
when the time came, "giving England
miss."

He did not see the horror that was
Europe and did not guess that he wo

He had surprisingly little to say ab
Greece, perhaps because his imprₑ
were swept away by the overwhel
the bright and intense colors he saw
and teeming bazaars during a loₙ
their infant son Fred in Ankara ₁

He arrived in Egypt in early ₁
the Pharoahs delightful beyond
the home of the British High C
wife Camilla was the daughtₑ
patient Jay Lippincott. He m
been so helpful to him duriₙ
fourteen years before. He aₜ

soon—implying that he thought Webb was not in good health.

And Aldous Huxley, running into Webb in California two weeks later, wrote his brother Julian that their friend the good doctor was looking old. Gerald was sixty-six at the time.

In mid-April he received a cable from Constance Pulitzer Elmslie. She had been taken ill while following his footsteps in Egypt and asked him please to meet her at Doctors Hospital in New York. He took the train east again immediately, writing Frank enroute, "I have been a shuttle between the Atlantic and the Pacific these last six weeks. Train life is getting tiresome."

Too much so this time. While having lunch with Constance in her hospital room he was struck with a severe pain in his chest and arms and collapsed.

The diagnosis was coronary thrombosis. Dr. James. A. Miller put him to bed in Room 803 of Doctors Hospital and summoned Dr. Robert Levy, an eminent Park Avenue cardiologist, to take care of him. Dr. Levy kept him flat on his back for three weeks, then gradually allowed him a few minutes, an hour, two hours a day of sitting up.

Word of his illness spread with the wind. He was showered with "a staggering amount of mail" and gifts galore. Flowers and books overflowed into other rooms. Constance, worried and feeling guilty, ordered a swank outfit of pajamas and robe in maroon velvet delivered to his room. And Betty Hare, living in New York again after Meredith's death, with her usual imaginative flair sent him a live anthill under glass. He loved it; his nurses hated it. They were sure "those nasty crawly things" would find a way to get out of their confining dome.

When he was not sleeping or reading—he said he found *Lawrence of Arabia* and Churchill's *Marlborough* "engrossing"—or scribbling notes of thanks, he was carrying on a dialogue in doggerel with his nurses. They entered into the verse game with a will and skill, and a merry flirtatious time was had by all.

After six weeks in Room 803 he was released from the hospital. Several of his doctor friends offered their homes or yachts for his further recovery and he chose the summer cottage of Dr. Joseph "Joe" Wheelright, Betty Hare's physician-friend, on the dunes at Southhampton. Marka came on from Colorado to take care of him during an additional month of lazy convalescence by the sea.

The Wheelright cottage was a cozy haven as Gerald described it on postcards home to grandsons Gerry and Chuck, playfully assigning names to its furnishings. The iron ducks that served as andirons in the fireplace he christened Socrates and Xantippe.

He and Marka returned to 1222 North Cascade in early July. But to a strange new way of life for Gerald Webb. Dr. Levy had forbidden him all work, driving a car, tennis, hikes, cold showers, air baths, night life! He was to rise late, nap after lunch, retire at six o'clock, and take only the lightest of exercise. "It is as if a high-powered car had been knocked suddenly into reverse," he said.

He could accept this restrictive regimen the more easily because he still suffered a good deal of pain. He said nothing about it even to Frank at the time, wrote only of an occasional spell of gout, but three years later when Betty Hare, recovering from a heart attack in her turn, wrote to him seeking comfort for her limited activity and continuing physical distress, he told her that for him too it had been more than a year before he was free from "a mean pain"—and from "those blue devils that I suppose must always haunt a person after an affaire de coeur."

Of course. He had suffered the psychological shock that comes with the first clear warning of one's own mortality. Not only had he lost—forever, given the cardiac therapy of the time—most of the diversions that had made his life vital; he had lost too his previous sense of secure wellbeing, his confident expectation of splendid adventures in his tomorrows. He was himself acquainted now with the near prospect of death.

Twice during the late months of 1938 in writing to friends he quoted what Thomas Huxley once wrote to John Morley: "It flashes across me with a sort of horror that in 1900 I shall know no more of what is going on than I did in 1800."

He chased away such dark thoughts by keeping his mind busy. He sent to Boston for books about butterflies and dragonflies and in quiet hours outdoors made a study of these creatures, eventually ordering nets and mounting pins and other such paraphernalia to help his grandsons begin a collection of the gossamer lovelies. And he spent many hours in his study pasting into scrapbooks the big bundles of clippings that had accumulated since Varina's death, along with the hundreds of snapshots and picture postcards he had brought home from Greece, Turkey, and Egypt.

Onlookers may have smiled at such incongruous occupations for a man who had been voted an honorary doctor of science degree by the University of Colorado. The committee in charge of such matters had accepted Dr. Spencer's suggestion and the degree was to have been conferred at the university's commencement in June. Now President Norlin proposed it be awarded at the summer commencement in August, but he did so anxiously. He did not want to overtax Dr. Webb's strength but he did want him to receive the degree as soon as possible lest he die without getting it!

Marka and Joel took their father to Denver for the ceremony, at which Dr. James Waring made the presentation in a delightfully informal and affectionate style. There was no pretentious Latin this time. Waring even told the audience about the neighborhood cats the boy Gerald was suspected of spiriting away for dissection.

As always in such biographical sketches of Dr. Webb there were some inaccuracies in Waring's remarks. For example, there is no evidence, and the circumstances make it extremely unlikely, that Webb was ever offered a teaching post at Guy's Hospital as Waring said he was—thinking perhaps of the offers he had received from Michigan and Harvard—and his postdoctoral study in Europe lasted nine months, not Waring's two years.

But those were trifles. Waring included the important things: Webb's research interests and achievements, his insistence on treating mind and spirit as well as body, and the testimony of a professional colleague who knew whereof he spoke that "in our medical world Colorado Springs has become synonymous with Gerald Webb."

Of the letters that kept coming to wish Dr. Webb a speedy recovery none were so cheering as those from his son Gerry, who had now arrived in his proper niche as editor of the *Chronicle*, a horseman's and hunting journal in Middleburg, Virginia. The young man had learned to write as well as he rode and his activities gave him plenty to write about.

For instance, screen tests were under way for the role of Rhett Butler in the motion picture of *Gone with the Wind* and Gerry, egged on by his friends who thought it would be hilariously fitting for the great-grandson of Jefferson Davis to play the part, took the test. He had a lot of fun in the process of losing and shared that fun in a vivid letter to his father.

He saw the completed picture in a pre-release screening at the White House. Franklin Roosevelt Jr. was studying law at the University of Virginia and he and his wife Ethel joined the fox-hunting crowd in which young Webb was popular. So Gerry was among the thirty friends the junior Roosevelts invited to dinner and the screening afterward in the dining and ball rooms of the White House. He was also one of the six invited to join the President and Mrs. Roosevelt for cocktails in FDR's private study upstairs before dinner.

Gerry made a lively tale of the experience in a seven-page letter to his father, describing all he had seen and heard, from the scrutiny by the Secret Service when he arrived to his night on the town with Franklin Jr. and Ethel after the movie. He had expected it to be "a sticky sort of party" but was reassured by FDR's affable informality as he shook up martinis and dispensed them from his wheelchair. "He does win you."

Gerry was awed by the "sniffy hauteur" of the President's mother and expressed pity for Eleanor Roosevelt's "lack of joy" and her "impatience to break up the drinking and chatting and get on to the dinner downstairs. The President was in no hurry. I think he was enjoying himself with us. He offered to shake up another round but Mrs. Roosevelt's frown made us all refuse."

The dinner was more formal. "The food was plain—good old roast beef etc., but the room and the service were so splendid they gave me goose bumps." The movie was "a work of genius," he thought; it kept them all sitting on the edge of their hard ballroom chairs for its full four hours. "The fiery Scarlett is a real stunner."

Gerald reciprocated these entertaining, heartening letters by slowly gathering together the notes he had been making since seeing the paintings of primitive horses in the caves of the Dordogne and writing them up in an article on "The Evolution and Extinction of the Horse in America" for Gerry to publish in the *Chronicle*. He claimed no originality for this piece; he candidly listed the books on the subject he had acquired over the years from the American Museum of Natural History, along with the fossils he had seen in that museum, the Philadelphia Zoo, and the Colorado shale deposits.

He was filled with wonder at the expanse of time covered by his story, which was then thought to have been fifty or so million years, and by the numerous stages of evolution from five-toed animals the size of a collie dog to hooved creatures reaching thirteen hands. Reporting that these horses had disappeared from the American continents before the Indians arrived, probably at about the time of the second Pleistocene ice age that did in the dinosaurs, he clearly preferred to think the cause of their extinction was not the freezing out of their fodder as generally assumed but instead an epidemic of fatal sickness carried by the tsetse fly.

XVIII

Gentle Slope

As the year 1938 came to an end Dr. Webb said he was, like Sam Weller in *Pickwick Papers*, "reasonably convalescent." When his local cardiologist, Dr. John L. McDonald, reported that the T-wave of his electrocardiogram had remained upright for eight weeks Dr. Levy gave him permission to drive his car again and go back to work for half of each day.

He made light of the continuing limits on his activity. "I'm learning late that I can make an adequate living in half a day and do what I want to the rest of the time." But he still tired quickly and recovered from fatigue more slowly. And he yielded noticeably to melancholy at the news of deaths that came trickling in.

His brother Harold died in 1939 and Wilfred soon thereafter. He was disheartened for weeks over the deaths of Harvey Cushing and Livingston Farrand, also in 1939, and by the illness and death of Spencer Penrose the same year. He had worked with Penrose on the boards of numerous projects including the Foundation and they had become friends, though never social buddies.

Spencer was struck with an attack of hoarseness while he and Julie were in Hawaii and it would not go away. Stopping off in Philadelphia on the way home he telephoned Dr. Webb to ask what he could do about it and Gerald advised him to see his friend Dr. Chevalier Jackson, the eminent bronchoscopist.

While Spec and Julie were awaiting the doctor's verdict, Dr. Webb and Marka arrived to stay overnight on their way to the convention of the Association of American Physicians in Atlantic City.

The four were having lunch in the Penroses' hotel suite when Dr. Jackson came to tell them the diagnosis was inoperable cancer of the larynx. There was a moment of stunned silence, then as tears appeared in Julie's eyes, Spencer jumped to his feet and said, "Let's all go to the Zoo." And they did.

Spencer died eight months later after many weeks in bed at his Broadmoor home El Pomar. His benefactions to Colorado Springs were continued, and extended to the entire state of Colorado, by the El Pomar Foundation which he established and to which he willed his immense fortune.

At that 1939 convention in Atlantic City Dr. Webb was handed the blue ribbon of his blue ribbon: he was elected president of the Association of American Physicians.

It was not a surprise; he had been elected vice-president the year before and in the AAP succession from second to first was the rule. But by Jove, it *was* gratifying to join the company of previous presidents he had so much admired: Osler, Welch, Hermann Biggs, Victor Vaughan, Simon Flexner, William Thayer, Henry Sewall among them.

The badge of his office was a special gavel made from the wood of Sir William Osler's house in Canada. It was a beautifully crafted piece but possession of it was as much burden as pleasure for Dr. Webb. When James Waring told him near the end of his term that the AAP had plenty of the Osler wood for the making of more gavels, Webb said, "They might have told me that! Then I wouldn't have been scared to death all the time that something would happen to the gavel while I had it."

The congratulatory festivities attending his election tired him out. On the train to New York he told Marka he thought it would be wiser for him to stay in the city only long enough for a checkup by Dr. Levy and then go home, forgoing the NTA convention in Boston he had planned to attend. The coming summer would be a strain, he thought; Sir Bruce Bruce-Porter, the father-in-law of Nell's son Geoffrey was coming for a visit in late May and that would mean entertaining and sightseeing; then on 25 July would come Joel's marriage to Barbara Shove Palmer, the New Jersey niece of his friend Eugene P. Shove. There were sure to be many guests from out of town and lots of parties for Joel and Bobbie; he had better rest to be ready for them.

So it was from the newspaper at home that Dr. Webb learned the NTA had awarded him its highest honor, the Trudeau Medal.

Dr. Boissevain was present at the meeting and accepted the medal on Webb's behalf. The presentation, a laudatory recital of Webb's achievements in research, his principles of therapy, and his many honors, concluding with a warm tribute to "his charming personality reinforced by a gentle but firm authority," was made by Dr. Charles J. Hatfield, the executive secretary to whom he had clung while president of the association.

In his presidential address to the AAP the next spring Dr. Webb did not make the mistake of trying to impress by profundity. He spoke briefly, simply, in his usual engaging way.

Eyebrows went up probably at sight of his topic on the program, "Prescribing the Scrap-Book," but he disarmed his audience by telling them at once that he knew they were saying "My God!"— like that athletic patient when he suggested she replace her tennis with keeping a scrapbook. Saying he was offering them "a trifle, but trifles make perfection," he explained why he thought the unimportant scrapbook "a means to great ends, a major weapon against the ennui of long illness and convalescence."

To illustrate the universal interest in scrapbooks he told of attending a "tea party" given recently by a recovered patient of his from twenty years ago. When, thinking ahead to this paper, he asked her if she remembered the scrapbook she made when she was ill, she exclaimed, "I've been making them ever since!" and pointed to the long row of them on her bookshelves.

"She pulled some of them down to show me, and in no time at all the whole party was on the floor poring over them. The joy those adults took in those scrapbooks is something I wish every physician could see. A simple thing, you may say, but nonetheless an important reminder of the sad fact that too often we physicians learn the medical textbook by rote but fail to acquire any knowledge of the human heart."

He then began to show and tell. He had lugged along one of his own scrapbooks and leafed through its pages to demonstrate the personal choice and variety it permitted its maker—and not incidentally the wide range of his own interests.

Here was an article about the fossils of the tsetse fly found in the Florrisant shale near his home, and next a piece by Julian Huxley, "an old friend and patient," arguing that man had only begun to develop a brain. Following notes on the evolution of the horse in America and a clipping about his cougar hunt with the late Theodore Roosevelt came medical pictures from Egypt.

Next appeared in sequence a newspaper report of casualties in the Great War, notes on nesting robins, cartoons from *Punch*, an article by the noted American anthropologist Ales Hrdlicka stating his conviction that there had been no tuberculosis in the New World before the white man arrived, a column of wartime poems, a newspaper account of the chess match Webb won from Emanuel Lasker in New York, a picture of his son Gerry astride the famous jumper "Easy Mark," a speech by Lord Halifax on Hitler and the Nazis.

On that last item Dr. Webb commented, "The great democracies of Europe, finding they had been playing in a diplomatic poker game with pickpockets and gangsters, are now trying to make the world safe for decency."

For some time Gerald had been watching events in Europe with foreboding. He and Frank had argued at length whether Prime Minister Neville Chamberlain's concessions to Hitler in the Munich Pact were appeasement or a wise compromise to keep the peace. When the Germans crushed Czechoslovakia and swept through Poland and then into Belgium, Frank said, "Now we know. You were right. He sold us out." Gerald answered merely, "The cave men are on the loose again over there. It makes me anxious."

As the Allies suffered initial reverses on all fronts, he grew impatient. He did not consider the evacuation from Dunkirk an admirably executed operation, only an inglorious defeat, and he wrote the Post Wheelers to that effect, adding a sharp thrust, "I think it's time England turned her affairs over to be managed by the U.S., with apologies for the shape they're in."

But he was upset by the government's insistence on American neutrality and by the vociferous isolationism of the Midwest and West. He went in person to the editor of the local *Gazette* to protest the paper's anti-involvement stand, wrote his senator, Alva B. Adams, to urge that the United States sell its reconditioned destroyers to Great Britain, and, overcoming his antipathy to begging for money, collected enough from his friends and acquaintances to purchase an ambulance and send it from Colorado Springs to the American Field Service in France.

He also requested reinstatement as a member of the American Legion, from which he had resigned in the 1920s "because I did not approve of some of your policies."

When the Battle for Britain began and the papers told of severe rationing in England, he and the girls started sending parcels of food regularly to Frank and Amy. At first Frank stood stiff on his dignity: "You need not take the trouble. We have all the food we need." But soon, and on until well after the war's end, he was truly grateful, carefully reporting to whom he had given each item in the parcel and even sometimes asking that the next one include more sugar or chocolate or tea or soap or whatever was in shortest supply at the moment.

Meanwhile a group of Colorado Springs entrepreneurs, Chase Stone at their head, all certain the United States would enter the conflict sooner or later, foresaw the disappearance of the city's income from tourists and invalids and the depopulation of the place when the young men left for military service and the workmen for jobs in war industries.

Well, there would be many thousands of soldiers moving around. The men thought they ought to try to secure some of them to keep life and dollars flowing in Colorado Springs. They launched an ingenious campaign to dispel the myth prevailing in Congress and the Army that the Pikes Peak region was snowbound nine months of the year and prove instead that it was perfect in climate and location for a military training camp.

The result was Camp Carson, named for the legendary mountain man Kit Carson, a $30,000,000 installation for housing upwards of 40,000 draftees on 35,000 acres the city had acquired adjoining Broadmoor. (This camp, later Fort Carson, was the forerunner of a succession of even juicier military plums handed to Colorado Springs as the years rolled along.)

When the Japanese bombing of Pearl Harbor impelled the United States into the war, Dr. Webb, apparently forgetting he was now seventy and in impaired health but remembering what were perhaps the most satisfying years of his life, itched to get into the action again. Confident of acceptance he wrote the Surgeon General offering his services in the Medical Corps and suggesting he be assigned to duty as a consultant at Camp Carson.

The words of the Surgeon General's reply were kindly; its message was not. It told Dr. Webb the Medical Corps preferred to enroll young men for active service; old men like himself could serve best by staying home to look after the civilian population.

Though this was hardly a surprising official policy, it really jolted Dr. Webb. For the first time he began expressing the common feelings of the retired and the old. He was no longer wanted. They thought him useless. They were putting him away on the shelf. All his experience and achievements were forgotten, ignored as unimportant. Self-pity crept into a carbon-copied letter he wrote to the scattered members of his family: "You are the ones out in the world doing its work now, while I must sit here idle and watch."

When Gerry, resurrecting his dream of flying, enlisted in the Army Air Corps and was sent for training as a pilot to a base near New York, he wrote to ask his father for a letter of introduction to his friends in that area. Gerald refused it. "A letter from me would be of no use to you. Nobody there knows me anymore."

That was absurd of course. True, many of his old friends were dead or ill and others were losing their status and power to younger men, but just as many retained influence in medical circles and kept in touch with him—Jim Miller, Simon Flexner, Reginald Fitz, Lewis Hamman, Hugh Young among others. Dr. Young, the Baltimore surgeon whom Webb had guided through a spell of incipient tuberculosis and who had just published his autobiography and was hopscotching around the country to promote the sale of it, kept sending Gerald bulletins like this one from Pittsburgh, "I just ran into another devoted former patient of yours. They are everywhere!"

Webb himself was not devoid of influence. He was asked to serve as adviser to the panel charged with appointing physicians to high offices in the Medical Corps and was thanked effusively for "your inestimable help in our work." The NTA named him chairman of the committee appointed to choose the next recipient of the Trudeau Medal. And he remained active on the Board of Regents and the Board of Governors of the American College of Physicians and on the editorial board of the *Annals of Medicine*, the official organ of the College. Here he made new and younger friends who became as devoted to him as any he had ever had—notably a fellow editor of the *Annals*, Dr. Oliver H. Perry-Pepper of Philadelphia and his wife Lalite.

When Gerald loaned Perry-Pepper his first edition copies of the works of Laënnec, Lalite, not knowing the value of original bindings however worn, returned the books rebound in exquisite French papers she had gone to enormous trouble to find. Gerald must have been dismayed but he thanked her affectionately: "It is a great joy to receive this gift from your hands."

In his black mood all this was stale crumbs in comparison with the days when he had known everyone of significance in his medical world and was often the man in charge. He could only accentuate the negative. When the Association of American Physicians and the New York Academy of Medicine, for which he had been a perennially favorite speaker and which had voted him an honorary life membership, solicited papers from him for their annual programs, he refused them both. To Dr. Hugh Morgan of the AAP he said, "I am too far out of the scientific mainstream. I prefer to let my talk on the scrap-book be my swan song." To the secretary of the Academy, Dr. Iago Galdston, he excused himself because "I have nothing to say."

Dr. Galdston's response was warm: "I can't think of a better reason for refusing to speak than because you have nothing to say. But we don't believe it. We shall ask you again, you may be sure. We covet your presence and your wise words."

Straitening circumstances may have fed Gerald's blue devils. The number of his private patients had dwindled to no more than eight, in addition to sixty tuberculous men at the Printers Home. He complained of "this terrific jump in the income tax. I shall have to cut down hard to save up for it."

Nor could he get away for diversion. In 1940 and 1941 he had felt strong enough, with Marka at his side, to journey east in the spring for the usual conventions. Now the trains were again overloaded with military traffic in men and supplies and journeying by civilians was discouraged and made difficult; they were ruthlessly bumped and left stranded enroute.

At home Gerald's life and family were set awry by the war and he no longer had the resilience to adjust readily. He worried about Gerry who wrote that he was slated for service in the Far East, and about Robine until the State Department moved Vevy from the danger zone in Istanbul to a safer station in Montreal. Leila, thank goodness, was nearer home, having moved with her two sons Timothy and Michael to Denver when the military claimed her pilot husband. Joel, refused for military service because of the stiffness in his back, was sent to manage the branch the First National Bank opened at Camp Carson, and Marka went to work full time at the main bank in town to help out her Uncle Jeff who was left shorthanded by the manpower drain into the armed forces.

There was not even the relief of Frank's acerbic humor. His wife Ann died in early spring 1942 and he wrote now almost wholly of his awful sense of loss and his desperate loneliness in the hotel room into which he had moved.

Like Varina before him, Gerald fell back on the cheery companionship of Opal Wojtacha. "Come on, Opal, let's drive out to see the spring wildflowers," he would say.

And he escaped into the major task he had undertaken just before the war began. He had said yes when Mrs. Henry Sewall asked him to write a biography of her husband. He felt honored, not least because he knew several others had sought Mrs. Sewall's permission to do this story and she had refused them.

He had a plethora of sources to work from in addition to his own memories of the man. Mrs. Sewall turned over to him a sizable collection of letters, manuscripts, notebooks, and photographs, and he wrote to mutual friends to ask for their recollections of Sewall and any letters of his they had kept. Florence Sabin and Allen Krause, with both of whom Dr. Sewall had corresponded voluminously for decades, both sent him bundles of letters.

But now as Gerald worked through these materials and Sewall's published papers, especially those of his later years when he had turned reflective and philosophical, they added to his gloom.

Dr. Sewall had not found much to praise in the coming of old age. He scoffed at the notion that it brings "poise and peace and placidity. What it brings are prostatectomy, boils, and plaster casts and other such miseries...and loneliness—no one around any more to let the mind roam with—when it is up to roaming. I whistle that I may not weep." Looking back, Sewall concluded he had ordered his life all wrong, that he had spent too much time experimenting in search of a few not very important facts and "not enough in searching for truth by the use of my mind alone."

Gerald wondered, had he made a similar mistake? Had he given too much time to activity, too little to thought? "Did it do any good for me to hurtle around so much?"

All in all, it is hardly surprising that in late fall 1942 Dr. Webb was stricken with a second heart attack.

Weeks in bed again. This time his mind turned often to recollections of times past and to longing for the mountains, and when Marka sought his help in devising the family Christmas card for that year he suggested she order reproductions of an old photograph of Webb Peak in the San Juan Mountains where he had often gone to climb.

It is a lovely picture of a snowcapped symmetrical peak framed by a virgin stand of tall pines on the shore of Emerald Lake below.

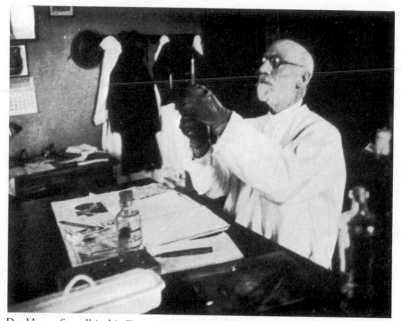

Dr. Henry Sewall in his Denver laboratory—"his work with the snakes was the beginning of immunology"

Percy Hagerman had christened it Webb Peak one time when he and Gerald were climbing it together and the name appears on old maps of the region. But stuffy bureaucrats in the U.S. Geological Survey persistently refused to make the name official because Webb was "just a doctor." What did he do to deserve a mountain named after him?

By his own choice Gerald spent his additional month of convalescence this time, during the deep winter of January 1943, in the company of old friends Phil and Fanny Stewart at a comfortable lodge in the mountain wilderness of Montana. There was no clambering up and down the canyons and ravines this time, no cougar-hunting, not even fishing. But the sounds and silences, the crystalline air, the "unsullied snow and sweet wind song in the trees" were healing.

For his rebellious spirit as well as his damaged heart. Or it may have been the second coronary attack itself that effected the change. Whichever, from this time on Gerald seems to have accepted his lot, quit lamenting it, made the best of the limitations it imposed.

When he resumed his work part time in the late spring of 1943 the biography of Sewall became, as he said, "a millstone around my neck." He felt pressed to get on with it. Mrs. Sewall was not well and he must finish it before she died. Or he did.

Sewall's adult decades, the years when Gerald had known him well, visited and talked with him often, were not difficult to recapture. But Webb found in his materials little information about Sewall's life before the 1890s and he could hardly go journeying to dig it out.

Remembering Desmond Powell, a professor at Stanford who had been his patient and very helpful while he was compiling facts for his *Tuberculosis*, he wrote to ask if Powell would be free for the summer and would help him again. The professor would, so Gerald "commissioned" him to search out the facts about Sewall's forebears and early years in Virginia, Maryland, New York, and Michigan and write them up in rough draft for the early chapters of the book. Gerald himself filled in the necessary medical background and carried the story on from the time of Sewall's experiments with snake venom at the University of Michigan.

With a great sense of release in the spring of 1944 he mailed the completed manuscript to the Johns Hopkins University Press which had agreed to publish it. It took the edge off his satisfaction, though, that Mrs. Sewall died and never saw the book because the wartime shortage of paper delayed publication until the spring of 1946.

Why Paul Hoeber did not publish the biography we do not know. Mrs. Sewall or her close friend James Waring may have suggested, even requested, publication by the Johns Hopkins press because of Dr. Sewall's early association with that university.

Webb's relations with Paul Hoeber were not strained. At this very time Hoeber wrote him cordially that his and Ryder's *Overcoming Tuberculosis* was still selling well, that his *Tuberculosis* was being reprinted again, in "a miniature edition" because of the paper shortage, but that Hoeber was having to put his *Laënnec* out of print. It had actually been out of stock since 1941 and Dr. Webb had been answering at least one request a month for a copy of it with the word that none was available.

Henry Sewall, Physiologist and Physician was the equal of *Laënnec* in engrossing readability, re-creating an extraordinary person in Webb's anecdotal, sensitively human way. It won acclaim in general magazines, including the *New York Times Book Review*, as well as in medical journals, and it has recently been rediscovered—

and abundantly used as I have used it—by pulmonary specialist Dr. L. Fred Ayvasian in writing an article about the Trudeau medalists for the *American Review of Respiratory Disease*. Dr. Ayvasian found Sewall to be "the most unknown today" of the medalists and remarked in an accent of surprise that Webb's book on Sewall is "a neglected and well-written, an excellent biography."

Webb said he wrote the book "in the hope of garnering for Sewall's original researches a recognition denied them while he was living." He made a plausible case, not only for Sewall as the unacknowledged source for the work of Von Behring and Roux and even perhaps of Koch, but also as the uncredited laboratory assistant who suggested the experiments that first made Edward Trudeau famous: "no subsequent work from Trudeau had so great a spark of originality."

Webb bolstered his case with the German recognition reported by Roger Morris in his letter of 1905 and clinched it, to his way of thinking, with the testimony of Dr. William Henry Howell, the preeminent American physiologist of his generation, in a letter to Mrs. Sewall: "Henry's work with the snakes was the beginning of the science of immunology."

Gerald put a great deal of his own medical life and experience into his biography of Sewall. Dr. Walter Palmer, a friend at the University of Chicago, writing to congratulate him on "a grand achievement," added: "I see in many a sentence and many a paragraph, behind the figure of Henry Sewall, the lineaments of Gerald Webb."

So it was with some justification that Gerald, when his children kept urging him to write his autobiography now, dismissed their pleas with "There's no need for that; it's all in the book on Sewall."

They could not be expected to allow for the diminished energy that comes with age, to understand how impossible it would be for their father, having got rid of "the millstone round my neck," to face the prolonged labor of producing another book.

His writing now was all in letters. Ever since Varina's death he had taken upon himself her task of sending a weekly letter to all the members of the family who were not at home, including the relatives in England. He gave his Sunday afternoons to pounding out on his Corona, with carbon copies often numbering as many as eight, a digest of what he had been reading that week. The variety of topics and information was impressive but his abstracts were uncharacteristically dull and juiceless, bearing all the marks of a chore to be got through. He himself called them his "weakly" letters. Any life in them was reserved for the personal postscript he penned on each copy.

Much livelier were the two additional letters he wrote each week to Gerry, who was now in a bomber group stationed in India and flying dangerous daily missions over the Hump in Burma. These bulletins of family news were often tinged with reminiscence — for example, "What you write about the heavy rains reminds me of the downpours we used to have at Tall Timbers. And do you remember our battle against all the rattlesnakes? And that old skinny cow that came nosing around to peek in the window?"

It was a great joy to have Gerry, after more than two years' absence, come home for a ten-day furlough in February 1945. But by then grandson Gerry, Marka's older boy, had enlisted in the Navy at seventeen and gone off to the naval training base in San Diego. "Please God the war will end before he is sent to sea."

There was the constant problem of keeping the Printers Home staffed with doctors and Dr. Webb was continually writing here and there to locate someone to fill a vacancy. He usually had to make do with ailing oldsters, most of them tuberculous themselves and able to work only part time.

And there was the Foundation laboratory to be watched over.

Charles Boissevain, chafing at the thought of the German yoke upon his native Holland but refused admission to the Medical Corps because of his asthma, in 1943 enlisted in the Sanitary Corps as a means of entry to service. As he hoped, he was soon transferred to the Medical Corps as a major and was stationed at a base hospital in England.

With him away, with Dr. Drea still clinging to his dental practice as income assurance, with no younger doctors coming along in search of laboratory experience, and with contributions drying up to drips, the animals had to be sacrificed and experimentation geared way down. Dr. Webb placed the staff physiologist, Dr. Mary Alice Hamilton of the Colorado College faculty, in custodial charge. He went regularly to the Foundation library to use its incoming journals to keep himself abreast of developments in tuberculosis research.

In 1940 he had written what was to be his farewell editorial for the *Journal of Laboratory and Clinical Medicine* on "Tuberculosis

—Present and Future." He began it by reporting what the statisticians had proved, that in parts of the world where records were kept the mortality rate from tuberculosis had been declining throughout the century, that since 1900 it had dropped by 76 percent in the United States, to fewer than 45 per 100,000. But, he warned, historical studies showed that the disease had waxed and waned in about two-hundred-year cycles. "We are now approaching the lower level of a declining cycle, and with what we know today a new cycle should never begin—though wartime shortage of food may again increase the number of tuberculous victims on the continent of Europe."*

In diagnosis, he said, the improved use of X-ray had largely supplanted physical examination, which he thought was still important nonetheless. And in treatment "the trend is against climate therapy and the long rest regime, although both those methods have been of definite value and it is possible that the pendulum has swung too far in the direction of radical surgery."

He doffed his hat to biochemistry in research but thought discoveries as to factors in the growth of the tubercle bacillus were more important than study of the chemical composition of the bacillus itself. "All efforts to discover a chemotherapy have failed. Many laboratories have investigated the value of the sulfa drugs but with no success."

As to prevention he thought vaccination with BCG might still prove effective, but, he concluded, "With the continued decline in the death rate a form of vaccination might not be necessary."

What a sad conclusion that was to the quest and hope of his life. And it was a false one, because it was too narrow in outlook. Dr. Webb had forgot the millions upon millions in undeveloped countries whom poverty and famine make susceptible to pestilence. They still cry aloud for a preventive vaccine against tuberculosis.

Dr. Webb himself had ordered a supply of sulfanilamide when it at last came to market in the late 1930s but found it of no help to his tuberculous patients. And when the demands of the military finally sped the manufacture and distribution of Fleming's penicillin

---

*As I write, in the midst of a severe recession, grievously high and prolonged unemployment, and sharply declining concern for our unfortunates, the newspapers are reporting an alarming increase in the incidence of tuberculosis in such big cities as New York and Chicago.

he wrote for some of that and was disappointed to discern no benefit from it. But it alerted him to the potential in fungi and when he came across a report form two biologists at the University of Buffalo saying they had discovered a mold that seemed to inhibit the growth of the tubercle bacillus in the laboratory, he wrote urgently to Dr. Boissevain suggesting that a therapeutic oil or serum might be made from such a mold.

In his army hospital in England Charles began research on molds in a hurry. In less than two years he devised a method for testing the properties of such fungi and found a promising strain of them. Then a severe attack of asthma put him to bed in the hospital.

Neither Webb nor Boissevain had any idea of what had been happening in the laboratory of Dr. Selman Waksman at Rutgers University. Why should they? Waksman was a *soil* microbiologist. Since getting his degree at Rutgers in 1915 he had been studying the organisms that live in soil and humus and had succeeded in classifying them into bacteria, fungi, and an intermediate group called actinomycetes. Who would have guessed that microbes whose business is to reduce plant residues to humus could have anything to do with bacteria that produce disease in man?

Waksman himself did not guess it until late in the 1930s when a suggestive speculation from his former student, Dr. René Dubos of the Rockefeller Institute, and the work of two other former students at Buffalo set him on the track. He decided actinomycetes were more likely than bacteria or fungi to produce an effective antibiotic, a word he coined in 1941. He quickly settled on the products of a subgroup called streptomyces and by 1943 was able to announce his discovery of streptomycin. It shriveled bacteria in the laboratory; would it do so in human beings?

Waksman turned the clinical testing of streptomycin over to the Mayo Clinic and the Cornell University Medical Center. At the NTA meeting in Buffalo in June 1946 a team of doctors from these two places confirmed what Dr. H. Corwin Hinshaw of the Clinic had told the New York Academy of Medicine in January: streptomycin worked against the human tubercle bacilli. It was "the first effective chemotherapeutic remedy for tuberculosis!"

Dr. Webb was not present to hear this electrifying announcement but he had been told it was coming by Dr. Esmond R. Long, whom the Mayo Clinic had asked to check its cases and findings.

Webb's reaction is unrecorded but we may be sure he was hopeful but skeptical. He had lived through so many announced "cures" that produced only disillusionment.

In fact streptomycin was not the perfect cure; it proved to have serious limitations. It would take a decade more of disappointments and further research before chemotherapy supplanted the rest regime and surgery in tuberculosis.

Meanwhile World War II had ended in Europe and in response to Dr. Webb's urgent request to the Surgeon General, Dr. Boissevain had been released from the Medical Corps and come home in July 1945, bearing the cultures of two precious molds—and shocking news: The hospital doctors had found a cancer growing in his colon.

He was operated on at Denver's Fitzsimons Hospital in October, but he had waited too long; the surgeons could promise him only a short while longer to live. When he returned to his Foundation laboratory he said to Dr. Webb, "You *must* keep me alive, by whatever means, until I've finished my tests on those molds." Dr. Webb used a painkiller called dilaudid.

Some days Charles could be out of bed and at the laboratory for only an hour or two, but he hung on until the scientist in him was sure the metabolic products of his fungus did inhibit the growth of the tubercle bacillus in the laboratory. Dr. C. B. Sherbakoff, plant pathologist at the University of Tennessee, helped him by identifying the molds as *Fusarium scirpi*.

Charles wrote a brief report of his methods and conclusion and mailed it in for publication in the *Proceedings* of the Society for Experimental Biology just a few days before his death on 18 October 1946, his fifty-third birthday.

Boissevain's going was a personal as well as professional loss to Gerald Webb. He had come to love Varina's Flying Dutchman almost as a son. And Charles's death soon took away the lovely Ruth too. After going to Denver with Marka to deliver cultures of Charles's molds to Professor Florian Cajori of the University of Colorado in the hope that he might do something further with them, Ruth fled from the constant reminders of Charles in Colorado Springs and moved with her children Menso and Marie to Santa Barbara, California.

There had been many other deaths to sadden Gerald in the war years: Allen Krause in 1941, Frank's wife Ann in 1942, their sister

Amy in 1944, and in the year between, Harriet and Arnold Klebs.

Arnold's last letter to Gerald was a harrowing tale of the cold and hunger he was suffering in his Geneva apartment while he sought to keep his crippled invalid Harriet alive. "I do not see how we can survive another year of this cursed war—no fuel and too little food." He died soon after Harriet, of a heart attack.

Helen Morley had gone too, at age ninety. Although her lifelong hypochondria had sometimes been a nuisance to Gerald, he was fond of her, usually calling her Gadmother (she was Marka's godmother) and sending her innumerable cheery bits of word-play in verse, the last of them this: "There's a He in Heaven / And another He in Hell. / Whichever is the livelier He / With him, be sure, our Helen will dwell."

Hardest of all for Gerald perhaps was the death of Frances Stewart in 1945, just two years after he had gone to celebrate hers and Phil's golden wedding anniversary, taking them as a whimsical mark of the occasion a live goldfish.

The war's end brought relief and eventually a return to normal life. Gerry Bennett came home from San Diego and Gerry Webb miraculously unharmed from Burma to take up again his editorship of the *Chronicle*. Joel returned from Camp Carson and Marka resumed her role as full-time homemaker. Leila and Tim continued to live nearby in Denver but Robine and Vevy went to a new station in Cairo.

About the atomic bomb Gerald could only shake his head. Now he learned what Edward Meade Earle and James Phinney Baxter had been so excited about when they stopped to see him on their way home from an inspection trip for the government to a laboratory at Los Alamos, New Mexico. He had been somewhat irritated by the mystery they made of what they had gone to inspect. They told him it was all very hush-hush but it was big, big enough maybe to put an end to war. Now that he knew what "it" was, he wondered. "The physicists seem to have let hell loose on earth," he wrote Frank. "What possible good can come of it?"

He got a "well, maybe" answer when he ventured to go with Marka to Philadelphia for a meeting of the Board of Regents of the American College of Physicians in 1946. David Lilienthal, outgoing director of the Tennessee Valley Authority and soon to be director of the Atomic Energy Commission, spoke to the men about the possible peaceful uses of atomic power. He predicted among these

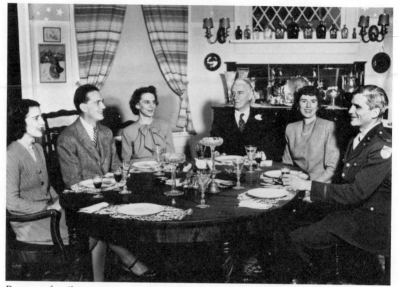

Postwar family reunion

the production of various radioactive isotopes that could be useful in medical research, diagnosis, and therapy.

Lilienthal's prediction has come magnificently true but at the time Dr. Webb could only wonder whether such benefit could be great enough to outweigh the destructive power science had unleashed.

That meeting was Dr. Webb's farewell to the American College of Physicians. He was quietly withdrawing from his responsibilities. He resigned from the editorial board of the *Journal of Laboratory and Clinical Medicine*, declined doing another revision of his chapter on tuberculosis in Cecil's *Textbook of Medicine* which he had been writing since the 1920s, refused to serve when he was elected Foundation Advocate by the state medical society: "I can no longer undertake the required journeys to Denver or to Foundation offices in the East."

He did, after a leisurely three-month study of the subject, address the local garden club on "Medicinal Herbs." But he no longer attended meetings of the El Paso Club or the Winter Night Club. To the monthly notices that came from those groups, as to almost all social invitations, he replied, "I do not go out at night anymore." His one regular departure from this rule was a weekly evening of bridge at the Cheyenne Mountain Country Club, which had voted him a life membership.

He began his day by turning on the radio to hear the news at six o'clock. By eight or eight-thirty he was ready to start on his rounds, sprucely dressed and wearing the fresh daily carnation for which Gerry Jr. maintained a standing order at the florist's. After visiting his private patients, only three or four at times now, and making his rounds at the Printers Home, he would go to his office to tend to correspondence until noon, then after lunch retreat into his study to read the *New York Times*, which was delivered daily only twenty-four hours late. He usually found much in it to clip for enclosing in letters on the morrow.

As he did in *Punch*, which he had always read for chuckles. He sometimes clipped cartoons from *Punch* and pasted them into small laugh-a-day scrapbooks for his men at the Printers Home. He often sent contributions of jokes, spoonerisms, or what he called portmanteau words to the magazine. One of them that was accepted and published was about his grandson Chuck who, upon coming home from school with a black eye, said to his mother, "Teacher tells me if I get into a fight again I'll be expended."

Or Gerald might spend the afternoon outdoors, potting up mariposa lilies for his patients or working with the Colorado wildflowers he was trying to grow in his rock garden. In this he had the help of an enthusiastic amateur botanist, Dr. John B. Hartwell, who had done much of his surgery for him in later years. When he persuaded Hartwell into trying some birdwatching with him, the surgeon gave up in frustration. "At least the flowers stand still," he said, providing Gerald with a hearty laugh and a joke for retelling.

On another afternoon Gerald might drive out with Opal into the near countryside to continue his observation of robins' nests. In time he made notes on five hundred such nests and concluded that the wary birds smartly chose nesting sites that were open for watching out on three sides and closed in on only one. He theorized that in town the robins nested above streets and sidewalks so as to take advantage of the extra heat rising up from the cement.

Sometimes enroute to the Printers Home he would stop at Prospect Lake and wander around its wooded shores to see what birds and flowers were in season, then bring his ambulatory patients to see the furry anemones or black-eyed susans or migrating warblers or shore birds he had found.

One summer season his earlier investment in equipment to inveigle his grandsons into an interest in butterflies paid off. Young Chuck discovered that when the gorgeous Monarchs first appeared they were torpid and if you approached them gently they would let you softly stroke their iridescent wings. When he demonstrated this fact to his grandfather, Gerald found the stroking such an exquisite pleasure he hurried to the Home to bring his patients out to share it.

Gerald's study—he called it his "den"—crossed the grain of Marka's housewifely instincts. Let her describe it: "His den was chaotic. His desk was piled high with papers, bits of things he had picked up from the fields and brought back to be looked up and identified, letters, reprints, books, and magazines. When I tried occasionally to tidy it up he would remonstrate, saying now he couldn't find a thing. He apparently had a photographic memory and could always put his finger at once on what he wanted despite the utter confusion. No one could find a place to sit down as the couch and chairs were strewn with everything imaginable.

"The net effect was attractive, though, I must admit—with a cozy fire of piñon logs burning in the fireplace, the window behind his desk letting in the sun from the south, and bookcases lining the walls. Pictures of eminent physicians and scientists were hung around the room and his little Peruvian silver hunchback and small copper statuette of the Egyptian god of medicine Imhotep stood on the mantel, next to a framed leaf from Hippocrates' island of Cos."

Gerald often retreated to that den when the house was full of people. He told Betty Hare that Marka kept too busy, "being called upon by everyone to entertain the universe, but she thrives on it." Once it was for the Daughters of the Confederacy who were conventioning in town and he agreed to be present awhile to greet the guests. He managed to keep a courteously straight face when one of them gushed that she could tell right off he was a southerner from his accent.

He was more sadly amused as he watched the ladies "finger with reverence" the old Worth gowns that Winnie Davis had worn, which Marka had brought down from the attic and spread around on chairs and sofas.

Sometimes the entertaining was for those who came to see him. Notable among them was the novelist Thomas Mann, who came to reminisce over tuberculosis sanatoriums of yore and stayed to pour out his distress over the demonic behavior of his native Germany under Hitler. He said he was sure the German intellectuals could have averted the war if they had tried.

Another visitor was the poet and biographer of Abraham Lincoln, Carl Sandburg, inquisitive still about the South during the Civil War. He left behind a copy of his *Prairie Years* inscribed to Marka with this puzzling wish: "May the peace of great phantoms be for you."

Dr. Boissevain's terminal illness heightened Dr. Webb's disquieting sense that death could come to him too at any time. He should put his affairs in order.

There was the partnership. It had endured for thirty-two years with Dr. Gilbert and for only a decade less with Dr. Sevier. They both said they were quite ready to retire and with declarations of mutual affection and gratitude the three signed the papers dissolving their legal relationship on 2 February 1946. Dr. Webb was not willing to give up entirely. He reduced his space in the Burns Building to one office and cut his staff to a single secretary; what little clinical laboratory work he needed thereafter was done at Glockner Hospital.

And what was he to do about the Foundation? He had been assuming that Dr. Boissevain would carry its work on, but now? Dr. Drea, even if he could be weaned from his dental practice, was not the sort of person to administer a laboratory or research projects beyond his own, especially not since he had just accepted an invitation to collaborate with Dr. A. Andrejew of the Pasteur Institute in Paris on an exhaustive study of the metabolism of the tubercle bacillus. And Gerald could think of no one at Colorado College who had knowledge or interest enough to keep the Foundation on the track of tuberculosis.

His thoughts turned to the University of Colorado. He had always wanted a vitalizing academic alliance for the Foundation. Perhaps it could be achieved after he was gone. He wrote to Dr. Ward Darley, dean of the medical school at the university, and to James Waring and Florence Sabin, suggesting that the University take over management of the Foundation after his death.

When Dr. Darley replied that the University certainly would want to consider doing so, Dr. Webb dropped the matter. Let Jim and Florence carry forward arrangements with the Foundation's trustees as they saw fit. He would be leaving them an institution with a solid record of achievement in research and an endowment fund of $172,000.

The American Clinical and Climatological Association was to hold its fall 1947 meeting in Colorado Springs and asked Dr. Webb to address it. He hesitated for several weeks but finally said yes because since the 1930s he had been building a case for the existence of pre-Columbian tuberculosis in the Americas and thought this would provide an occasion for getting it into print.

He worked desultorily on assembling his notes through the early months of 1947.

On the evening of 18 April he was enjoying his weekly game of bridge at the Cheyenne Mountain Country Club when he was urgently summoned home to take a long-distance telephone call. It came from Baltimore. His son Gerry had been severely injured that afternoon when his mount in a steeplechase balked at a hurdle and threw him; he was in critical condition in a Baltimore hospital.

Gerald had barely absorbed this alarming news when a second call came: Gerry was dead.

It could not be. That spirited, adventurous, gifted son who had flown dozens of missions over the Hump without a mishap had been killed by a fall from his famous horse Easy Mark in a sport he had loved since boyhood. When he was just at the prime age of forty.

It was decided that Marka and Joel should go east the next morning to bury Gerry in the Davis family plot in the Richmond cemetery. Robine, at home on vacation, would stay with their father. They left him slumped in grief.

He could not rouse himself from it. Gerry's death drained all spirit from him, all interest in anything. When Robine persuaded him to go with her to one of their favorite birdwatching spots, "out near Sinton's Dairy," he remained indifferent to what they saw. He walked through his days and chores blankly, absentmindedly.

What forced him from this apathy was the previously planned visit from his brother Frank in July and August. Ida's death in the nursing home earlier in the year had left the two youngest brothers the sole survivors from the big brood William John and Frances Susannah had reared at Heimat and the men had looked forward to their reunion.

Frank was surprised by Gerald's condition. He learned for the first time of his brother's heart attacks and restricted schedule and saw for himself the devastating melancholy that gripped him. Having fought through his own illnesses, his own bereavement and loneliness, he set about drawing Gerald out of depression.

Frank had traveled little outside Great Britain since his youth, so this trip to America was an exhilarating adventure for him. Entering with vim into the many plans for entertaining him, he dragged Gerald with him to luncheons and dinners, to picnics and barbecues on nearby ranches, on sightseeing trips as far as Santa Fe. And above all to the Opera Festival at Central City.

This Festival had become an annual summertime event that drew thousands of opera lovers from throughout Colorado and beyond. Dr. Webb was a regular visitor and had got to know many in the casts imported from New York. He introduced Frank to them, especially to Gladys Swarthout, who had grown to be a warm friend through their mutual affection for Vincent Youmans. The two courtly old English gentlemen who were so appreciative of the singing and the staging became pets of the singers.

All this was good mental therapy and Gerald was himself again when Frank reluctantly said goodbye and left for England, having won the enduring affection of his nieces Marka and Leila.

Gerald resumed work on his paper for the meeting of the Climatological.

In the mid-1930s while he was reading for his book *Tuberculosis* in the Surgeon General's library he would take occasional breaks to go see exhibits in the Smithsonian Institution. He was struck by the similarity between the ancient Peruvian drawings and ceramic statuettes he saw there and those of ancient Egypt reproduced in the books he was reading. Both portrayed men with hunched backs and pigeon breasts and exaggerated chins, which together were considered a sure sign of Pott's disease, i.e. tuberculosis of the spine.

There was no doubt that tuberculosis was widespread in old Egypt but it was thought not to have existed in the Americas until it was brought in by the white men. Now Gerald wondered whether this was true.

He paid a call on Ales Hrdlicka the noted anthropologist who was working in the Smithsonian at the time. Hrdlicka declared there could not possibly have been any tuberculosis in pre-Columbian America and gave Webb a reprint of an article that set forth the reasons for his conviction.

Webb was not convinced by the anthropologist's arguments; he thought they rested more on abstract logic than on observation of physical facts. He stated his own position in *Tuberculosis* and Hrdlicka took him vigorously to task for his daring.

From that time on Dr. Webb was a hound on the trail. He collected every report he could find about the peoples of early North and South America and went through them for archeological descriptions and pictures. He got the curators of half a dozen anthropological museums to keep on the lookout for new evidence for him. They sent him dozens of pictures of ancient artifacts but he put a good many of these aside as representations of "kephosis of the aged," a disorder that produced the knuckle spine but not the peculiar breast and chin. Still, he gathered enough—from Venezuela, Peru, Mexico, and various spots in Arizona, New Mexico, and Colorado, from the Maya and the Incas down to the Anasazi and the Zuni—to convince him that tuberculosis existed widely in America before the Conquest.

All his friends knew of his obsessive interest in the subject. Betty Hare once made him a Christmas present of a silver statuette of a hunchback she had found in a curio shop in New York with certification from the dealer that it was from Peru and the twelfth century. He kept it on his mantel with Imhotep. And when Dorothy Jones, a patient who flew her own airplane, heard of a new dig in an Indian mound in Kansas she offered to fly him to Salina to see it. Despite his deep dislike of flying, he went with her but was disappointed to find nothing that added to his evidence.

When Professor Earnest A. Hooton, the well-known Harvard anthropologist, arrived in Colorado Springs to take part in a symposium on archeology, he found at his hotel desk a note from Dr. Webb asking for an hour of his time to review the controversial matter. Hooton amiably agreed, spent an evening at 1222 North Cascade going over the Doctor's evidence, and said it convinced him that Webb was right.

Sylvanus G. Morley, the renowned expert on the early peoples of Middle America and the civilization of the Maya, also reviewed Webb's case and wrote him afterward, "To me you have certainly proved the existence of Pott's disease in pre-Columbian America."

The missing clincher for his argument, Dr. Webb well knew, was the absence among the finds of any ancient bones carrying the typical cavities left by tuberculosis. He was not deterred by this lack; he knew few such bones had been found even in Egypt.

Then in quick succession, in 1945 and 1946, such cavity-bearing bones were found in Venezuela and in New Mexico. Webb thought his case was complete.

This was the story, attended by much lore about hunchback flute players and jesters at the court of Montezuma and about migrations across the Bering Straits, that he prepared for the Climatological, along with many slides to illustrate it. He faced only the final problem of what to wear!

His wardrobe had got a mite shabby during the war years when he could not order clothes as usual from Thomas the Tailor in Cheltenham and he had not bothered to replenish it since. His youngest suit, more than ten years old, was a gray worsted in reasonably good condition but he did not like the cut of it. He would rather wear an older double-breasted dark-blue serge that fit him better but it was unmistakably shiny from use.

He consulted Marka. She thought either suit would do well enough. Finally he decided: "I'll wear the blue. I'm showing slides so the room will be dark most of the time and they won't see the shine."

He was seventy-six when he rose to address the Climatological, standing tall without the slightest hint of stoop, in his blue suit with a white carnation in his buttonhole. His hair was unmistakably white now and the skin was stretched taut over the bones of his face. He had lost most of the rosy color in his cheeks but his English accent and baritone voice remained strong as ever.

He was applauded vigorously when he finished speaking and his paper was published in the association's *Proceedings* for that year. The question of pre-Columbian tuberculosis in America has remained somewhat controversial but the consensus among anthropologists today is that Dr. Webb had the right of it.

December was occupied with the chores of Christmas. For the family's greeting card that year Gerald agreed to the use of his portrait painted by Boardman Robinson. "I've never liked it, and neither has anyone else who knows me," he wrote Frank, "but Mike is dying and it will make him feel good to have us use it. See if you can find any look of me in it."

It took him most of January 1948 to reply to the greetings and good wishes for the new year he had received, and he was relieved to finish the annual chore on the morning of 27 January — with letters, among others, to Clarence Lieb, who had retired and was living in Tucson, Arizona; to Mrs. Gregg, all three of whose sons had worked in the Webb Laboratory when they were boys, congratulating her on Alan's rise to power in the Rockefeller Foundation; and to Donald Gregg, whose esophageal stricture as an adolescent Webb had cured with Plummer's graduated bulbs and who was now a doctor on the staff of a hospital in the Philippines.

It was a day of subzero cold and Gerald was glad to get into the warm house when he went home for lunch. He turned on the radio to listen to the news while he ate. When the announcer reported that a flock of evening grosbeaks had been spotted in a grove on the edge of town, Marka offered to drive him out to see them. He said no, he'd see them another day. He was feeling tired and would rather stay by the fire with a book.

He went to bed early that night.

At midnight he awoke with that heavy searing pain in his chest. He knew what it meant. He made his way haltingly down the dark hall to Marka's room and asked her to call Joel and Dr. McDonald.

She ran downstairs to the telephone, then to unlock the front door for the men. When she got back to her father's room, he was lying quiet on the bed, neat in pajamas and dressing gown. Too quiet. Too still. He was dead.

Gone was the adored father. Gone was the beloved physician. Gone was the cherished friend, the admired colleague. But he had left behind myriad words of vivid record, many heartwarming memories, a rippling sigh of sorrow for the loss of an extraordinary human being.

Epilogue: Memorial

THE STORY of Dr. Webb did not end with his death.

When the period of interment (beside Varina in Evergreen Cemetery), obituary, condolence, and eulogy had passed, and while Dr. Webb's home of fifty years at 1222 North Cascade Avenue was being dismantled and the house sold, and while his thousands of books were being dispersed among various libraries, personal and public, the trustees of his Colorado Foundation took up the question of its future. As a first step on the way to university affiliation he had prepared for them, they elected Dr. James J. Waring to succeed him as president and research director.

Dr. Waring was then in his sixty-fourth year. He had been chairman of the department of medicine in the University of Colorado's medical school for fifteen years and was widely admired and loved for, in the words of a colleague, "his humanity, wisdom, wit, and trailblazing spirit."

Because of his always uncertain health he had to choose what tasks he would undertake. Now he unhesitatingly resigned his chairmanship of medicine and, it is said, refused election as president of the American College of Physicians, in order to take on responsibility for developing the Foundation. He shared Dr. Webb's vision of what the medical school and the Foundation might do for each other.

He struck at once, before memories of Webb could fade, for tribute from the Committee on Research of the NTA in honor of its founder, and the Committee responded with a substantial grant to the Foundation in 1949.

The research program of the Foundation was in need of resuscitation. Dr. Drea still held the title of associate research director but never looked beyond his own investigations with Dr. Andrejew of

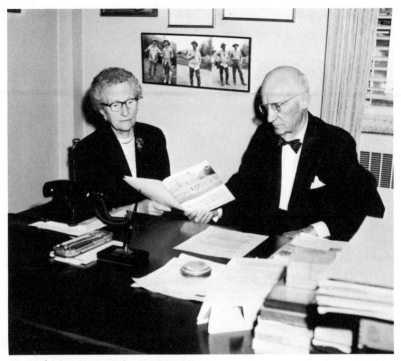

Dr. and Mrs. James Johnston Waring

Paris, which were shortly to produce a prize-worthy book on *The Metabolism of the Tubercle Bacillus*.

The other laboratories stood vacant, their equipment idle. The animal quarters too were empty; the animals had all been sold. There was only the loyal Dr. Mary Alice Hamilton to provide custodial care.

The one other piece of Foundation research was being done in Denver, where Dr. Florian Cajori Jr. was working with Dr. Boissevain's Fusarium molds. He had eliminated one of the two as useless but still had hope that the other might produce an antibiotic effective against tubercle bacilli.

Dr. Waring could hardly expect to involve other members of his medical faculty and their graduate students in the research of the Foundation if its laboratories and equipment remained an hour or more away in Colorado Springs. The trustees understood this fact and urged Waring to negotiate with university officials the transfer of the Foundation's laboratory work to the campus in Denver.

This move was arranged in 1950. Only an office for the trustees and the financial headquarters in the suite of the dedicated secretary-treasurer, Morris A. Esmiol, in the First National Bank Building were to remain in Colorado Springs. Dr. Drea would transfer his work to the laboratory at Glockner Hospital and the old machine shop so handsomely remade into laboratories would be returned to Colorado College.

Now Waring's problem was to find space in Denver. The medical school itself was growing fast and could spare no laboratories for the Foundation's work. Never a piker in planning, Dr. Waring convinced his university superiors and the Foundation's trustees that the only solution was to construct a separate building for the Foundation's laboratories.

As Dr. Webb had foreseen, alliance with the university made possible what he as an individual could not command. Philanthropic foundations were willing to consider an application for support when it was backed by the prestige and permanence of a university. Several of them in concert promised to contribute $75,000 if private donors would provide the remainder of the $150,000 it was estimated the building would cost.

The required amount was quickly pledged, the university designated a site adjoining its newly constructed Florence R. Sabin Research Building, and on 22 April 1953 Joel Webb laid the cornerstone in the presence of a host of his father's remembering friends and patients. Ruth Boissevain came back from California for the ceremony and Fanny Robbins the candymaker conferred the baptism of her tears.

Eleven months later the structure of red brick was ready for occupancy. It was modest in size, only two stories high and providing just 5,000 square feet of space, but its foundations had been made strong enough to support more floors when needed. It was named the Gerald B. Webb Memorial Building.

Dr. Waring saw to it that hung above its portals was the motto Dr. Webb had chosen from Henry Sewall's copy of Descartes' *Discours* thirty years before: FAC ET SPERA.

The principal speaker at the dedication ceremony on 12 March 1954 was Dr. René Jules Dubos, renowned bacteriologist of the Rockefeller Institute (later Rockefeller University). In speaking of the man the new building memorialized, Dr. Dubos said it was conversations with Dr. Webb and hearing one of his talks to medical

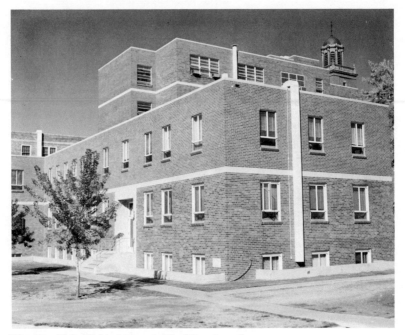

The Gerald B. Webb Memorial Building in 1961

students at Rutgers that had first turned his own attention to tuberculosis.

With significant consequence. Dubos's work in that field had won him the Trudeau Medal two years before and he had just published, in collaboration with his wife Jean Porter, *The White Plague*, a bestselling account of interrelationships between tuberculosis and society through the ages.

Dr. Dubos's main topic that bright blue-and-gold spring day was the current state of chemotherapy for tuberculosis. It would soon, he thought, provide a reliable cure at last.

It had been learned that streptomycin alone was only temporarily effective. Too many strains of tubercle bacilli became resistant to it. It had to be reinforced with supplementary anti-tuberculosis drugs. One of these, called PAS, had been discovered long before streptomycin and another, isoniazid, had become available in 1952. (Several more would come along in the next few years.) The investigation occupying research doctors at the time Dubos spoke was field testing on a grand scale to determine the most effective combinations of these drugs with streptomycin—the right dosages and the right frequencies and sequences of administration.

When this wide testing was completed in the early 1960s chemotherapy made all other therapies for tuberculosis obsolete. Gone for good was the need for Dr. Webb's long rest cure, for artificial pneumothorax and all forms of radical surgery. And gone too was the usefulness of sanatoriums; they closed by the hundreds throughout the Western world. Young physicians soon were entering practice with no knowledge of what a killing plague tuberculosis had been; to them it was just another disease that required a short stay in the hospital and treatment with an established formula of curative drugs.

The organizations long dedicated to control of tuberculosis did not fade away with its decline; they just changed their names and turned their efforts upon other pulmonary diseases, notably emphysema, asthma, and lung cancer. The National Tuberculosis Association, for instance, became the American Lung Association. And in 1961 the Colorado Foundation for Research in Tuberculosis was renamed the Webb Institute for Medical Research—though still "dedicated to study of the diseases of the lungs."

It was flourishing. Dr. Waring was still its president but no longer its research director. When he took emeritus status at the university in 1954 and wanted to cement for the future the bond between the medical school and the Institute, he sought a man who could wear his own two hats, teaching in the medical school and directing research in the Institute.

He was lucky. The great Trudeau Sanatorium was closing its doors that year and thus releasing its clinical director, Dr. Roger S. Mitchell, whom a colleague called "the foremost authority in the country on pulmonary diseases." A native of Pennsylvania and a graduate of the Harvard medical school, Dr. Mitchell had acquired substantial experience both in university teaching and in specialized practice. He became head of the division of pulmonary diseases in the medical school and director of the Institute in 1955. (In 1980 he became the fifth physician from Colorado—following Henry Sewall, Gerald Webb, Florence Sabin, and James Waring—to win the Trudeau Medal.)

Life in the Institute jumped. By 1961 it had added a third floor to the Webb Memorial Building and was amassing the $250,000 needed to build fourth and fifth floors in 1964. Its endowment fund had passed the milestone of one million dollars; its maintenance funds were approaching half a million dollars annually. In addition it was tapping, in the amount of some $150,000 a year, the multiplying government sources for grants-in-aid: the U.S. Public Health Service, the National Science Foundation, the National Institutes of Health.

The research staff had grown to twenty-five, including six principal investigators, organized in five divisions. They all held teaching appointments on the medical school faculty and together were addressing some fifty professional societies and publishing more than twenty-five books and papers each year. Several of them were also acting as consultants to government health agencies.

This was an explosion of growth in only a decade that Dr. Webb could not have imagined in his rosiest fantasies.

Watching it all with gratification were the members of his family, especially Marka and Joel. Marka, now Mrs. John Wolcott Stewart (she had married the son of her father's cherished friends Phil and Frances Stewart), had served as trustee and vice-president since her father's death, and Joel, elected to the board later in the decade, was a continuing member of the finance committee.

The two of them felt strongly that Dr. Waring's immense contribution to developments should be officially recognized and when the change from Foundation to Institute was being considered they urged that Waring's name be added to Webb's in the new appellation.

But Dr. Waring would not have it so. He wrote them, "I am honored by your suggestion, and grateful for it, but I think it would be better in every way to let Gerald's name stand alone."

Death came to Dr. Waring the next year, in 1962, when he was seventy-eight years old. The trustees then expressed their devotion and sense of loss by accepting Marka's and Joel's recommendation: they renamed their institution the Webb-Waring Institute for Medical Research. A decade later it became the Webb-Waring Lung Institute, which it remains today.

It has grown steadily bigger and stronger — in financial resources, in physical plant, in expanding education and training programs of several sorts, in research personnel and investigations. Remaining dedicated to basic research and emphasizing cooperation and exchange of ideas among its many specialists, it has made significant contributions of new knowledge on several advancing frontiers of medical science.

One phase of its work has special relevance to the story of Dr. Webb.

In 1959 a young Ph.D. in bacteriology from Stanford University, Dr. Alfred J. Crowle, was appointed assistant professor of microbiology in the medical school and head of the Division of Immunology in the Webb Institute. He was already interested in the persisting problems of immunity and now, with the strong encouragement of Dr. Waring, tackled the thorny challenge of producing an anti-tuberculosis vaccine.

However close a reliable cure was in the Western world at the time, the white plague was still a devastating killer elsewhere on the planet; its victims in the third world were estimated to number ten or twelve million. BCG was still the nearest thing to an effective vaccine available, but it was not always reliable, it caused the tuberculin test to become positive, and some authorities would not approve the use of it.

By applying the knowledge of tubercle bacilli painstakingly accumulated bit by bit in previous decades and by using new methods in biochemistry and microbiology, Dr. Crowle and his associates, after a decade of unremitting labor, were able to announce on 8 September 1969, at an international conference on tuberculosis, the development of a new vaccine. It was described as "a non-living antigen extracted by the action of the enzyme trypsin on killed tubercle bacilli," and it had the virtue of not producing a positive reaction to the tuberculin test. It had proved extremely effective in animals and was ready for large-scale testing in human beings.

Such is the snail's pace in these matters that Dr. Crowle is still waiting for these human trials. They were at last to be authorized at a session of the Pan American Health Organization in Argentina in 1982 but the Falklands War erupted just in time to cancel the meeting.

Dr. Crowle and his assistants have in the meantime made notable discoveries in other aspects of immunology, some having to do with transplant rejection and the growth of cancer. But validation of his revolutionary anti-tuberculosis vaccine remains first on his and the Institute's agenda.

It does seem likely that Dr. Webb's passionate dream will become reality, that his long quest will end in success at last, achieved by a laboratory doctor working in a traceable line of descent from Dr. Webb himself. In the perspective of the centuries it will be another long stride forward for man when we can, as Dr. Webb always hoped, put tuberculosis alongside smallpox and polio on the list of conquered infectious diseases.

Sources and Acknowledgments

When I am reading a book for its story I do not like to face a blanket of fine print at the bottom of the page or the impediment of reference symbols in the text, and I assume more readers are like than unlike me in this. So I chose to rely on internal documentation rather than footnotes to assure the reader that this biography is not fiction. But some further description of my sources is in order, and here it is.

Among unpublished sources the trove of highest yield was Dr. Webb's correspondence. I have not counted the letters but there must be several thousand of them. Roughly two thirds are professional — to anxious patients and their relatives and hometown doctors and to colleagues in the national effort to control tuberculosis — and one third are personal, to family and friends.

The surviving professional letters came to me in thick annual folders as filed by Webb's secretaries from 1907 on. They were typewritten and dated but badly mixed up within each year. Owing to Gerald Webb's confessed "besetting sin" of procrastination, a letter he got and his reply to it might lie months, in a few cases a year or two, apart. I reassembled them in usable order.

His personal letters arrived in my study in a dismaying jumble that filled a huge cardboard carton. All, until after Varina bought him that Corona portable when he went off to the war in Europe, were handwritten in the Doctor's small, often hard-to-decipher script. Separated pages, continuations on odd scraps of paper, postscripts scribbled on prescription blanks were loose in the scrambled lot. And rarely was a date set down anywhere. It took a lengthy spell of eyestrain to put them together in sequence according to their contents.

What then appeared was a remarkably vivid record of much that Dr. Webb did and thought from 1891, when he first left Heimat, to the day of his death in 1948. I have quoted freely from the letters to let the reader share the flavor of them and to let the Doctor speak for himself.

We are fortunate that two of Webb's womenfolk had the keeping habit. Mater was the first. She made Gerald's letters a means of linking her scattered brood, sending each one on, sometimes after scratching down a comment or newsy tidbit of her own at top or bottom, till it had made the rounds of the siblings in England. When it got back to her she tossed it into some drawer or box.

She did this with no eye to biography or history; it was just that Heimat's fourteen rooms allowed such keeping. Her lot of letters from Gerald included a few from Jenny Webb too. But none of Mater's own survived. What she wrote I had to infer from Gerald's replies.

Varina's hoard of her husband's letters overlapped Mater's for two years, until Mater's death in 1906. Since Gerald did so much traveling and wrote home almost every day while he was away, that hoard is huge. It includes quite a few sporadic letters from his sisters Nell, Amy, and Ida but almost none from his brothers. Who threw away Varina's letters and the children's I do not know; only a scattered few of them remain.

Invaluable were some five hundred additional letters kept by Francis Webb and brought to me from England by Marka Webb Stewart. Thanks to the meticulous habits of the lawyer, these were in perfect order and almost all typewritten. Frank even included postcards and cables, and copies or abstracts of his own letters to which Gerald was replying. His file was sparse in the 1890s and early 1900s but grew fat as the years passed. It reveals Frank as a man of quick intelligence, acerbic wit, and admirable literary verve.

I had the use also of three manuscript histories of the Webb family: a short one by Frank, who set down important dates of births, deaths, and the like; a much longer one by his son Denis, who ferreted out the ancestries of William John and Frances Susannah and proved by official records that the former's father became a man of substance despite his bastard birth; and the third by Harold's son John, who traced the history of Webb Brothers Limited's business in coal and bricks and tiles.

The younger generation in America helped me immeasurably. I enjoyed informative conversations with Mrs. Stewart and her brother Joel A. H. Webb and found much to use in letters of remi-

niscence and comment from Mrs. Stewart, Robine Webb Farnsworth, and Leila Webb Collins Davidson. I say a heartfelt thank-you
to them all.

Some of those letters of reminiscence and comment, especially
from Marka Stewart and Leila Davidson, were written to Mrs.
Judith Hannemann. As a writer on the editorial staff of the *Denver
Medical Society Bulletin*, Mrs. Hannemann got interested in Dr.
Webb when she included a brief biographical sketch of him in her
article, "Four Physicians and Their Bookplates," published in the
Fall 1969 issue of the *University of Colorado Quarterly*. Recognizing
the unusual quality of the man and sensing a good and significant
story in his life, Mrs. Hannemann did some further research and
expanded her sketch into a manuscript, "Gerald Bertram Webb,
M.D., a Biography." (Unpublished, 124 typewritten pages, 1970.)
She has generously allowed me to make use of this manuscript and
the materials she assembled for it. I am warmly grateful to her for
this professional courtesy.

Mrs. Stewart and Mr. Webb allowed me to use family photograph albums and some of Dr. Webb's scrapbooks that are in their
possession. The clippings in those scrapbooks saved me many
hours of research in newspaper files and other assorted memorabilia
pasted into them pointed the way to some of the most important
episodes in Dr. Webb's life.

An instance: In one scrapbook a blank letterhead bearing the
name of the American Association of Immunologists and listing
Dr. Webb as president started me on the trail of his participation in
founding that organization. No one, not even his family or the
officers of the Association, knew anything about this until I was
able to tell them of it.

I got valuable word-pictures of Dr. Webb in his prime from con-
versations and correspondence with three men who knew him then:
Dr. William Francis Drea, Dr. William Corr Service, and Marshall
Sprague. More information, and chuckles too, came from manu-
script copies of informal talks Mr. Sprague gave to various clubs in
Colorado Springs. I express deep appreciation to all three men.

Among published sources the richest mine again was Dr. Webb's
own writings. His highly personal and anecdotal style made even
his scientific papers a good source for incidents in his life. His book
Henry Sewall, Physiologist and Physician, contained facts about
his own experience that I found nowhere else.

He was a forgetful recorder of his bibliography but I was able to compile a list of one hundred forty-six papers and books he wrote and to collect copies or photocopies of all but fourteen of them. For assistance in the latter task I am indebted to Mrs. Stewart, Mrs. Hannemann, Dr. William C. Service, Dr. David W. Talmage of the Webb-Waring Lung Institute, Dr. Joanne Finstead-Good of the Sloan-Kettering Institute, and Mrs. Blanche B. Reines of the American Association of Immunologists.

Besides referring to articles in many medical journals and society Proceedings of Webb's years, I made a systematic survey of the *Transactions* of the National Tuberculosis Association, 1904–1948; the same society's *Journal of the Outdoor Life*; its *American Review of Tuberculosis*, 1917–1925; and the *Journal of Immunology* for its initial year, 1916. Equally helpful were Dr. Webb's files of Cragmor Sanatorium's *Ninety-eight-Six*, 1924–1932, and *Annual Reports* of the Colorado Foundation for Research in Tuberculosis, 1924–1946, and of its successors, 1949–1982.

Many books gave me the background I needed on one phase or another of Dr. Webb's life. I list here a few that were especially helpful.

On the national anti-tuberculosis movement: S. Adolphus Knopf, *A History of the National Tuberculosis Association* (1922) and Richard H. Shryock, *National Tuberculosis Association, 1904–1954* (1957). Dr. Knopf's book is long out of print and I owe thanks to Mr. Jules Saltman of the American Lung Association for lending me a copy from the Association's archives.

On Colorado Springs: Marshall Sprague, *Newport in the Rockies* (1971) and *Money Mountain: The Story of Cripple Creek Gold* (1953). Manly D. and Eleanor Ormes, *The Book of Colorado Springs* (1933). Charlie Brown Hershey, *Colorado College, 1874–1949* (1952).

On developments in bacteriology and immunology: A. C. Abbott, *Principles of Bacteriology* (1915). William Osler, *Principles and Practice of Medicine* (1892). Esmond R. Long, *History of Pathology* (1928). William Bulloch, *History of Bacteriology* (1938). Fielding H. Garrison, *Introduction to the History of Medicine* (1929). Richard H. Shryock, *The Development of Modern Medicine* (1936). Paul De Kruif, *Microbe Hunters* (1926). Hans Zinsser, *Resistance to Infectious Diseases* (1914) and *As I Remember Him* (1940). Theodore Sourkes, *Nobel Prize Winners in Medicine and*

Physiology, 1901–1965 (1966). Selman A. Waksman, *Streptomycin* (1949) and *My Life with Microbes* (1954). Ronald J. Glasser, *The Body Is the Hero* (1976).

To those I must add the *Encyclopaedia Britannica*, eleventh edition, 1910. Histories sweep so fast through the centuries they rarely stop to provide a close-up description of a particular year. Although the *Britannica* of 1910 carried no entries under *immunity* or *immunology*, I could gather details of how things stood when Dr. Webb began his research from entries under *blood*, *bacteria*, *vaccine*, *Metchnikoff*, *Wright*, and the like.

On the history of tuberculosis: Edward D. Otis, *The Great White Plague* (1909). Gerald B. Webb, *Tuberculosis* (1936). Lawrason Brown, *The Story of Clinical Pulmonary Tuberculosis* (1941). René and Jean Dubos, *The White Plague: Tuberculosis, Man, and Society* (1952).

On working with Sir Almroth Wright: Leonard Colebrook, *Almroth Wright* (1954) and André Maurois, *The Life of Sir Alexander Fleming* (translated from the French by Gerard Hopkins, 1959).

On Webb's colleagues and friends: H. C. Cameron, *Mr. Guy's Hospital, 1726–1948* (1954). Edward L. Trudeau, *Autobiography* (1916). Simon Flexner and James Thomas Flexner, *William Henry Welch and the Heroic Age of American Medicine* (1941). Harvey Cushing, *Life of Sir William Osler* (1925) and *From a Surgeon's Journal 1915–18* (1936). Elizabeth H. Thomson, *Harvey Cushing: Surgeon, Author, Artist* (1950). Helen Clapesattle, *The Doctors Mayo* (1941). Victor C. Vaughan, *A Doctor's Memories* (1926). John M. T. Finney, *A Surgeon's Life* (1940). Gustav Eckstein, *Noguchi* (1931). Loyal Davis, *J. B. Murphy, Stormy Petrel of Surgery* (1933). Elinor Richey, *Eminent Women of the West* (1975) for a biographical sketch of Florence R. Sabin. Douglas R. McKay, *Asylum of the Gilded Pill* (1983) for the story of Dr. Alexius M. Forster and Cragmor Sanatorium.

I want to express my deepest gratitude to the members of Dr. Webb's family for not trying to shape or censor my biography of their father. Mrs. Stewart in particular graciously answered my many questions, sent me materials, and read the biography in manuscript, but she never dictated what it should or should not include. She allowed me to make my own assessment and interpretation, though these must differ at many points from her own.

Although Dr. Roger S. Mitchell, emeritus director of research at the Webb-Waring Lung Institute, read the manuscript for the publisher, I should like to add my personal thanks to him for saving me from errors that as a nonspecialist in medicine and medical science I ran the risk of making.

And I happily acknowledge my great debt to my husband, Professor Roger W. Shugg, not just for his caring advice and criticism and his encouragement when the road got rough, but for cheerfully accepting Dr. Webb as a third member of our household while this work was in progress.

Helen Clapesattle

Albuquerque   New Mexico
October 1983

Peter Bent Brigham Hospital, 185, 310
Peters, LeRoy S., 210
Pfeiffer, Richard, 154
Pfeiffer bacillus, 165
Phagocytes, 154, 159, 166, 193, 199, 282
Phagocytosis, *see* Phagocytes
Philadelphia, 13, 14, 26; *see also* Zoo
Philadelphia North American, 168
Philip, Sir Robert, 358, 360, 361, 369
Phipps, Henry, 212; Research Institute, 212, 342
Phipps, Hubert, 426
Phipps, Lawrence, 426
Phrenicectomy, 254
Pthisiophobia, 237, 238–40. *See also* Tuberculosis, phobia
Pthisis, 24, 28, 33, 34, 35. *See also* Tuberculosis
Pikes Peak, 38, 39, 41, 42, 53, 72, 190; Highway, 351, 426; Hill Climb, 351
Pikes Peak Avenue, 72, 80
Piness, George, 414–15
Pine trees, 28; as mistletoe carriers, 202, 272
Piney Woods Hotel, 27, 28–29, 30
Pipettes, 157, 179
Pirquet, Clemens von, 179, 270
Pius X (pope), 212
Platelets, 193, 197
Pleurisy, 11, 30–31, 32, 256, 409
Pliny the Elder, 28, 32
Plummer, Henry, 111, 210, 257
Pneumococcus, 168
Pneumonia, 165, 317
Pneumothorax, 212–13, 252–56, 311, 364, 397
Pobschell, Sister Ida, 241, 244
Poe, Edgar A., 406
Poker, 69, 421
Polio, 151, 484
Polo, 114, 120, 145, 147, 175, 279, 352
Porgy, 423
Porter, Ruth (Mrs. J. J. Waring), 234
Postural rest, 255–56, 301, 370
Potter, Ashton, 147, 350, 352
Potter, Grace Goodyear, 147, 352
Pott's disease, 116, 473–75
Pourtales, James, 45, 87, 351
Powell, Desmond, 461
Powers, Charles W., 70, 71, 148, 161, 262, 263, 280, 283, 320, 369
Praed Street laboratories, *see* St. Mary's Hospital
Prairie Years, 471

"Prescribing the Scrap-Book" (Webb), 454
Prescription of books, 403, 404–08
"Prescription of Literature, The" (Webb), 382, 413
Princeton University, 394
Printers Home. *See* Union Printers Home
Prior discovery problem, for Sewall, 60, 191, 434, 462; for Webb, 191–92, 214, 438
Prospect Lake, 469
Protein Split Products, 199
Prudential, insurance, 399
Public Health Service, U.S., 327-28
Puerperal fever, 92, 242
Pulitzer, Constance, 245, 246–48, 262, 267, 289, 369, 447
Pulitzer, Joseph, 245, 247, 390–91
Pulitzer, Kate Davis, 245, 246, 247
Pullman, Mrs. George, 110
Pullman, John Sanger, 37, 104
Punch, 46, 411, 454, 469
Puy de Dome, 306
Pyorrhea, 156, 163

Queen's Head, 4
Quimper, 305, 376

Rabbits, 176, 184, 189, 237
Rabelais, François, 413
Rabies, 242
Rackemann, Francis, 414
Radio, 404
Rainbow Falls, 39
Râles, 256; *see also* Auscultation
Rampart Range, 72
Rats, Lice, and History, 204
Ravenel, Mazÿck P., 167, 168, 178, 180, 189, 209, 211, 242, 279, 339
Recovery Record, 375
Recovery Road, 376, 385
Red Cross, 302, 335
Red tape, 295
Reed, Mrs. A. J., 172
Reed, Jacob, 114, 115
Reed, Margery, 121–22, 373
Reed, Mrs. Verner Z., 121, 373
Reed, Verner Z., 121, 122
Reeves-Smith, ——, 359
Renfraw brothers, 12
Rest cure, 50, 93, 94, 141, 143, 205, 249–50, 251–52, 301, 396, 397, 402, 464, 481; postural, 255–56, 301, 370